Next-Generation Interstitial Lung Disease

Editors

KERRI A. JOHANNSON
HAROLD R. COLLARD
LUCA RICHELDI

CLINICS IN CHEST MEDICINE

www.chestmed.theclinics.com

June 2021 • Volume 42 • Number 2

ELSEVIER

1600 John F. Kennedy Boulevard • Suite 1800 • Philadelphia, Pennsylvania, 19103-2899

http://www.theclinics.com

CLINICS IN CHEST MEDICINE Volume 42, Number 2
June 2021 ISSN 0272-5231, ISBN-13: 978-0-323-75783-6

Editor: Joanna Collett
Developmental Editor: Karen Justine Solomon

Clinics in Chest Medicine (ISSN 0272-5231) is published quarterly by Elsevier Inc., 360 Park Avenue South, New York, NY 10010-1710. Months of issue are March, June, September, and December. Periodicals postage paid at New York, NY and additional mailing offices. Subscription prices are $396.00 per year (domestic individuals), $1009.00 per year (domestic institutions), $100.00 per year (domestic students/residents), $423.00 per year (Canadian individuals), $1075.00 per year (Canadian institutions), $484.00 per year (international individuals), $1075.00 per year (international institutions), $100.00 per year (Canadian Students), and $230.00 per year (International Students). International air speed delivery is included in all Clinics subscription prices. All prices are subject to change without notice. **POSTMASTER:** Send address changes to Clinics in Chest Medicine, Elsevier Health Sciences Division, Subscription Customer Service, 3251 Riverport Lane, Maryland Heights, MO 63043. **Customer Service: Telephone: 1-800-654-2452** (U.S. and Canada); **1-314-447-8871** (outside U.S. and Canada). **Fax: 1-314-447-8029. E-mail: journalscustomerservice-usa@elsevier.com (for print support); journalsonlinesupport-usa@elsevier.com (for online support).**

Reprints. For copies of 100 or more of articles in this publication, please contact the Commercial Reprints Department, Elsevier Inc., 360 Park Avenue South, New York, NY 10010-1710. Tel.: 212-633-3874; Fax: 212-633-3820; E-mail: reprints@elsevier. com.

Clinics in Chest Medicine is covered in *MEDLINE/PubMed (Index Medicus), Current Contents/Clinical Medicine, EMBASE/ Excerpta Medica, Science Citation Index,* and *ISI/BIOMED.*

Contributors

EDITORS

KERRI A. JOHANNSON, MD, MPH
Associate Professor, Departments of Medicine
and Community Health Sciences, University of
Calgary, Calgary, Alberta, Canada

HAROLD R. COLLARD, MD
Associate Vice Chancellor of Clinical Research,
Professor, Department of Medicine, University
of California, San Francisco, San Francisco,
California, USA

LUCA RICHELDI, MD, PhD
Professor of Respiratory Medicine,
Department of Medical and Surgical Sciences,
Università Cattolica del Sacro Cuore, Head of
Pulmonary Medicine, Fondazione Policlinico
Universitario A. Gemelli IRCCS, Rome, Italy

AUTHORS

AYODEJI ADEGUNSOYE, MD, MS, FCCP
Assistant Professor of Medicine, Section of
Pulmonary and Critical Care, The University of
Chicago Medicine, Chicago, Illinois, USA

HAYLEY BARNES, MBBS, MPH
Department of Respiratory Medicine, Alfred
Hospital, Central Clinical School, Monash
University, Melbourne, Australia

HAROLD R. COLLARD, MD
Associate Vice Chancellor of Clinical Research,
Professor, Department of Medicine, University
of California, San Francisco, San Francisco,
California, USA

BRIDGET F. COLLINS, MD
Clinical Assistant Professor, Department of
Medicine, Center for Interstitial Lung Diseases,
University of Washington Medical Center,
Seattle, Washington, USA

TAMERA J. CORTE, MD, PhD
Department of Respiratory Medicine, Royal
Prince Alfred Hospital, The University of
Sydney Central Clinical School, Sydney,
Australia; NHMRC Centre of Research
Excellence in Pulmonary Fibrosis, Australia

VINCENT COTTIN, MD, PhD
Department of Respiratory Medicine, National
Coordinating Reference Center for Rare
Pulmonary Diseases, Louis Pradel Hospital,
Hospices Civils de Lyon, Claude Bernard
University Lyon 1, INRAE, IVPC, Member of
OrphaLung, RespiFil, Radico-ILD and ERN-
LUNG, Lyon, France

SONYE K. DANOFF, MD, PhD
Associate Professor of Medicine, Co-Director,
ILD/IPF Program, Associate Director, Myositis
Center, Division of Pulmonary and Critical Care
Medicine, Johns Hopkins Medicine, Baltimore,
Maryland, USA

ERICA FARRAND, MD
Assistant Professor of Medicine, University of
California, San Francisco, San Francisco,
California, USA

JOLENE H. FISHER, MD, MSc
Department of Medicine, University Health
Network, University of Toronto, Toronto,
Ontario, Canada

SABINA A. GULER, MD, MHSc
Department of Pulmonary Medicine,
Inselspital, Bern University Hospital, University
of Bern, Bern, Switzerland

ERICA L. HERZOG, MD, PhD
Professor, Section of Pulmonary, Critical Care,
and Sleep Medicine, Department of Medicine,
Yale School of Medicine, Yale University, New
Haven, Connecticut, USA

KERRI A. JOHANNSON, MD, MPH
Associate Professor, Departments of Medicine
and Community Health Sciences, University of
Calgary, Calgary, Alberta, Canada

MELANIE KÖNIGSHOFF, MD, PhD
Research Unit Lung Repair and Regeneration,
Helmholtz Zentrum München, Member,
German Center of Lung Research (DZL),
München, Germany; Division of Pulmonary,
Allergy and Critical Care Medicine, Department
of Medicine, University of Pittsburgh,
Pittsburgh, Pennsylvania, USA

LETICIA KAWANO-DOURADO, MD
HCor Research Institute, Hospital do Coracao,
Pulmonary Division, Heart Institute (InCor),
Medical School, University of Sao Paulo, Sao
Paulo, Brazil; INSERM UMR 1152, University of
Paris, Paris, France

JOYCE S. LEE, MD
Department of Medicine, Division of Pulmonary
Sciences and Critical Care Medicine,
University of Colorado Denver – Anschutz
Medical Campus, Aurora, Colorado, USA

MAREIKE LEHMANN, PhD
Research Unit Lung Repair and Regeneration,
Helmholtz Zentrum München, Member,

German Center of Lung Research (DZL),
München, Germany

ANDREW H. LIMPER, MD
Professor of Medicine, Professor of
Biochemistry and Molecular Biology, Mayo
Clinic, Rochester, Minnesota, USA

FABRIZIO LUPPI, MD, PhD
Associate Professor, Department of Medicine
and Surgery, University of Milan Bicocca,
Pneumology Unit, Ospedale "S. Gerardo",
ASST Monza, Monza, Italy

CHAD A. NEWTON, MD, MSCS
Assistant Professor, Division of Pulmonary and
Critical Care Medicine, Department of Internal
Medicine, The University of Texas
Southwestern Medical Center, Dallas, Texas,
USA

JUSTIN M. OLDHAM, MD, MS
Department of Internal Medicine, Division of
Pulmonary, Critical Care and Sleep Medicine,
University of California, Davis, Sacramento,
California, USA

ANNA J. PODOLANCZUK, MD, MS
Assistant Professor of Medicine, Division of
Pulmonary and Critical Care Medicine, Weill
Cornell Medical College, New York, New York,
USA

RACHEL K. PUTMAN, MD, MPH
Instructor in Medicine, Division of Pulmonary
and Critical Care Medicine, Brigham and
Women's Hospital, Harvard Medical School,
Boston, Massachusetts, USA

LUCA RICHELDI, MD, PhD
Professor of Respiratory Medicine,
Department of Medical and Surgical Sciences,
Università Cattolica del Sacro Cuore, Head of
Pulmonary Medicine, Fondazione Policlinico
Universitario A. Gemelli IRCCS, Rome, Italy

CHRISTOPHER J. RYERSON, MD, FRCPC
Department of Medicine, University of British
Columbia, Centre for Heart Lung Innovation,
St. Paul's Hospital, Vancouver, British
Columbia, Canada

MARGARET L. SALISBURY, MD
Department of Medicine, Division of Allergy, Pulmonary and Critical Care, Vanderbilt University Medical Center, Nashville, Tennessee, USA

CARLO VANCHERI, MD, PhD
Department of Clinical and Experimental Medicine, University of Catania, Regional Referral Center for Rare Lung Diseases, University-Hospital "Policlinico -Vittorio Emanuele," Catania, Italy

MARLIES S. WIJSENBEEK, MD, PhD
Department of Respiratory Medicine, Centre for Interstitial Lung Diseases and Sarcoidosis, Erasmus Medical Center, University Medical Centre Rotterdam, Rotterdam, the Netherlands

ALYSON W. WONG, MD, MHSc
Clinical Instructor, Department of Medicine, University of British Columbia, Centre for Heart Lung Innovation, St. Paul's Hospital, Vancouver, British Columbia, Canada

Contributors

MARGARET L. SALISBURY, MD
Department of Medicine, Division of Allergy, Pulmonary and Critical Care, Vanderbilt University Medical Center, Nashville, Tennessee, USA

CARLO VANCHERI, MD, PhD
Department of Clinical and Experimental Medicine, University of Catania, Regional Referral Center for Rare Lung Diseases, University Hospital "Policlinico Vittorio Emanuele," Catania, Italy

MARLIES S. WIJSENBEEK, MD, PhD
Department of Respiratory Medicine, Centre for Interstitial Lung Diseases and Sarcoidosis, Erasmus Medical Center, University Medical Centre Rotterdam, Rotterdam, the Netherlands

ALYSON W. WONG, MD, MHSc
Clinical Instructor, Department of Medicine, University of British Columbia, Centre for Heart Lung Innovation, St. Paul's Hospital, Vancouver, British Columbia, Canada

Contents

> Interstitial lung diseases (ILDs) are heterogenous and complex chronic lung diseases that even today are challenging to diagnose and classify. The terminology and mechanistic understanding of specific ILDs have evolved substantially over the last centuries and decades, and clinicians, pathologists, radiologists, and researchers are continuously working to untangle the various ILDs of differing causes. Despite many drawbacks and negative clinical trials, the unremitting work of ILD researchers have resulted in great therapeutic successes over the last decade. In this chapter, the authors present historical aspects of ILD and build a foundation to understand current and emerging concepts in ILD.

> Cellular level changes that lead to interstitial lung disease (ILD) may take years to become clinically apparent and have been termed preclinical ILD. Incidentally identified interstitial lung abnormalities (ILA) are increasingly being recognized on chest computed tomographic scans done as part of lung cancer screening and for other purposes. Many individuals found to have ILA will progress to clinically significant ILD. ILA are independently associated with greater risk of death, lung function decline, and incident lung cancer. Current management recommendations focus on identifying individuals with ILA at high risk of progression, through a combination of clinical and radiological features.

> Interstitial lung diseases (ILDs) are challenging to diagnose, requiring integration of multiple complex features that are often difficult to interpret. This article reviews a pragmatic approach to ILD diagnosis and classification, focusing on diagnostic tools and strategies that are used to separate different subtypes and identify the most appropriate management. We discuss the evolution of ILD classification and the contemporary approach that integrates routinely used diagnostic tools in a multidisciplinary discussion. We highlight the increasing importance of taking a multipronged approach to ILD classification that reflects the recent emphasis on disease behavior while also considering etiopathogenesis and morphologic features.

> Idiopathic pulmonary fibrosis (IPF) is a devastating disease for patients and their loved ones. Since initial efforts to characterize this disease in the 1960s,

understanding of IPF has evolved considerably. Such evolution has continually challenged prior diagnostic and treatment paradigms, ushering in an era of higher confidence diagnoses with less invasive procedures and more effective treatments. This review details how research and clinical experience over the past half century have led to a rethinking of IPF. Here, the evolution in understanding of IPF pathogenesis, diagnostic evaluation and treatment approach is discussed.

Progress in the past 2 decades has led to widespread use of 2 medications to slow loss of lung function in patients with pulmonary fibrosis. Treatment of individual patients with currently available pharmacotherapies can be limited by side effects, and neither drug has a consistent effect on patient symptoms or function. Several promising new pharmacotherapies are under development. Comprehensive management of pulmonary fibrosis hinges on shared decision making. Patient and caregiver education, and early identification and management of symptoms and comorbidities, can help improve quality of life.

We are in the midst of transformative innovation in health care delivery and clinical trials in idiopathic pulmonary fibrosis (IPF). Health systems are uniquely positioned at the crossroad of these shifting paradigms, equipped with the resources to expand the research pipeline in IPF through visionary leadership and targeted investments. The authors hope that by prioritizing development of health information technology, supporting a broader range of clinical trial designs, and cultivating broad stakeholder engagement, health systems will generate data to address knowledge-evidence-practice gaps in IPF. This will continue to improve the ability to deliver high-quality, safe, and effective care.

The presence of interstitial lung disease (ILD) negatively affects prognosis among patients with an underlying connective tissue disease (CTD). The initial approach to care should determine whether the CTD-ILD needs pharmacologic treatment or not. There is little direct evidence to guide who and how to treat. At present, any severe, active, and/or progressive ILD should be pharmacologically treated. Immunosuppressants and/or corticosteroids are the mainstay of pharmacologic therapy for all CTD-ILDs, whereas antifibrotics may be beneficial in some scenarios. A comprehensive and multidisciplinary approach to management is also an important aspect of patient care.

Fibrotic hypersensitivity pneumonitis (fHP) is a chronic, often progressive fibrosing form of interstitial lung disease caused by inhaled antigenic exposures. fHP can lead to impaired respiratory function, reduced disease-related quality of life, and early mortality. Management of fHP should start with exposure remediation where possible, with systemic immunosuppression and antifibrotic therapy considered in patients with symptomatic or progressive disease. Nonpharmacologic and supportive management should be offered and, in cases of treatment-resistant, progressive illness, lung transplant should be considered.

Nonidiopathic pulmonary fibrosis (non-IPF) progressive fibrotic interstitial lung diseases (PF-ILDs) are a heterogeneous group of ILDs, often challenging to diagnose, although an accurate diagnosis has significant implications for both treatment and prognosis. A subgroup of these patients experiences progressive deterioration in lung function, physical performance, and quality of life after conventional therapy. Risk factors for ILD progression include older age, lower baseline pulmonary function, and a usual interstitial pneumonia pattern. Management of non-IPF P-ILD is both pharmacologic and nonpharmacologic. Antifibrotic drugs, originally approved for IPF, have been considered in patients with other fibrotic ILD subtypes, with favorable results in clinical trials.

There have been growing interest in and emphasis on health systems adopting a patient-centered care (PCC) approach, which focuses on providing care that is respectful and responsive to patient preferences, needs, and values. The features of PCC can fall into 3 domains: structure, process, and outcomes. These domains encompass the necessary infrastructure and culture required to facilitate respectful and compassionate care and patient engagement. This review discusses the features that characterize each of these PCC domains and how they can be applied specifically to clinical care and research within the field of interstitial lung disease.

Comprehensive Interstitial lung disease (ILD) care delivery models have several key components including diagnosis, treatment, monitoring, coordination with other health care providers, patient support/advocacy, education, and research. ILD is rapidly evolving, and specialized centers with ILD-specific expertise have emerged as ways to care for complex patients. The role of the specialized center in care delivery is multifaceted and aimed at improving patient care and advancing the field of ILD. Widespread access to specialized centers is a barrier to ILD care delivery worldwide. Creative and innovative strategies that leverage technology are needed to bridge gaps in ILD care.

Management of patients with interstitial lung disease (ILD) requires accurate classification. However, this process relies on subjective interpretation of nonspecific and overlapping clinical features that could hamper clinical care. The development and implementation of objective biomarkers reflective of specific disease states could facilitate precision-based approaches based on patient-level biology to improve

CLINICS IN CHEST MEDICINE

SERIES OF RELATED INTEREST

Cardiology Clinics
Available at: cardiology.theclinics.com

THE CLINICS ARE AVAILABLE ONLINE!
Access your subscription at:
www.theclinics.com

Preface
Progress and Innovation in Interstitial Lung Disease

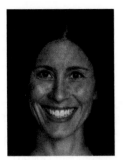
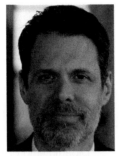
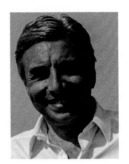

Kerri A. Johannson, MD, MPH   Harold R. Collard, MD   Luca Richeldi, MD, PhD

Editors

There have been important advancements in the field of interstitial lung disease (ILD) over the past decade. Our understanding of risk factors, pathobiology, and behavioral phenotypes has guided the diagnostic evaluation, while the identification of effective therapies and a deeper valuation of the patient experience continue to shape clinical care delivery. From preclinical disease to regenerative therapies, there is much to reflect upon and to synthesize. For this *Clinics in Chest Medicine* series, we have invited an international and diverse group of experts to share their discoveries and insights into a broad range of ILD topics. These insights are both practical and philosophical, offering novel frameworks for disease classification and biology. Overall, each article highlights recent developments, summarizes the current evidence, and outlines ongoing areas of uncertainty in key areas.

To contextualize our current ILD paradigm, Drs Guler and Corte introduce this series with a historical overview of ILD. From early clinical and histopathological descriptions to modern-day approaches, they lay the foundation for our current understanding of pulmonary fibrosis. Drs Podolanczuk and Putman introduce the concepts of "preclinical ILD" and interstitial lung abnormalities, an important and evolving area, as chest imaging is increasingly used, and at-risk individuals are screened for the presence of lung fibrosis. As our knowledge about ILD advances, so do our conceptual frameworks. In this context, Drs Adegunsoye and Ryerson present a clinically relevant approach to ILD that incorporates the latest advancements in disease behavior, etiopathogenesis, and morphology.

The subsequent 3 articles focus on idiopathic pulmonary fibrosis (IPF), starting with Drs Oldham and Vancheri summarizing the current understanding of IPF and how recent developments should guide the diagnostic evaluation. Drs Salisbury and Wijsenbeek follow this up, presenting a comprehensive approach to clinical care and management of patients with IPF. Drs Farrand and Limper identify the challenges that exist in our reliance on traditional randomized clinical trials to identify effective IPF therapeutics. They outline how health systems can contribute to and promote research in IPF, linking knowledge generation to evidence, and ultimately, to clinical practice. Addressing other important forms of ILD, Drs Kawano-Dourado and Lee provide an overview of connective tissue disease–associated ILD, with current data on epidemiology, risk factors, and treatment approaches. Drs Barnes and Johannson summarize the current approach to management of fibrotic hypersensitivity pneumonitis, an entity increasingly recognized as prevalent, and often, progressive. Drs Collins and Luppi provide an overview of the management of patients with non-IPF fibrotic ILD, incorporating data from recent clinical trials supporting new indications for antifibrotic therapy.

The next 4 articles focus on broad approaches to clinical care and scientific discovery in ILD. In their article, Drs Wong and Danoff define patient-centered care, highlight its critical importance, and provide frameworks for its implementation

Clin Chest Med 42 (2021) xiii–xiv
https://doi.org/10.1016/j.ccm.2021.03.015
0272-5231/21/© 2021 Published by Elsevier Inc.

into research and clinical care. Drs Fisher and Cottin discuss care delivery models and the importance of specialized ILD centers to provide accurate diagnoses, gold-standard management, education, and collaborative shared-care models for patients with pulmonary fibrosis. They further explore how technological advancements can be leveraged to improve access to specialty ILD centers. Drs Newton and Herzog present a state-of-the-art overview of omics-based discoveries, presenting a roadmap toward precision-based approaches to disease management. Finally, Drs Lehmann and Königshoff round out this series with the latest developments in our understanding of pulmonary fibrosis, and the hope for a cure through antiaging and regenerative therapeutic approaches.

In the final article, we summarize the current and future state of ILD management with an overview of short-term priorities for action and longer-term areas for discovery and innovation. All together, we hope that this *Clinics in Chest Medicine* series engages readers with a passion for ILD clinical care and research. The developments seen in recent years are stepping stones for further advancements in the field, toward goals of early disease identification, efficient provision of patient-centered care, and ultimately, curing lung fibrosis.

Kerri A. Johannson, MD, MPH
6th Floor, Pulmonary Diagnostics
4448 Front Street SE
Calgary AB T3M-1M4, Canada

Harold R. Collard, MD
490 Illinois Street, 6th Floor
San Francisco, CA 94158, USA

Luca Richeldi, MD, PhD
Dipartimento di Scienze Mediche e Chirurgiche
Largo Agostino Gemelli 1
00168 Roma, Italy

E-mail addresses:
kerri.johannson@ahs.ca (K.A. Johannson)
harold.collard@ucsf.edu (H.R. Collard)
luca.richeldi@unicatt.it (L. Richeldi)

Interstitial Lung Disease in 2020: A History of Progress

Sabina A. Guler, MD, MHSc[a],*, Tamera J. Corte, MD, PhD[b]

KEYWORDS

- Interstitial lung disease • Idiopathic pulmonary fibrosis • History of medicine

KEY POINTS

- The understanding of underlying mechanisms of interstitial lung diseases has changed drastically over the last centuries.
- Changing terminology over the past decades has complicated communication and collaborative research, whereas progressively detailed clinical guidelines have been provided.
- Therapeutic successes over the last decade have been substantial.

INTRODUCTION

Our understanding of interstitial lung diseases (ILDs) has evolved drastically over the last 2 centuries, and today ILD is viewed as a large, heterogenous group of distinct diseases that affect the lung parenchyma via inflammation and fibrosis.[1] Patients with ILD suffer from frequently progressive dyspnea, cough, and impaired physical function affecting their quality of life. In addition, mortality in patients with ILD can be as high as in some types of cancer. Patients with idiopathic pulmonary fibrosis (IPF), the most common of the idiopathic ILDs, have a median life expectancy of only 3 to 5 years from the time of diagnosis, although there is considerable heterogeneity with some patients living longer than 10 years after diagnosis.[2] Symptoms at presentation are typically nonspecific, which may lead to initial misdiagnosis and subsequent delay in specific ILD diagnosis. Furthermore, different ILD subtypes have overlapping pathophysiological and morphologic features, which makes ILD classification challenging.[1]

In the last decade, there have been major developments in our understanding of ILD, and consequently, our approach to its diagnosis and management. The frequently changing ILD terminology has limited communication between clinicians and researchers, and today agreement on diagnostic and management standards is still not optimal. Knowledge of underlying mechanisms of specific ILDs has grown substantially over the last few years, and particularly for IPF, effective therapies have been identified.[3–5] In this chapter, the authors aim to elucidate historical aspects of ILD and build a foundation to understand current and emerging concepts in these complex diseases. The history of ILD is intertwined with the history of anatomy, physiology, and chemistry, with changes in society, occupational developments, technical achievements, and emerging infectious diseases that have influenced the epidemiology and identification of the ILDs.

EVOLUTION OF INTERSTITIAL LUNG DISEASE CLASSIFICATION AND TERMINOLOGY

Early descriptions of "chronic interstitial pneumonia" were quite different from our current understanding of ILD, and physicians mostly referred to chronic nonresolving pneumonia, post-tuberculosis lung damage, and pneumoconiosis. Even though infectious pulmonary sequelae and occupational pulmonary fibrosis are still important causes of restrictive lung disorders, today there

[a] Department of Pulmonary Medicine, Inselspital, Bern University Hospital, University of Bern, Switzerland Freiburgstrasse 18, 3010 Bern, Switzerland; [b] Respiratory Department, Royal Prince Alfred Hospital, Missenden Rd, Camperdown, NSW, 2050, Australia
* Corresponding author.
E-mail address: sabina.guler@insel.ch

Clin Chest Med 42 (2021) 229–239
https://doi.org/10.1016/j.ccm.2021.03.001
0272-5231/21/© 2021 The Author(s). Published by Elsevier Inc. This is an open access article under the CC BY-NC-ND license (http://creativecommons.org/licenses/by-nc-nd/4.0/).

are many other idiopathic, autoimmune, and exposure-associated ILDs described.[1]

The terminology and classification of ILD has evolved steadily since its first descriptions (**Figs. 1** and **2**).

Idiopathic Interstitial Pneumonias

Early descriptions

In 1872, Von Buhl, a German physician, reported cases of *desquamative pneumonia* and *chronic interstitial pneumonia* where he described spindle and star cells and excessive connective tissue. His letters to a friend might have been one of the first descriptions of pulmonary fibrosis.[6] In 1892, Osler mentioned in his medical textbook the evolution of acute infectious pneumonia into a *chronic interstitial pneumonia* or *cirrhosis of the lung*, and this emphasizes that many of the chronic ILDs of that time were nonresolving pneumonias. In 1898, Rindfleisch reported a case of a 40-year-old man with progressive cough and dyspnea, who had a large right ventricle and small stiff lungs on autopsy, with multiple cystic spaces that Rindfleisch called *cirrhosis cystica pulmonum*.[7]

The clinician Louis Hamman and the pathologist Arnold Rich reported in 1933 and 1935, respectively, fulminating *diffuse interstitial fibrosis of the lungs*,[8] coining the term Hamman-Rich syndrome. Somewhat surprisingly, at that time acute and chronic cases were not distinguished, and cases were labeled Hamman-Rich syndrome as long as the typical pathologic features of diffuse alveolar damage were found (usually on autopsy). In 1957, Rubin reviewed 15 cases with Hamman-Rich syndrome[9] and found that presentations were more heterogenous than previously thought.

Some patients had systemic illness, which were likely signs of connective tissue diseases. Furthermore, not all cases were rapidly progressive, and a distinction between acute and chronic forms was made. From the 1950s, *chronic Hamman-Rich syndrome* was synonymously used for chronic interstitial pulmonary fibrosis and in the 1960s this phenomenon was renamed as cryptogenic fibrosing alveolitis (CFA) (see **Fig. 2**).

In the 1960s case reports and series on conditions that were named *cystic pulmonary cirrhosis, bronchiolar emphysema, muscular cirrhosis of the lung*, and *pulmonary muscular hyperplasia* were published in the United States, Canada, Mexico, Scandinavia, France, and Britain.[10–12] Patients were reported to have suffered from dyspnea for at least a year before presentation, with little cough and sputum, a few presenting with clubbed fingers and the majority with crepitations on lung auscultation. When pulmonary function tests were performed, patients had reduced forced vital capacity and diffusion capacity of the lung for carbon monoxide. On autopsy the pulmonary tissue showed honeycombing, and replacement of alveolar tissue with smooth muscle, but little evidence of active inflammation. A few of the patients described were coal miners and others had lymph node involvement; consequently, some of these cases may have had what are now classified as pneumoconiosis and sarcoidosis.

Around that time the conceptualization of ILD (Hamman-Rich syndrome) as a chronic disease was further supported: Gross hypothesized that acute Hamman-Rich syndrome might be an acute exacerbation of the chronic Hamman-Rich syndrome,[13] and Sheridan found that patients

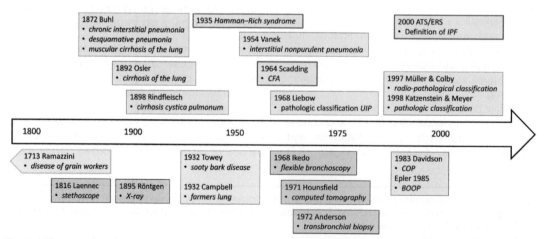

Fig. 1. Milestones for idiopathic interstitial pneumonias (*blue*), hypersensitivity pneumonitis (*green*), organizing pneumonia (*red*), and for relevant technical achievements (*gray*). BOOP, bronchiolitis obliterans organizing pneumonia; COP, cryptogenic organizing pneumonia; UIP, usual interstitial pneumonia.

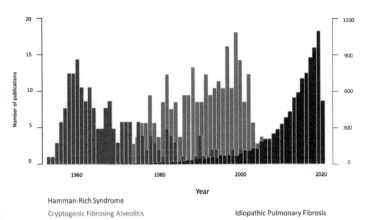

Fig. 2. Number of PubMed publications by year for Hamman-Rich syndrome, cryptogenic fibrosing alveolitis, and IPF.

Hamman-Rich Syndrome

Cryptogenic Fibrosing Alveolitis   Idiopathic Pulmonary Fibrosis

survived on average for several years with this chronic lung disease.[14]

Modern descriptions

In 1968 to 69, Liebow and Carrington provided the first pathologic classification of chronic ILDs.[15] They introduced the term *usual interstitial pneumonia (UIP)*, which was called *usual* because it was the most commonly observed pattern. Furthermore, they described bronchiolitis obliterans organizing pneumonia (BOOP), diffuse alveolar damage, desquamative interstitial pneumonia (DIP), lymphocytic interstitial pneumonia, and giant cell interstitial pneumonia. In the 1970s the clinical disease associated with UIP was called CFA (sometimes idiopathic). In 1980, Turner-Warwick discussed CFA with underlying pathologic patterns of DIP or UIP (end-stage fibrosis) depending on the stage and severity of the clinical CFA.[16]

With increasing use of chest computed tomography (CT) scans in the 1990s, the modern differentiation between IPF and other idiopathic interstitial pneumonias (IIPs) was further refined. In 1997, Müller and Colby published the first radiological-histological classification of IIPs and proposed radiological criteria for UIP, acute interstitial pneumonia (AIP), DIP, nonspecific interstitial pneumonia (NSIP), and BOOP/ cryptogenic organising pneumonia (COP).[17] The pathologists, Katzenstein and Myers, described the 1998 criteria for the pathologic classification of AIP, UIP, DIP/ respiratory bronchiolitis-ILD, and NSIP,[18] which led to the definition of IPF and its discrimination from other IIPs in the American Thoracic Society (ATS)/European Respiratory Society (ERS) 2000 consensus statement.[19] The 2002 ATS/ERS multidisciplinary consensus classification of IIPs discriminated IIPs from diffuse parenchymal lung diseases of known cause and granulomatous

ILDs. In addition, a diagnostic algorithm and sets of radiological and pathologic classification criteria were proposed.[20] The 2011 ATS/ERS/JRS/ALAT statement on IPF diagnosis allowed for a confident IPF diagnosis without surgical lung biopsy if a definite radiological UIP pattern was present.[21] Seven years later, the 2018 ATS/ERS/JRS/ALAT Clinical Practice Guideline further specified the radiological patterns as UIP, probable UIP, indeterminate for UIP, and alternate diagnosis.[2] At the same time the Fleischner Society published similar diagnostic criteria for IPF and further strengthened the role of CT by allowing a clinical-radiological IPF diagnosis in cases with a probable radiological UIP pattern (**Table 1**).[22]

Hypersensitivity Pneumonitis

In 1713, Ramazzini described grain workers in Italy who frequently developed dyspnea, cachexia, and finally edema attributed to right heart failure. Ramazzini also wrote what is thought to be the first book on occupational medicine (De Morbis Artificum Diatriba [Diseases of Workers]) wherein he described health hazard associated with different occupations.

Not until the 1930s was "farmers lung" mentioned again in more detail: Campbell reported an acute respiratory disease in North English farmers working with mouldy hay. Workers had developed severe dyspnea and cyanosis that persisted for several weeks with development of fibrosis in some cases.[23] At the same time Towey described severe dyspnea, cough, night sweats, and weight loss in railroad workers near Lake Michigan. The patients were all exposed to "black dust" on maple bark from which fungus spores were isolated (*Cryptostroma corticale*). Towey and colleagues conducted a variety of animal and human experiments with the putative antigen and concluded that the railroad workers had

Table 1
Landmark papers and guidelines for interstitial lung disease classification

Classifications and Guidelines	IIP—ILD	IPF
Historical	Liebow & Carrington 1968/69[15] Katzenstein 1998[18] Müller & Colby 1997[17]	ATS/ERS Consensus 2000 (diagnosis and treatment)[19]
Previous	*ATS/ERS 2002 (classification)*[20]	*ATS/ERS/JRS/ALAT 2011*[21]
Current	*Update ATS/ERS 2013*[1] *Hypersensitivity Pneumonitis ATS/JRS/ALAT 2020 (diagnosis)*[25]	*ATS/ERS/JRS/ALAT 2018 Clinical Practice Guideline*[2] *Fleischner 2018*[22]

Abbreviations: ALAT, Latin American Thoracic Association ATS; American Thoracic Society; ERS, European Respiratory Society; ILD, interstitial lung disease; IIP, idiopathic interstitial pneumonia; IPF, idiopathic pulmonary fibrosis; JRS, Japanese Respiratory Society.

developed an immunologic disease with sensitization to proteins and foreign body reaction to the fungal spores.[24]

Today, hypersensitivity pneumonitis (HP) is considered an immune-mediated inflammatory and fibrotic reaction of the lung to an inhaled antigen in sensitized individuals. Potentially inciting antigens are usually organic, including avian and microbial antigens; however, in up to half of cases at ILD referral centers, the antigen cannot be identified.[25] Traditionally, acute, subacute, and chronic forms of HP have been distinguished, depending on the duration, frequency, and intensity of the exposure.[26] Because of the challenging differentiation of these forms, it had also been suggested to classify HP as active or residual disease for clinical purposes.[27] The most recently published clinical practice guideline categorizes HP into nonfibrotic and fibrotic phenotypes, deeming this classification more objective and clinically relevant (see **Table 1**).[25]

Organizing Pneumonia

In the early twentieth century, autopsy descriptions of patients deceased from nonresolving pneumonia emerged. Intraalveolar exudates with proliferation of fibroblasts and production of connective tissue described in cases of congestion and hepatization, the classic Laennec stages of pneumonia, were not followed by resolution. Von Hansemann described "Lymphangitis reticularis" in 1915 as a morphologic pattern that destroyed the lung progressively after tuberculosis but could also develop without previous infectious disease.[28]

The perception that organizing pneumonia (OP) was always a sequela of pulmonary infection has changed to the current understanding, suggesting that OP may arise due to a variety of toxic or autoimmune triggers, or can be idiopathic. In 1986, Basset reported on intraluminal organizing and fibrotic changes occurring in a variety of ILDs, including pneumoconiosis, sarcoidosis, and hypersensitivity pneumonitis.[29] Around the same time, Davidson introduced the term "cryptogenic organising pneumonia,"[30] and Epler introduced "idiopathic bronchiolitis obliterans with organising pneumonia" (BOOP).[31]

Katzenstein and Myer did not include BOOP in their pathologic classification of *idiopathic interstitial pneumonias* (1998) because of its mainly intraluminal and not interstitial fibrosis.[18] In 2002 the ATS/ERS IIP Consensus Classification suggested using the term "cryptogenic organizing pneumonia" (COP) to avoid confusing BOOP with airways diseases, for example, bronchiolitis obliterans.[19] Currently, in the 2013 updated IIP classification guideline, COP is listed as 1 of the 6 major IIPs (see **Table 1**).[1]

Recent Developments

Combined pulmonary fibrosis and emphysema was proposed as a distinct clinical entity in 2005.[32] The combination of upper lobe emphysema and lower lobe fibrosis typically occurs in current or former smokers. Patients frequently have preserved lung volumes but severely reduced diffusion capacity for carbon monoxide and hypoxemia. The prevalence of pulmonary hypertension is estimated at 50% in this population and is an important clinical feature, as it is also prognostic.

Around 12% of patients with ILD remain unclassifiable despite the modern approach to ILD diagnosis and classification.[33] Phenotyping these patients might facilitate management decisions, and phenotyping according to specific clinical features and/or according to disease behavior is becoming increasingly popular. Occasionally ILD is the first manifestation of a connective tissue disease (CTD). Terminology for these cases has been inconsistent including "forme fruste" CTD, lung-dominant CTD, and more recently interstitial pneumonia with autoimmune features (IPAF).[34,35] In 2015 ATS and ERS released a research statement for the IPAF concept to facilitate future research in this area. Patients with an unclassifiable ILD who did not fulfill criteria for a CTD but demonstrate clinical, serologic, and morphologic signs of autoimmunity were labeled IPAF.[34] Currently, the therapeutic implications of the IPAF phenotype are still unclear.

The approach to classifying fibrotic ILD according to disease behavior has culminated in large clinical trials investigating the safety and efficacy of antifibrotic medications in patients with progressive fibrosing ILD. A recent placebo controlled study of nintedanib included progressive ILDs of different etiologic subtypes,[36] and a study of pirfenidone recently focused on patients with unclassifiable ILD with a progressive disease behavior.[37] Lumping patients with distinct ILDs is appealing, given their frequently overlapping clinical and morphologic characteristics and the potential management implications that have been demonstrated by recent clinical trials. However, we learned from past that a detailed characterization of patients with ILD can enable the development of targeted therapies. Currently, classification according to cause and disease behavior is complementary and should not compromise a thorough, multidisciplinary ILD diagnosis.

PATHOGENESIS

In 1965, Meyer and Liebow discussed the pathogenetic mechanisms leading to honeycombing in patients with chronic interstitial pneumonia. Because of their observation that some patients had honeycombing and lung cancer, they suspected a connection between honeycombing, atypical cells, and "scar cancers." Furthermore, they stated that "Interstitial pneumonia can result from damage by a great variety of agents, of which only a few are known." Viruses; chemical exposures; collagen diseases, for example, rheumatoid arthritis; and genetic factors (familial pulmonary fibrosis) were suspected to cause honeycombing and chronic interstitial pneumonia.[38]

In the 1970s and 1980s, the accepted framework of IPF pathogenesis was of a chronic inflammatory alveolitis caused by repetitive harmful stimuli. Therapeutic efforts were aimed at stopping the inflammatory process in the hopes of preventing irreversible fibrosis.[39] Unfortunately, long-term treatment with corticosteroids did not usually prevent the hypothesized progression from inflammation to fibrosis.

Later, the hypothesis of fibrosis as a result of abnormal wound healing emerged. Fibrosis was interpreted as a result of activated macrophages that produce growth factors, which in turn stimulate fibroblasts to produce extracellular matrix.[40]

The theory of impaired restoration of alveolar epithelial cells after repetitive lung injury leading to fibrosis[41] was supported by electron microscopy studies that emphasized the role of epithelial cells in the pathogenesis of pulmonary fibrosis.[42] After 2000, UIP was recognized as a distinct pathologic entity and not only a common final pathway of inflammatory ILDs. The paradigm changed from a model of inflammation leading to fibrosis to a model of repetitive alveolar epithelial injury and abnormal wound healing with predominant fibrosis and minimal inflammation.[43]

EPIDEMIOLOGY

There has been an increase in reporting of ILD overall, as well as IPF over the second half of the twentieth century. Aside from changes in the diagnostic guidelines, and the availability of high-resolution CT scans, this also coincides with increased cigarette smoking, an established risk factor for IPF.[44] However, unlike in lung cancer and COPD it is less clear if increasing IPF prevalence developed as a direct consequence of the smoking epidemic.[45] More likely, an interaction between smoking, genetic predisposition, age, and male sex underlies the increasing prevalence of IPF.[46] In 1994 in Bernalillo County (New Mexico, half a million inhabitants), Coultas recorded all new cases of ILD over 2 years and estimated an incidence and prevalence of 31.5/100,000/y and 80.9/100,000 in men and 26.1/100,000/y and 67.2/100,000 in women, respectively.[47] Between 1991 and 2003, the incidence of IPF increased by 11% annually in the United Kingdom,[48] reflecting the increasing overall burden of IPF.

DIAGNOSIS

Clinical examination of patients with pulmonary fibrosis has always been considered important, but pathognomonic signs of the specific ILDs are lacking. In 1816 Laennec invented the stethoscope and correlated the auscultation sounds with autopsy findings. He described the fine crackles and velcro rales, which are still valuable clinical clues for advanced ILDs. In 1945 Eder described clubbing of the fingers and toes as a clinical sign of IPF.

In 1895, Röntgen discovered radiography and later received the first Nobel Prize in physics for this invention. Röntgen techniques were quickly adopted, and after World War II radiography became widely available. In 1933, Kerley described a thickening of the pulmonary septa, sometimes observed in ILD.[49] Scadding proposed a radiographic staging of sarcoidosis and demonstrated that the 4 stages were predictive of survival in patients with sarcoidosis.[50] MRI was used commercially from 1979 but did not contribute significantly to the diagnosis of ILDs. Similarly, gallium scans were used to detect "active alveolitis" and stage IPF/CFA, HP, and sarcoidosis between 1980 and 1990[51,52] but were not used widely after this period. Only the discovery of CT paved the way for modern ILD diagnosis and classification. After the discoveries of Hounsfield, the first CT scans were used on patients in the 1970s. The Fleischner Society proposed a first glossary of terms for CT of the lungs in 1984 and defined the radiological criteria for honeycombing.[53] The glossary was updated in 1996[54] and in 2008 when honeycombing was listed as a key criterion for radiological UIP.[55] In the latest expert opinion of the Fleischner Society, the role of CT imaging was further strengthened by allowing for a confident IPF diagnosis in cases with a definite or probable UIP pattern, when clinical features were compatible with IPF but surgical lung biopsy was not available.[22]

Flexible bronchoscopy was introduced in clinical practice from 1968, and bronchoalveolar lavage (BAL) fluid has been used as both a research tool and in clinical practice for various ILDs.[56] Today, BAL is a very safe procedure and BAL cellular analysis can provide valuable data for ILD diagnosis. Furthermore, BAL can be helpful to exclude infections or detect malignancy in patients with suspected ILD.[25,57] The first transbronchial lung biopsies (TBB) were performed by Anderson and colleagues in 1972.[58] Today, histologic samples from TBB are frequently performed if sarcoidosis is suspected, whereas their diagnostic value is limited for other ILDs.[1]

Transbronchial lung cryobiopsy has emerged as a new diagnostic tool for ILD over the last 10 years,[59] with higher diagnostic yield but also higher complication rate compared with conventional TBB.[60] Transbronchial lung cryobiopsy might replace surgical lung biopsy in some scenarios, and the technique continues to be used and studied in clinical practice.[61,62]

The current pathologic sampling standard for ILD diagnosis is surgical lung biopsy, which has been performed for this purpose since 1952, when Rubin performed a thoracotomy in a patient with suspected pulmonary fibrosis.[63] In 1964, Gaensler reported on 105 patients after surgical lung biopsy for suspected Hamman-Rich syndrome, concluding that the procedure can be performed safely in this population.[64] Today the 30-day mortality after elective surgical lung biopsy is estimated to be 2%, with significantly higher risk of death in nonelective procedures and high-risk patients.[65]

Multidisciplinary cancer conferences have long been an integral component of cancer care.[66] For ILD, multidisciplinary team (MDT) discussions have emerged as the diagnostic reference standard over the last few decades. The 2002 ATS/ERS consensus paper recommended a clinico–radiological–pathological case discussion for patients with unclassifiable ILD,[19] and the 2013 update proposed that MDT discussion should replace histologic diagnosis as the reference standard for ILD diagnosis.[1] Walsh and colleagues then demonstrated in 2016 an improved diagnostic accuracy with the integration of an MDT in the diagnostic process.[67] Current MDTs consist of experienced ILD physicians, thoracic radiologists, pathologists, and occasionally thoracic surgeons or rheumatologists. All available clinical, radiological, and pathologic information are synthesized in a structured manner. Ideally the patient's history (including exposures and occupation), symptoms, and clinical signs and results from pulmonary function and physical performance tests including oxygenation, echocardiography, and serologic tests for CTD should be available. Furthermore, high-quality chest CT scans with inspiratory and expiratory images, and if available results from BAL, and histologic sampling are discussed.

MANAGEMENT
Nonpharmacological Treatment

One of the earliest treatments for chronic postinfectious pulmonary fibrosis was "collapse therapy," which was used from 1930s for the treatment of tuberculosis. By artificial pneumothorax, phrenic paralysis, or thoracoplasty the lung was "set at rest to heal."[68]

In 1963 Hardy successfully completed the first human lung transplant in a patient with lung cancer.[69] However, only the introduction of potent immunosuppressive drugs along with improved surgical techniques led to long-term survival of patients after lung transplant. One of the first long-term survivors after single-lung transplant in 1986 was a man with pulmonary fibrosis.[70] Implementation of the lung allocation score in 2005, ex-vivo lung perfusion, and extracorporeal membrane oxygenation as a bridge to transplant have further advanced the potential of lung transplantation.[71] Today, IPF is the leading indication for lung transplant in many countries; however, given the high number of comorbidities and typically advanced age of patients with IPF, lung transplant remains a treatment option that is only available to a minority of the patients.

Supplemental oxygen has been used to improve oxygenation and relieve dyspnea since 1926 when Barach demonstrated its application in a patient with pneumonia.[72] He later introduced portable oxygen systems for patients with emphysema.[72] Today, long-term oxygen therapy is well established for hypoxemic patients with chronic lung diseases, and at least some patients with fibrotic ILD experience an improvement in health-related quality of life by using ambulatory supplemental oxygen therapy.[73]

Ramazzini, the founder of occupational medicine, already warned in the seventeenth century that "sitting can lead to an early death," and "sedentary workers" were on the list of occupations with particular hazards. However, until the middle of the twentieth century patients with pulmonary diseases were advised to avoid physical activity as a mean to manage dyspnea. In 1969 a group from Denver demonstrated that patients with COPD improved their exercise tolerance and well being by participation in a comprehensive, multidisciplinary outpatient program.[74] A few years later the term "pulmonary rehabilitation" was defined by the American College of Chest Physicians and in 1981 the first ATS statement on pulmonary rehabilitation was published.[75] Patients with IPF and other ILDs benefit from pulmonary rehabilitation in terms of exercise performance and health-related quality of life,[76] and today pulmonary rehabilitation is recommended for the management of IPF.[21]

Pharmacologic Treatment

Since the 1940s corticosteroids have been used with the goal of preventing the progression of inflammation to irreversible fibrosis. Several case studies from the 1960s report improvement after initiation and worsening after stopping corticosteroids. These patients likely included cases with NSIP and CTD-associated ILD, fibrotic HP, and organizing pneumonia. In 1959 Rubin and Lubliner reported that only a minority of the patients treated with corticosteroids for Hamman Rich Syndrome improved after 1 year.[9] Similarly, in a case series from 1962 only 2 of 9 patients with "interstitial pulmonary fibrosis" had a slight subjective improvement, whereas the others did not respond to corticosteroid treatment.[77]

In the 1980s phenotypes of pulmonary fibrosis were identified that responded well or did not respond to corticosteroids. Carrington found that 50% and 14% of patients with DIP and UIP on pathology responded to corticosteroids, respectively.[78] Furthermore, patients with higher cellularity on biopsy were found to have better clinical responses to corticosteroids.[79] The notion at that time was that highly cellular DIP represented early CFA and needed to be treated with corticosteroids and immunosuppression.[80] A randomized controlled trial in 1991 concluded that azathioprine combined with prednisone was likely more efficacious than prednisone alone for the treatment of IPF.[81] It was thought, however, that the 27 patients included in that trial represented a mixture of NSIP, COP, and CTD-associated ILDs. Following these studies, the 2000 ATS/ERS consensus group suggested treating patients with IPF with corticosteroids and cytotoxic agents such as azathioprine or cyclophosphamide.[19]

In the early 2000s the exploration of therapies against antifibrotic processes improved the knowledge on the natural history of IPF substantially but did not produce therapeutic success. None of the randomized controlled trials were able to demonstrate efficacy of the investigated drugs including interferons beta/gamma, etanercept, imatinib, and endothelin receptor antagonists. Subsequently, the 2011 ATS/ERS/JRS/ALAT statement no longer recommended any specific therapy for IPF, acknowledging the lack of evidence at that time.[21] Shortly after, the National Institutes of Health–sponsored PANTHER trial completely changed the approach to IPF treatment by demonstrating detrimental effects of combined N-acetylcysteine, azathioprine, and prednisone for patients with IPF.[81]

In the meantime, the role of immunosuppression for the treatment of non-IPF ILDs was further clarified by the Scleroderma Lung Studies. The Scleroderma Lung Study I in 2006 and II in 2016 established cyclophosphamide and mycophenolate mofetil as treatment options for systemic sclerosis–associated ILD.[82,83]

Antifibrotic treatment had already been investigated in 1999, when Raghu reported stabilization of pulmonary function in 29 of 46 patients treated with the antifibrotic, pirfenidone.[84] In 2014, 3 large, randomized-controlled placebo-controlled trials demonstrated a slowed decline in forced vital capacity in patients with IPF treated with either pirfenidone or nintedanib compared with a placebo group.[3–5] Following these trials pirfenidone and nintedanib are now approved for the treatment of

IPF. In addition, Nintedanib has recently been approved by Food and Drug Administration and European Medicine Agencies for the treatment of systemic sclerosis–associated ILD and for progressive fibrosing ILD following the SENSCIS and INBUILD trials.[36,85]

SUMMARY

Historically, we have seen recurring challenges concerning the terminology, classification, and staging of the ILDs. Since the Hamman-Rich era, clinicians, radiologists, pathologists, and researchers have used emerging data to untangle the ILDs arising from different causes and with differing prognoses and treatment approaches. Although controversies and challenges persist, tremendous progress has been made over the last decade

CLINICS CARE POINTS

- The understanding of underlying mechanisms of interstitial lung diseases has changed drastically over the last centuries.
- Changing terminology over the past decades has complicated communication and collaborative research, whereas progressively detailed clinical guidelines have been provided.
- Therapeutic successes over the last decade have been substantial.

DISCLOSURE

The authors have no conflicts of interest related to this work.

REFERENCES

1. Travis WD, Costabel U, Hansell DM, et al. An Official American Thoracic Society/European Respiratory Society statement: update of the international multidisciplinary classification of the idiopathic interstitial pneumonias. Am J Respir Crit Care Med 2013; 188(6):733–48.
2. Raghu G, Remy-Jardin M, Myers JL, et al. Diagnosis of idiopathic pulmonary fibrosis. An official ATS/ERS/JRS/ALAT clinical practice guideline. Am J Respir Crit Care Med 2018;198(5):e44–68.
3. King TE Jr, Bradford WZ, Castro-Bernardini S, et al. A phase 3 trial of pirfenidone in patients with idiopathic pulmonary fibrosis. N Engl J Med 2014; 370(22):2083–92.
4. Noble PW, Albera C, Bradford WZ, et al. Pirfenidone in patients with idiopathic pulmonary fibrosis (CAPACITY): two randomised trials. Lancet 2011; 377(9779):1760–9.
5. Richeldi L, du Bois RM, Raghu G, et al. Efficacy and safety of nintedanib in idiopathic pulmonary fibrosis. N Engl J Med 2014;370(22):2071–82.
6. Buhl L. Lungenentzündung, Tuberkulose und Schwindsucht: zwölf Briefe an einen Freund. Bayrische Staatsbibliothek München: Oldenbourg; 1873.
7. Rindfleisch G. Ueber cirrhosis cystica pulmonum. Zentralbl Pathol 1897;8:864–5.
8. Hamman L, Rich AR. Fulminating diffuse interstitial fibrosis of the lungs. Trans Am Clin Climatol Assoc 1935;51:154–63.
9. Rubin EH, Lubliner R. The Hamman-Rich syndrome: review of the literature and analysis of 15 cases. Medicine (Baltimore) 1957;36(4):397–463.
10. Burman SO, Kent EM. Bronchiolar emphysema (cirrhosis of the lung). J Thorac Cardiovasc Surg 1962;43:253–61.
11. Davies D, MacFarlane A, Darke CS, et al. Muscular hyperplasia ("cirrhosis") of the lung and bronchial dilatations as features of chronic diffuse fibrosing alveolitis. Thorax 1966;21(3):272–89.
12. Hirshfield HJ, Krainer L, Coe GC. Cystic pulmonary cirrhosis (bronchiolar emphysema). (Muscular cirrhosis of the lungs). Dis chest 1962;42:107–10.
13. Gross P. The concept of the Hamman-Rich syndrome. A critique. Am Rev Respir Dis 1962;85: 828–32.
14. Sheridan LA, Harrison EG Jr, Divertie MB. The current status of idiopathic pulmonary fibrosis (HAMMAN-RICH syndrome). Med Clin North Am 1964; 48:993–1010.
15. Liebow A, Carrington C, Simon M, et al. Frontiers of pulmonary radiology. In: Alveolar diseases: the interstitial pneumonias. New York: Grune & Stratton; 1969. p. 102–41.
16. Turner-Warwick M, Burrows B, Johnson A. Cryptogenic fibrosing alveolitis: clinical features and their influence on survival. Thorax 1980;35(3):171–80.
17. Müller NL, Coiby TV. Idiopathic interstitial pneumonias: high-resolution CT and histologic findings. Radiographics 1997;17(4):1016–22.
18. Katzenstein AL, Myers JL. Idiopathic pulmonary fibrosis: clinical relevance of pathologic classification. Am J Respir Crit Care Med 1998;157(4 Pt 1): 1301–15.
19. American Thoracic Society. Idiopathic pulmonary fibrosis: diagnosis and treatment. International consensus statement. American Thoracic Society (ATS), and the European Respiratory Society (ERS). Am J Respir Crit Care Med 2000;161(2 Pt 1):646–64.
20. American thoracic society/European respiratory society international multidisciplinary consensus classification of the idiopathic interstitial pneumonias. This joint statement of the American thoracic society (ATS), and the European respiratory society (ERS) was adopted by the ATS board of directors, June

2001 and by the ERS Executive Committee, June 2001. Am J Respir Crit Care Med 2002;165(2): 277–304.

21. Raghu G, Collard HR, Egan JJ, et al. An official ATS/ERS/JRS/ALAT statement: idiopathic pulmonary fibrosis: evidence-based guidelines for diagnosis and management. Am J Respir Crit Care Med 2011;183(6):788–824.

22. Lynch DA, Sverzellati N, Travis WD, et al. Diagnostic criteria for idiopathic pulmonary fibrosis: a Fleischner society white paper. Lancet Respir Med 2018; 6(2):138–53.

23. Campbell JM. Acute symptoms following work with Hay. Br Med J 1932;1143–4.

24. Towey JW, Sweany HC, Huron WH. Severe Bronchial asthma apparently due to fungus spores found IN maple bark. J Am Med Assoc 1932; 99(6):453–9.

25. Raghu G, Remy-Jardin M, Ryerson CJ, et al. Diagnosis of hypersensitivity pneumonitis in adults. An official ATS/JRS/ALAT clinical practice guideline. Am J Respir Crit Care Med 2020;202(3):e36–69.

26. Richerson HB, Bernstein IL, Fink JN, et al. Guidelines for the clinical evaluation of hypersensitivity pneumonitis. Report of the Subcommittee on Hypersensitivity Pneumonitis. J Allergy Clin Immunol 1989; 84(5 Pt 2):839–44.

27. Lacasse Y, Selman M, Costabel U, et al. Clinical diagnosis of hypersensitivity pneumonitis. Am J Respir Crit Care Med 2003;168(8):952–8.

28. von Hansemann D. Die Lymphangitis reticularis der Lungen als selbständige Erkrankung. Arch Path Anat 1915;220(3):311–21.

29. Basset F, Ferrans VJ, Soler P, et al. Intraluminal fibrosis in interstitial lung disorders. Am J Pathol 1986;122(3):443–61.

30. Davison AG, Heard BE, McAllister WA, et al. Cryptogenic organizing pneumonitis. Q J Med 1983; 52(207):382–94.

31. Epler GR, Colby TV, McLoud TC, et al. Bronchiolitis obliterans organizing pneumonia. N Engl J Med 1985;312(3):152–8.

32. Cottin V, Nunes H, Brillet PY, et al. Combined pulmonary fibrosis and emphysema: a distinct underrecognised entity. Eur Respir J 2005;26(4):586–93.

33. Guler SA, Ellison K, Algamdi M, et al. Heterogeneity in unclassifiable interstitial lung disease. A systematic review and meta-analysis. Ann Am Thorac Soc 2018;15(7):854–63.

34. Fischer A, Antoniou KM, Brown KK, et al. An Official European Respiratory Society/American Thoracic Society research statement: interstitial pneumonia with autoimmune features. Eur Respir J 2015;46(4): 976–87.

35. Fischer A, West SG, Swigris JJ, et al. Connective tissue disease-associated interstitial lung disease: a call for clarification. Chest 2010;138(2):251–6.

36. Flaherty KR, Wells AU, Cottin V, et al. Nintedanib in progressive fibrosing interstitial lung diseases. N Engl J Med 2019;381(18):1718–27.

37. Maher TM, Corte TJ, Fischer A, et al. Pirfenidone in patients with unclassifiable progressive fibrosing interstitial lung disease: a double-blind, randomised, placebo-controlled, phase 2 trial. Lancet Respir Med 2020;8(2):147–57.

38. Meyer EC, Liebow AA. Relationship of interstitial pneumonia honeycombing and atypical epithelial proliferation to cancer of the lung. Cancer 1965;18: 322–51.

39. Crystal RG, Fulmer JD, Roberts WC, et al. Idiopathic pulmonary fibrosis. Clinical, histologic, radiographic, physiologic, scintigraphic, cytologic, and biochemical aspects. Ann Intern Med 1976;85(6): 769–88.

40. Bitterman PB, Adelberg S, Crystal RG. Mechanisms of pulmonary fibrosis. Spontaneous release of the alveolar macrophage-derived growth factor in the interstitial lung disorders. J Clin Invest 1983;72(5): 1801–13.

41. Witschi H, Haschek WM, Meyer KR, et al. A pathogenetic mechanism in lung fibrosis. Chest 1980;78(2 Suppl):395–9.

42. Katzenstein AL. Pathogenesis of "fibrosis" in interstitial pneumonia: an electron microscopic study. Hum Pathol 1985;16(10):1015–24.

43. Selman M, King TE, Pardo A. Idiopathic pulmonary fibrosis: prevailing and evolving hypotheses about its pathogenesis and implications for therapy. Ann Intern Med 2001;134(2):136–51.

44. Baumgartner KB, Samet JM, Stidley CA, et al. Cigarette smoking: a risk factor for idiopathic pulmonary fibrosis. Am J Respir Crit Care Med 1997;155(1): 242–8.

45. Cordier JF, Cottin V. Neglected evidence in idiopathic pulmonary fibrosis: from history to earlier diagnosis. Eur Respir J 2013;42(4):916–23.

46. Steele MP, Speer MC, Loyd JE, et al. Clinical and pathologic features of familial interstitial pneumonia. Am J Respir Crit Care Med 2005;172(9):1146–52.

47. Coultas DB, Zumwalt RE, Black WC, et al. The epidemiology of interstitial lung diseases. Am J Respir Crit Care Med 1994;150(4):967–72.

48. Gribbin J, Hubbard RB, Le Jeune I, et al. Incidence and mortality of idiopathic pulmonary fibrosis and sarcoidosis in the UK. Thorax 2006;61(11):980–5.

49. Kerley P. Radiology IN heart disease. Br Med J 1933;2(3795):594–612, 593.

50. Scadding JG. Prognosis of intrathoracic sarcoidosis in England. A review of 136 cases after five years' observation. Br Med J 1961;2(5261): 1165–72.

51. Line BR, Hunninghake GW, Keogh BA, et al. Gallium-67 scanning to stage the alveolitis of sarcoidosis: correlation with clinical studies, pulmonary

function studies, and bronchoalveolar lavage. Am Rev Respir Dis 1981;123(4 Pt 1):440–6.

52. Vanderstappen M, Mornex JF, Lahneche B, et al. Gallium-67 scanning in the staging of cryptogenetic fibrosing alveolitis and hypersensitivity pneumonitis. Eur Respir J 1988;1(6):517–22.

53. Tuddenham WJ. Glossary of terms for thoracic radiology: recommendations of the nomenclature Committee of the Fleischner society. AJR Am J Roentgenol 1984;143(3):509–17.

54. Austin JH, Müller NL, Friedman PJ, et al. Glossary of terms for CT of the lungs: recommendations of the nomenclature Committee of the Fleischner society. Radiology 1996;200(2):327–31.

55. Hansell DM, Bankier AA, MacMahon H, et al. Fleischner Society: glossary of terms for thoracic imaging. Radiology 2008;246(3):697–722.

56. Reynolds HY. Use of bronchoalveolar lavage in humans–past necessity and future imperative. Lung 2000;178(5):271–93.

57. Meyer KC, Raghu G, Baughman RP, et al. An Official American Thoracic Society clinical practice guideline: the clinical utility of bronchoalveolar lavage cellular analysis in interstitial lung disease. Am J Respir Crit Care Med 2012;185(9):1004–14.

58. Andersen HA, Fontana RS, Harrison EG Jr. Transbronchoscopic lung biopsy in diffuse pulmonary disease. Dis chest 1965;48:187–92.

59. Babiak A, Hetzel J, Krishna G, et al. Transbronchial cryobiopsy: a new tool for lung biopsies. Respiration 2009;78(2):203–8.

60. Johannson KA, Marcoux VS, Ronksley PE, et al. Diagnostic yield and complications of transbronchial lung cryobiopsy for interstitial lung disease. A systematic review and metaanalysis. Ann Am Thorac Soc 2016;13(10):1828–38.

61. Hetzel J, Maldonado F, Ravaglia C, et al. Transbronchial Cryobiopsies for the diagnosis of diffuse parenchymal lung diseases: expert statement from the cryobiopsy working group on safety and utility and a call for standardization of the procedure. Respiration 2018;95(3):188–200.

62. Troy LK, Grainge C, Corte TJ, et al. Diagnostic accuracy of transbronchial lung cryobiopsy for interstitial lung disease diagnosis (COLDICE): a prospective, comparative study. Lancet Respir Med 2020;8(2): 171–81.

63. Rubin EH, Kahn BS, Pecker D. Diffuse interstitial fibrosis of the lungs. Ann Intern Med 1952;36(3): 827–44.

64. Gaensler EA, Moister VB, Hamm J. Open-lung biopsy in duffuse pulmonary disease. N Engl J Med 1964;270:1319–31.

65. Fisher JH, Shapera S, To T, et al. Procedure volume and mortality after surgical lung biopsy in interstitial lung disease. Eur Respir J 2019;53(2): 1801164.

66. Wright FC, De Vito C, Langer B, et al. Multidisciplinary cancer conferences: a systematic review and development of practice standards. Eur J Cancer 2007;43(6):1002–10.

67. Walsh SLF, Maher TM, Kolb M, et al. Diagnostic accuracy of a clinical diagnosis of idiopathic pulmonary fibrosis: an international case-cohort study. Eur Respir J 2017;50(2):1700936.

68. Miller AF, Schaffner VD. The results of phrenic nerve paralysis in the treatment of pulmonary tuberculosis. Can Med Assoc J 1939;40(1):55–63.

69. Hardy JD, Webb WR, Dalton ML Jr, et al. Lung homotransplantation IN man. JAMA 1963;186:1065–74.

70. Unilateral lung transplantation for pulmonary fibrosis. N Engl J Med 1986;314(18):1140–5.

71. Panchabhai TS, Chaddha U, McCurry KR, et al. Historical perspectives of lung transplantation: connecting the dots. J Thorac Dis 2018;10(7): 4516–31.

72. Barach AL. Ambulatory oxygen therapy: oxygen inhalation at home and out-of-doors. Dis chest 1959;35(3):229–41.

73. Visca D, Mori L, Tsipouri V, et al. Effect of ambulatory oxygen on quality of life for patients with fibrotic lung disease (AmbOx): a prospective, open-label, mixed-method, crossover randomised controlled trial. Lancet Respir Med 2018;6(10):759–70.

74. Petty TL, Nett LM, Finigan MM, et al. A comprehensive care program for chronic airway obstruction. Methods and preliminary evaluation of symptomatic and functional improvement. Ann Intern Med 1969;70(6):1109–20.

75. Hodgkin JE, Farrell MJ, Gibson SR, et al. American thoracic society. Medical section of the American lung association. Pulmonary rehabilitation. Am Rev Respir Dis 1981;124(5):663–6.

76. Dowman L, Hill CJ, Holland AE. Pulmonary rehabilitation for interstitial lung disease. Cochrane Database Syst Rev 2014;(10):CD006322.

77. Herbert FA, Nahmias BB, Gaensler EA, et al. Pathophysiology of interstitial pulmonary fibrosis. Report of 19 cases and follow-up with corticosteroids. Arch Intern Med 1962;110:628–48.

78. Carrington CB, Gaensler EA, Coutu RE, et al. Usual and desquamative interstitial pneumonia. Chest 1976;69(2 Suppl):261–3.

79. Scadding JG, Hinson KF. Diffuse fibrosing alveolitis (diffuse interstitial fibrosis of the lungs). Correlation of histology at biopsy with prognosis. Thorax 1967; 22(4):291–304.

80. Turner-Warwick M. Staging and therapy of cryptogenic fibrosing alveolitis. Chest 1986;89(3):148S–50S.

81. Raghu G, Depaso WJ, Cain K, et al. Azathioprine combined with prednisone in the treatment of idiopathic pulmonary fibrosis: a prospective double-blind, randomized, placebo-controlled clinical trial. Am Rev Respir Dis 1991;144(2):291–6.

82. Tashkin DP, Elashoff R, Clements PJ, et al. Cyclophosphamide versus placebo in scleroderma lung disease. N Engl J Med 2006;354(25):2655–66.

83. Tashkin DP, Roth MD, Clements PJ, et al. Mycophenolate mofetil versus oral cyclophosphamide in scleroderma-related interstitial lung disease (SLS II): a randomised controlled, double-blind, parallel group trial. Lancet Respir Med 2016; 4(9):708–19.

84. Raghu G, Johnson WC, Lockhart D, et al. Treatment of idiopathic pulmonary fibrosis with a new antifibrotic agent, pirfenidone: results of a prospective, open-label Phase II study. Am J Respir Crit Care Med 1999;159(4 Pt 1):1061–9.

85. Distler O, Highland KB, Gahlemann M, et al. Nintedanib for systemic sclerosis-associated interstitial lung disease. N Engl J Med 2019;380(26): 2518–28.

Clinical Relevance and Management of "Pre–Interstitial Lung Disease"

Anna J. Podolanczuk, MD, MS[a], Rachel K. Putman, MD, MPH[b],*

KEYWORDS

- Preclinical ILD • Interstitial lung abnormalities • At-risk individuals • Early detection • CT imaging

KEY POINTS

- Interstitial lung abnormalities (ILA) are radiologic abnormalities that are incidentally found on chest computed tomography (CT) imaging; they are independently associated with a decline in pulmonary function, incident lung cancer, and an increased risk of death.
- Preclinical interstitial lung disease (ILD) are any radiologic, physiologic, molecular, and/or histopathologic abnormalities suggestive of ILD in individuals that are asymptomatic or undiagnosed.
- Both ILA and preclinical ILD are more common than clinical ILD, a subset of patients with ILA and/or preclinical ILD will progress to ILD; risk of progression can be stratified by clinical and radiologic characteristics.
- While additional studies are needed, the current recommendation is that individuals with ILA or preclinical ILD at high risk for progression to ILD are actively monitored for disease progression.

INTRODUCTION

Interstitial lung disease (ILD) has been defined by the presence of cellular proliferation, cellular infiltration, and/or fibrosis of the lung parenchyma not owing to infection or neoplasia.[1] Cellular level changes that lead to ILD may take years to become clinically apparent and have been termed preclinical ILD. In practice, preclinical ILD often refers to incidentally identified interstitial lung abnormalities (ILA) on chest computed tomographic (CT) scan in individuals without an established diagnosis of ILD, although these terms are not synonymous. Widespread adoption of CT imaging to screen for lung cancer and other diagnoses has led to greater recognition of incidental CT findings, although until recently, there were no guidelines or uniform definitions for reporting of ILA on clinical CT scans. The 2020 Fleischner Society Position Paper addressed this gap by standardizing the definition of ILA and proposing a clinical algorithm for evaluation of patients found to have ILA.[2]

Given the progressive nature of many ILDs, there has been a growing interest in the detection of preclinical ILD, and in the identification of individuals at highest risk of progression to clinically relevant disease, who may benefit from early initiation of therapies aimed at slowing disease progression. However, to date, there have been no prospective studies to investigate the appropriate diagnostic evaluation and optimal management strategies of individuals with preclinical ILD. This review describes the current state of knowledge about preclinical ILD, with an emphasis on the clinical implications and consensus recommendations for management of ILA in asymptomatic individuals.

DEFINITIONS

The development and progression of ILD occur on a spectrum that ranges from individuals at increased risk for ILD to those with clinically apparent disease (**Fig. 1**). Idiopathic pulmonary

[a] Division of Pulmonary and Critical Care Medicine, Weill Cornell Medicine, 1305 York Avenue, Y-1053, Box 96, New York, NY 10021, USA; [b] Division of Pulmonary and Critical Care Medicine, Brigham and Women's Hospital, Harvard Medical School, 75 Francis Street, Thorn 908D, Boston, MA 02115, USA
* Corresponding author.
E-mail address: rputman@bwh.harvard.edu

Clin Chest Med 42 (2021) 241–249
https://doi.org/10.1016/j.ccm.2021.03.009
0272-5231/21/© 2021 Elsevier Inc. All rights reserved.

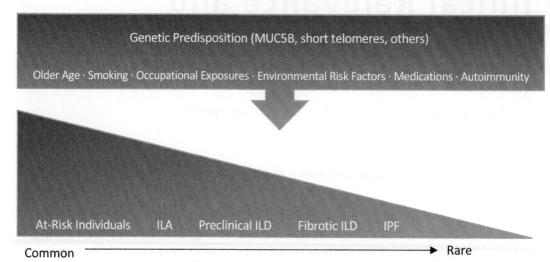

Fig. 1. Spectrum of ILD development and progression. Although IPF and other fibrotic ILDs are relatively rare in the general population, there is a larger number of at-risk individuals, a subset of whom will develop preclinical disease and then progress to clinical ILD. Risk factors for development and progression of preclinical and clinical ILD include several genetic, clinical, and environmental factors, as listed.

fibrosis (IPF) is 1 type of ILD, characterized by progressive pulmonary fibrosis without an identifiable cause.[3] IPF has been the focus of many studies, including those aimed at earlier detection and diagnosis, because of the large burden of morbidity and mortality associated with it. There is no uniform definition that distinguishes clinical from preclinical disease (**Table 1**).

Table 1
Definitions

	Definition	Comment
Preclinical ILD	• Any radiologic, physiologic, molecular, and/or histopathologic abnormalities suggestive of ILD • Asymptomatic or undiagnosed individuals	• Also referred to as subclinical ILD and early ILD • Can also refer to individuals at increased risk for ILD undergoing screening
ILA	• Nondependent abnormalities in the lung fields on CT scan ○ Reticular abnormalities ○ Ground-glass abnormalities ○ Lung distortion ○ Traction bronchiectasis ○ Honeycombing ○ Nonemphysematous cysts • Involve at least 5% of any lung zone • ILD is not suspected in the patient undergoing CT imaging	Excludes: • Findings identified during screening of high-risk individuals for ILD • Imaging findings limited to ○ Dependent lung atelectasis ○ Focal paraspinal fibrosis abutting spinal osteophytes ○ Isolated smoking-related centrilobular nodularity ○ Mild focal abnormality ○ Interstitial edema ○ Focal findings related to aspiration
Clinically significant ILD	• Symptoms of dyspnea, cough, or fatigue, either at rest or with exertion • Physical examination findings of crackles or clubbing • Resting or exertional hypoxemia • Decreased pulmonary function or gas transfer abnormalities • Extensive CT abnormalities, with findings involving 3 or more of the 6 lung zones	Lung zones refer to the right and left upper, middle, and lower lung zones, demarcated by the levels of the inferior aortic arch and right inferior pulmonary vein

Features suggestive of clinically significant disease include the following:

- Symptoms of dyspnea, cough, or fatigue, either at rest or with exertion
- Physical examination findings of crackles or clubbing
- Resting or exertional hypoxemia
- Decreased pulmonary function or gas transfer abnormalities
- Extensive CT abnormalities, with findings involving 3 or more of the 6 lung zones (lung zones refer to the right and left upper, middle, and lower lung zones, demarcated by the levels of the inferior aortic arch and right inferior pulmonary vein[2])

Preclinical ILD can be broadly defined as radiological, physiologic, molecular, and/or histopathologic abnormalities suggestive of ILD that are present in asymptomatic or undiagnosed individuals.[1,4] The terms subclinical ILD and early ILD have also been used in this context. Preclinical ILD has also been used to refer to individuals at increased risk for ILD found to have imaging findings suggestive of early ILD on screening CT scans.[5]

At-risk individuals and groups refer to those with particular genetic, molecular, demographic, radiological, and clinical characteristics that are known to increase the risk of preclinical and clinical ILD.[1] Examples are first-degree relatives of patients with fibrotic ILDs and adults with systemic sclerosis. Known risk factors for ILD are further discussed later.

ILA, as defined in the 2020 Fleischner Society Position Paper, are purely radiological findings and are indifferent to the presence or absence of symptoms, or physiologic impairment.[2] ILA are defined as the presence of nondependent abnormalities in the lung fields on CT scan, including reticular or ground-glass abnormalities, lung distortion, traction bronchiectasis, honeycombing, and/or nonemphysematous cysts in at least 5% of any lung zone (see **Table 1**). ILA are purely incidental findings, and their definition requires that the CT scan be done for reasons other than to screen or evaluate for ILD.[2] Before the 2020 Fleischner paper, the term ILA had been used more broadly in research to refer to interstitial changes suggestive of ILD in individuals without an established diagnosis of ILD.

ILA can be subcategorized based on their radiological distribution and features the following:

- Subpleural ILA have a predominantly subpleural localization

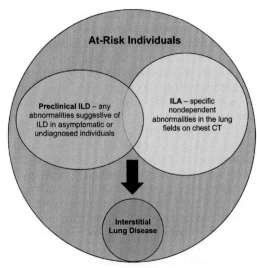

Fig. 2. Overlap between clinical preclinical ILD and ILA. A subset of individuals with ILA and preclinical disease will go on to develop clinical ILD.

- Fibrotic ILA are characterized by the presence of architectural distortion with traction bronchiectasis or honeycombing, or both[2]
- Subpleural fibrotic ILA are the subtype associated with the highest risk of progression[2,6,7]

The radiological findings of ILA may identify individuals at risk for ILD, may represent preclinical disease, or in some cases, may be incidental findings that do not progress to clinically significant findings (**Fig. 2**). A subset of individuals found to have ILA will have symptoms or evidence of functional impairment on objective testing. When clinically significant findings are present, ILA may represent early or mild ILD.

EPIDEMIOLOGY

Large cohort studies of individuals sampled without regard for respiratory symptoms or smoking, such as the Framingham Heart Study (FHS) and Age Gene Environment Susceptibility (AGES)-Reykjavik Study, have been used to examine the prevalence of ILA in the general population. ILA was found in 7% of both FHS and AGES-Reykjavik participants.[8,9] In other large cohorts that sampled higher proportions of smokers, older adults, and individuals with chronic obstructive pulmonary disease (COPD) (COPDGene study, lung cancer screening trials, and others), ILA prevalence ranged from 4% to 17%.[6,8–15]

Relatives of patients with familial interstitial pneumonia (FIP), defined as the presence of idiopathic interstitial pneumonia in 2 or more family members, are at increased risk for ILD. In 1 cohort,

14% of asymptomatic first-degree relatives of FIP patients had evidence of interstitial changes on high-resolution chest CT, and 35% had abnormalities on transbronchial biopsies.[16] In another study, 31% of first-degree relatives of patients with both familial pulmonary fibrosis and sporadic IPF were found to have radiological findings consistent with ILA.[17]

Adults with connective tissue disease represent another large group of individuals at risk for ILD. The prevalence of ILA has been reported in 30% to 50% of adults with rheumatoid arthritis and is associated with a spectrum of functional impairments and symptoms, that in some cases may represent undiagnosed ILD rather than preclinical disease.[18–20] Similarly, in a nationwide cohort of patients with systemic sclerosis, 50% had CT findings consistent with ILD, with a wide range of radiological patterns from ground-glass abnormalities to honeycombing.[21]

RISK FACTORS

Risk factors associated with preclinical ILD and ILA include many of the same clinical and demographic characteristics that are thought to be risk factors for ILD, and IPF in particular (see **Fig. 1**).

Older age has been consistently and strongly associated with increased likelihood of having ILA.[8,10,17,22] In the FHS, the prevalence of ILA in individuals younger than 50 years of age was 2%, compared with 9% for those 50 years of age and older.[8] In first-degree relatives of patients with FIP, each 1-year increase in age was associated with a 9% increase in the odds of ILA.[22]

Smoking has also been strongly linked to preclinical ILD and the presence of ILA.[8,10,23] Occupational exposure to vapors, gases, dusts, and fumes, and increased exposure to environmental traffic-related air pollution have also been shown to be associated with ILA.[24–26]

Family history of ILD, and pulmonary fibrosis in particular, has long been recognized as a strong risk factor for IPF and other idiopathic ILDs, suggesting that genetic predisposition has a critical role in the development of ILD.[27] The presence of the minor allele in the promoter of the MUC5B gene (rs35705950) is the strongest known risk factor for IPF and has been consistently associated with ILA, particularly subpleural fibrotic ILA.[8,28,29] Decreasing length of the telomere restriction fragment has also been shown to be associated with ILA.[22] A large genome-wide association study of individuals with ILA identified several loci that are strongly associated with both IPF and ILA (DPP9, DSP, FAM13A, IVD, MUC5B), supporting the idea that at least some ILA represent preclinical

ILD.[29] However, several other variants associated with ILA were not associated with IPF, suggesting that these radiological abnormalities represent a broad range of preclinical lesions.

Other clinical factors shown to be associated with preclinical ILD include higher levels rheumatoid arthritis–associated autoantibodies (rheumatoid factor and anti-cyclic citrullinated peptide), even in the absence of clinically evident RA, medications (statins, angiotensin-receptor blockers), and obstructive sleep apnea.[30–33]

PATHOLOGY

Few studies have looked at the histologic correlates of ILA. In 1 small study of 26 individuals with ILA undergoing lung nodule resections, the presence of ILA was associated with subpleural interstitial fibrosis, fibroblastic foci, honeycombing/usual interstitial pneumonia, and atypical adenomatous hyperplasia.[34] Although fibrosis was common among those with ILA (73%), so were respiratory bronchiolitis (71%) and pigment-laden macrophages (80%), suggesting that many of the findings in this study were smoking related.

Histopathologic examination of transbronchial biopsy specimens of at-risk relatives of patients with familial ILD revealed a range of abnormalities. Peribronchiolar fibrosis was most commonly seen, but other patterns included interstitial fibrosis, chronic inflammation, giant cells/granulomas, and respiratory bronchiolitis.[16] Notable, in this and other studies, histopathologic abnormalities were much more common than radiological abnormalities, suggesting that current methods of visual assessment of CT scans for preclinical disease may not detect early fibrosis in many cases.[16,34,35] However, the clinical significance of incidentally identified histologic fibrosis has not been investigated.

CLINICAL IMPLICATIONS

In large cohort studies, ILA have been shown to be associated with reduced lung volumes, respiratory symptoms, and diminished exercise capacity.[8,10,13] In the AGES-Reykjavik study, participants with ILA had poorer self-reported health, were less likely to participate in physical activity, or less likely to be independent with activities of daily living.[36] Increased lung attenuation measured by automated methods, suggestive of preclinical ILD, was also associated with lower forced vital capacity (FVC) and diminished exercise capacity on follow-up.[12] In first-degree relatives of familial ILD patients, those with ILA had normal lung function but diminished reduction in dead space ventilation at peak exercise.[27] These findings highlight the clinical significance of ILA, but also the difficulty in drawing a distinction between preclinical and clinical disease in individual patients.

Rates of radiological progression of ILA vary based on the clinical characteristics of the cohort and the definition of progression. ILA progression occurred in 20% of National Lung Screening Trial participants over 2 years, in 43% of FHS participants over 6 years, and in 73% of AGES-Reykjavik participants over 5 years.[6,7,37] However, it is still unclear what proportion of those with ILA develop IPF or other clinically significant ILD over time. Among individuals at risk for familial pulmonary fibrosis, 9% developed clinically significant ILD, and an additional 10% had radiological progression of ILA, over 5 years of follow-up.[22]

Risk factors for progression of ILA include increasing age, history of smoking, and increasing copies of the MUC5B minor allele.[37] Imaging patterns associated with progression include features of definite fibrosis (architectural distortion with traction bronchiectasis and/or honeycombing), the presence of basal and peripheral predominant reticular changes, and the subpleural fibrotic subtype of ILA.[2,6,7,20] The progressive ILA phenotype was associated with accelerated FVC decline and increased risk of death.[37]

The presence of ILA, regardless of progression, has been shown to be associated with all-cause mortality in 4 distinct cohorts of both smoking and non-smoking adults, with hazard ratios ranging from 1.3 to 2.7.[9] The increased mortality can in part be explained by increased respiratory mortality. However, deaths owing to cardiovascular disease and cancer are also common among those with ILA.[9,38]

Other studies have reported increased respiratory morbidity in those with ILA, including a 5-fold increase in the risk of being diagnosed with ILD, and approximately 2-fold increase in the risk of being diagnosed with COPD, pneumonia, and respiratory failure.[39] The presence of ILA is also associated with an increased incidence of lung cancer, and increased risk of death owing to lung cancer.[38,39]

Taken together, these findings suggest that both ILA and preclinical ILD have important clinical implications, in terms of progression to clinically established ILD and a greater risk of other clinically significant comorbidities and poor outcomes.

CLINICAL MANAGEMENT

The diagnostic evaluation and optimal management of individuals with incidental finding of ILA and preclinical ILD have not been investigated in any prospective studies to the authors' knowledge.

Consensus guidelines for the clinical evaluation of ILA, based on the opinion of an international group of pulmonologists, radiologists, and pathologists, were published in 2020.[2] They propose an initial evaluation and monitoring of incidentally identified ILA (**Fig. 3**).

Individuals found to have ILA should undergo an evaluation to determine if such findings represent clinically relevant ILD. Individuals should be assessed for respiratory symptoms and signs, resting or exertional hypoxemia, and abnormalities on pulmonary function testing (reduced lung volumes or gas transfer abnormalities). Anyone with respiratory symptoms or signs, abnormal lung function, physiologic abnormalities, or extensive disease by chest CT should be referred for a pulmonary evaluation, ideally at a center with ILD expertise and access to multidisciplinary discussion. Care of such patients should follow established guidelines for the diagnosis and treatment of patients with newly detected ILD.[40]

Individuals with ILA without clinically significant findings should undergo an assessment aimed at identifying potential causes of the ILA as well as risk factors for progression to clinically significant disease (see **Fig. 1**). A baseline evaluation should include an assessment of smoking history and occupational and environmental exposures that are known to cause ILD, drug toxicity, recurrent aspiration, occult connective tissue disease, family history of ILD, and signs of genetic syndromes associated with ILD (early graying, liver disease, bone marrow failure, oculocutaneous albinism, and easy bruising and bleeding).

Individuals with ILA should then be risk stratified based on the presence of clinical and radiological features associated with a high risk of progression.[2] Radiological risk factors for progression include the following:

- ILA with basal and peripheral predominance (both fibrotic and nonfibrotic)
- Fibrotic ILA
- Honeycombing

Individuals at high risk for progression should be actively monitored. Shared decision making should include a discussion about the risk of progression, clinical implications of ILA, and areas of uncertainty. There are no data on the optimal timing of reassessment and the role of lung biopsy in preclinical disease. Repeat pulmonary function testing should be considered at 3- to 12-month intervals. Repeat chest CT should be considered at

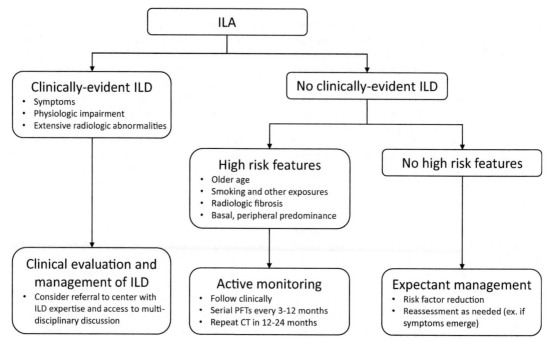

Fig. 3. Proposed algorithm for the clinical evaluation of individuals found to have ILA.

12 to 24 months, or sooner if there is other evidence of progression.[2]

Individuals with ILA without high-risk features or risk factors for progression should be counseled appropriately about the signs and symptoms of ILD, and can be followed as needed, if any new symptoms develop.

There are no data on optimal timing of initiation of treatment, and there is currently no recommendation for initiation of therapy, either antifibrotic or immune modulatory, for individuals with preclinical disease outside of a clinical research study. Referral to a center that specializes in ILD should be considered for any patient who develops signs of progression or clinically significant ILD. Therapeutic strategies in the preclinical stage should focus on risk reduction and mitigation of factors known to cause ILD, including smoking cessation, avoidance of pneumotoxic medication, environmental assessment for mold and other organic antigens, counseling on the use of masks in the setting of any ongoing inhalational exposures, treatment of recurrent aspiration or gastroesophageal reflux, as well as age-appropriate vaccination.

Appropriate screening for lung cancer in those that meet criteria should be strongly encouraged given the increased incidence of lung cancer in this population.[38] Patients with ILA undergoing surgical procedures are at increased risk for acute exacerbations, rapid progression of ILD, and acute respiratory distress syndrome. Care should be

taken to ensure lung-protective ventilation and avoidance of hyperoxemia in patients who need mechanical ventilation.

AREAS OF UNCERTAINTY AND FUTURE DIRECTIONS
Screening

The study of preclinical ILD and the clinical implications of ILA are still in its infancy. There is a dearth of evidence with respect to recommendations for screening of at-risk individuals. Groups at increased risk for ILD, in whom screening could be considered, include the following:

- Adults with connective tissue disease, including systemic sclerosis and rheumatoid arthritis
- First-degree relatives of patients with familial and sporadic pulmonary fibrosis
- People with specific, known genetic mutations and syndrome that carry a high risk of pulmonary fibrosis (short telomere syndrome, Hermansky-Pudlak syndrome, dyskeratosis congenita)
- Those with certain high-risk exposures and occupations (asbestos, silica)

The optimal modality for screening has not been established. However, symptom-based screening and pulmonary function testing have been shown to have poor sensitivity for detecting early disease.[41,42] High-resolution chest CT has better sensitivity and has been recommended by some groups for screening purposes in systemic sclerosis.[43] There are no consensus recommendations on the frequency of screening and the follow-up of any findings identified through screening. Screening for early or preclinical ILD is an area with many unanswered questions; in addition to those outlined above, perhaps the most important is whether early identification and initiation of treatment improve outcomes. Additional research is needed to answer this important question.

Automated Computed Tomography

Automated tools to detect increased lung attenuation have been developed, and in some cases may identify more subtle areas of lung injury and/or fibrosis that preceded clinically apparent ILD. However, normal ranges for these objective measures have not been published, and cutoffs for pathologic changes are not known. More advanced texture-based methods and deep learning algorithms hold promise as potential tools to identify preclinical disease. However, they are not widely available for clinical use, and at present, these automated tools are mainly applicable in research settings.

Blood Biomarkers

Blood biomarkers also hold promise as potentially useful tools to identify preclinical disease, especially in combination with imaging modalities. MMP-7, IL-6, GDF-15, and ICAM-1 have all been shown to be associated with preclinical disease, and in some studies, with increased risk of ILD death and hospitalization.[12,44–46] However, no biomarker has been validated for early detection of ILD or shown to be predictive of progression from preclinical to clinical disease, among those with ILA.

Risk Prediction

Further research studies are needed to better risk-stratify patients and create risk-prediction models for disease development and progression. Ideally, such risk-prediction models would incorporate high-risk genetic polymorphisms, clinical characteristics, blood biomarkers, and imaging features to create a risk score, which could inform recommendations for screening, follow-up, and early treatment. Such scores have been developed to stratify patients at risk for pulmonary embolism, cardiovascular disease, atrial fibrillation, and other life-threatening conditions, yet are lacking in ILD.

SUMMARY

Current evidence suggests that the presence of ILA, and in particular subpleural fibrotic ILA, is associated with poor clinical outcomes, including increased all-cause mortality and incident lung cancer, and that many individuals with ILA will progress. Current consensus guidelines recommend that individuals with ILA and high-risk features should undergo a clinical evaluation for ILD and should be actively monitored for disease progression. Reasonable management strategies include risk-reduction strategies and shared decision making.

CLINICS CARE POINTS

- Patients at risk for ILD include: older adults, smokers, relatives of patients with familial interstitial pneumonia, and adults with connective tissue disease.
- ILA is specific to abnormalities seen on chest CT scan, while preclinical ILD encompasses all abnormalities (radiologic, histopathologic, physiologic, and/or molecular) suggestive of ILD.
- Radiologic features or patterns of ILA that are more likely to progress include: subpleural ILA - characterized by subpleural reticulation, fibrotic ILA - characterized by traction bronchiectasis and/or honeycombing in any distribution, and subpleural fibrotic ILA - characterized by fibrotic changes in a subpleural distribution, which has the highest risk of progression.
- Patients with ILA and preclinical ILD and high risk features should be actively monitored for disease progression, however the duration and frequency of monitoring required is not known, current recommendations are based on expert consensus.
- There are no clear guidelines to support screening all high risk individuals for preclinical ILD or ILA.
- Preclinical ILD/ILA and ILD exist on a spectrum and it remains difficult to determine precisely when and if a patient will progress to clinically relevant ILD.

DISCLOSURE

Dr. Podolanczuk is supported by NIH grant K23 HL140199 and a grant from the American Lung Association. Dr. Putman is supported by NIH grant K08 HL140087.

REFERENCES

1. Rosas IO, Dellaripa PF, Lederer DJ, et al. Interstitial lung disease: NHLBI workshop on the primary prevention of chronic lung diseases. Ann Am Thorac Soc 2014;11(Suppl 3):S169–77.
2. Hatabu H, Hunninghake GM, Richeldi L, et al. Interstitial lung abnormalities detected incidentally on CT: a position paper from the Fleischner society. Lancet Respir Med 2020;8:726–37.
3. Raghu G, Collard HR, Egan JJ, et al. An official ATS/ERS/JRS/ALAT statement: idiopathic pulmonary fibrosis: evidence-based guidelines for diagnosis and management. Am J Respir Crit Care Med 2011;183:788–824.
4. Doyle TJ, Hunninghake GM, Rosas IO. Subclinical interstitial lung disease: why you should care. Am J Respir Crit Care Med 2012;185:1147–53.
5. Mathai SK, Humphries S, Kropski JA, et al. MUC5B variant is associated with visually and quantitatively detected preclinical pulmonary fibrosis. Thorax 2019;74:1131–9.
6. Jin GY, Lynch D, Chawla A, et al. Interstitial lung abnormalities in a CT lung cancer screening population: prevalence and progression rate. Radiology 2013;268:563–71.
7. Putman RK, Gudmundsson G, Axelsson GT, et al. Imaging patterns are associated with interstitial lung abnormality progression and mortality. Am J Respir Crit Care Med 2019;200:175–83.
8. Hunninghake GM, Hatabu H, Okajima Y, et al. MUC5B promoter polymorphism and interstitial lung abnormalities. N Engl J Med 2013;368:2192–200.
9. Putman RK, Hatabu H, Araki T, et al. Association between interstitial lung abnormalities and all-cause mortality. JAMA 2016;315:672–81.
10. Washko GR, Hunninghake GM, Fernandez IE, et al. Lung volumes and emphysema in smokers with interstitial lung abnormalities. N Engl J Med 2011;364:897–906.
11. Hoyer N, Wille MMW, Thomsen LH, et al. Interstitial lung abnormalities are associated with increased mortality in smokers. Respir Med 2018;136:77–82.
12. Podolanczuk AJ, Oelsner EC, Barr RG, et al. High attenuation areas on chest computed tomography in community-dwelling adults: the MESA study. Eur Respir J 2016;48(5):1442–52.
13. Doyle TJ, Washko GR, Fernandez IE, et al. Interstitial lung abnormalities and reduced exercise capacity. Am J Respir Crit Care Med 2012;185:756–62.
14. Sverzellati N, Guerci L, Randi G, et al. Interstitial lung diseases in a lung cancer screening trial. Eur Respir J 2011;38:392–400.
15. Tsushima K, Sone S, Yoshikawa S, et al. The radiological patterns of interstitial change at an early phase: over a 4-year follow-up. Respir Med 2010;104:1712–21.
16. Kropski JA, Pritchett JM, Zoz DF, et al. Extensive phenotyping of individuals at risk for familial interstitial pneumonia reveals clues to the pathogenesis of interstitial lung disease. Am J Respir Crit Care Med 2015;191:417–26.
17. Hunninghake GM, Quesada-Arias LD, Carmichael NE, et al. Interstitial lung disease in relatives of patients with pulmonary fibrosis. Am J Respir Crit Care Med 2020;201:1240–8.
18. Doyle TJ, Dellaripa PF, Batra K, et al. Functional impact of a spectrum of interstitial lung abnormalities in rheumatoid arthritis. Chest 2014;146:41–50.
19. Gochuico BR, Avila NA, Chow CK, et al. Progressive preclinical interstitial lung disease in rheumatoid arthritis. Arch Intern Med 2008;168:159–66.
20. Kawano-Dourado L, Doyle TJ, Bonfiglioli K, et al. Baseline characteristics and progression of a spectrum of interstitial lung abnormalities and disease in rheumatoid arthritis. Chest 2020;158:1546–54.
21. Hoffmann-Vold AM, Fretheim H, Halse AK, et al. Tracking impact of interstitial lung disease in systemic sclerosis in a complete nationwide cohort. Am J Respir Crit Care Med 2019;200:1258–66.
22. Salisbury ML, Hewlett JC, Ding G, et al. Development and progression of radiologic abnormalities in individuals at risk for familial interstitial lung disease. Am J Respir Crit Care Med 2020;201:1230–9.
23. Lederer DJ, Enright PL, Kawut SM, et al. Cigarette smoking is associated with subclinical parenchymal lung disease: the Multi-Ethnic Study of Atherosclerosis (MESA)-lung study. Am J Respir Crit Care Med 2009;180:407–14.
24. Rice MB, Li W, Schwartz J, et al. Ambient air pollution exposure and risk and progression of interstitial lung abnormalities: the Framingham Heart Study. Thorax 2019;74:1063–9.
25. Sack C, Vedal S, Sheppard L, et al. Air pollution and subclinical interstitial lung disease: the Multi-Ethnic Study of Atherosclerosis (MESA) air-lung study. Eur Respir J 2017;50:1700559.
26. Sack CS, Doney BC, Podolanczuk AJ, et al. Occupational exposures and subclinical interstitial lung disease. The MESA (Multi-Ethnic study of atherosclerosis) air and lung studies. Am J Respir Crit Care Med 2017;196:1031–9.
27. Rosas IO, Ren P, Avila NA, et al. Early interstitial lung disease in familial pulmonary fibrosis. Am J Respir Crit Care Med 2007;176:698–705.
28. Seibold MA, Wise AL, Speer MC, et al. A common MUC5B promoter polymorphism and pulmonary fibrosis. N Engl J Med 2011;364:1503–12.
29. Hobbs BD, Putman RK, Araki T, et al. Overlap of genetic risk between interstitial lung abnormalities and idiopathic pulmonary fibrosis. Am J Respir Crit Care Med 2019;200:1402–13.

30. Bernstein EJ, Barr RG, Austin JH, et al. Rheumatoid arthritis-associated autoantibodies and subclinical interstitial lung disease: the Multi-Ethnic Study of Atherosclerosis. Thorax 2016;71(12):1082–90.

31. Xu JF, Washko GR, Nakahira K, et al. Statins and pulmonary fibrosis: the potential role of NLRP3 inflammasome activation. Am J Respir Crit Care Med 2012;185:547–56.

32. Gannon WD, Anderson MR, Podolanczuk AJ, et al. Angiotensin receptor blockers and subclinical interstitial lung disease. MESA Study 2019;16:1451–3.

33. Kim JS, Podolanczuk AJ, Borker P, et al. Obstructive sleep apnea and subclinical interstitial lung disease in the Multi-Ethnic Study of Atherosclerosis (MESA). Ann Am Thorac Soc 2017;14:1786–95.

34. Miller ER, Putman RK, Vivero M, et al. Histopathology of interstitial lung abnormalities in the context of lung nodule resections. Am J Respir Crit Care Med 2018;197:955–8.

35. Hung YP, Hunninghake GM, Miller ER, et al. Incidental nonneoplastic parenchymal findings in patients undergoing lung resection for mass lesions. Hum Pathol 2019;86:93–101.

36. Axelsson GT, Putman RK, Araki T, et al. Interstitial lung abnormalities and self-reported health and functional status. Thorax 2018;73:884–6.

37. Araki T, Putman RK, Hatabu H, et al. Development and progression of interstitial lung abnormalities in the Framingham Heart Study. Am J Respir Crit Care Med 2016;194:1514–22.

38. Axelsson GT, Putman RK, Aspelund T, et al. The associations of interstitial lung abnormalities with cancer diagnoses and mortality. Eur Respir J 2020;56:1902154.

39. Hoyer N, Thomsen LH, Wille MMW, et al. Increased respiratory morbidity in individuals with interstitial lung abnormalities. BMC Pulm Med 2020;20:67.

40. Raghu G, Remy-Jardin M, Myers JL, et al. Diagnosis of idiopathic pulmonary fibrosis. An official ATS/ERS/JRS/ALAT clinical practice guideline. Am J Respir Crit Care Med 2018;198:e44–68.

41. Suliman YA, Dobrota R, Huscher D, et al. Brief report: pulmonary function tests: high rate of false-negative results in the early detection and screening of scleroderma-related interstitial lung disease. Arthritis Rheumatol 2015;67:3256–61.

42. Showalter K, Hoffmann A, Rouleau G, et al. Performance of forced vital capacity and lung diffusion cutpoints for associated radiographic interstitial lung disease in systemic sclerosis. J Rheumatol 2018;45:1572–6.

43. Hoffmann-Vold A-M, Maher TM, Philpot EE, et al. The identification and management of interstitial lung disease in systemic sclerosis: evidence-based European consensus statements. Lancet Rheumatol 2020;2:e71–83.

44. Armstrong HF, Podolanczuk AJ, Barr RG, et al. Serum matrix metalloproteinase-7, respiratory symptoms, and mortality in community-dwelling adults. MESA (Multi-Ethnic Study of Atherosclerosis). Am J Respir Crit Care Med 2017;196:1311–7.

45. McGroder CF, Aaron CP, Bielinski SJ, et al. Circulating adhesion molecules and subclinical interstitial lung disease: the Multi-Ethnic Study of Atherosclerosis. Eur Respir J 2019;54:1900295.

46. Sanders JL, Putman RK, Dupuis J, et al. The association of aging biomarkers, interstitial lung abnormalities, and mortality. Am J Respir Crit Care Med 2020. [Epub ahead of print].

Diagnostic Classification of Interstitial Lung Disease in Clinical Practice

Ayodeji Adegunsoye, MD, MS, FCCP[a], Christopher J. Ryerson, MD, FRCPC[b],*

KEYWORDS

• Interstitial lung disease • Diagnostic classification • Pulmonary fibrosis

KEY POINTS

- Interstitial lung disease (ILD) classification has evolved toward an integrated approach that is based on a multidisciplinary discussion of pertinent clinical, radiological, and pathologic data.
- Routinely used tools for diagnostic precision in ILD classification include the history and physical examination, chest imaging, lung function testing, serologic analyses, bronchoalveolar lavage, and histopathologic evaluation of surgical lung biopsy specimens.
- There is an increasing emphasis on disease behavior in classifying and directing management of fibrotic ILD.
- Management and prognostication of ILD is increasingly reliant on a multipronged classification approach that considers the etiology, morphology, and disease behavior.

BACKGROUND

Interstitial lung disease (ILD) includes many rare and often poorly understood heterogeneous diseases that cause fibrosis and/or inflammation of the lungs. ILDs are challenging to diagnose, requiring integration of multiple complex features that are often difficult to interpret. In this review, we discuss the approach to the diagnosis and classification of ILD, focusing on practical diagnostic tools and strategies that can be used by clinicians to separate different ILD subtypes and identify the most appropriate management. We further describe likely future approaches to ILD classification based on our evolving understanding of these diseases.

EVOLUTION OF INTERSTITIAL LUNG DISEASE CLASSIFICATION

ILD classification has evolved substantially since the first descriptions of pulmonary fibrosis more than a century ago. ILDs were often classified based on pathologic features until the turn of the century,[1–3] with increasing use and understanding of computed tomography (CT) ushering in a new era in which many people with ILD are more confidently diagnosed without histopathology. The contemporary approach to ILD classification has been established in a series of consensus statements and clinical practice guidelines produced over the past 2 decades (**Fig. 1**). A 2002 consensus statement provided an update on the classification of the

Final approval of the submitted article and accountability for all aspects of the work: All authors (A. Adegunsoye, C.J. Ryerson).

[a] Section of Pulmonary & Critical Care, The University of Chicago Medicine, 5841 South Maryland Avenue - MC6076 | M662, Chicago, IL 60637, USA; [b] Department of Medicine, University of British Columbia, Centre for Heart Lung Innovation, St. Paul's Hospital, Ward 8B, 1081 Burrard Street, Vancouver, British Columbia V6Z 1Y6, Canada

* Corresponding author.

E-mail address: Chris.Ryerson@hli.ubc.ca

Clin Chest Med 42 (2021) 251–261

https://doi.org/10.1016/j.ccm.2021.03.002

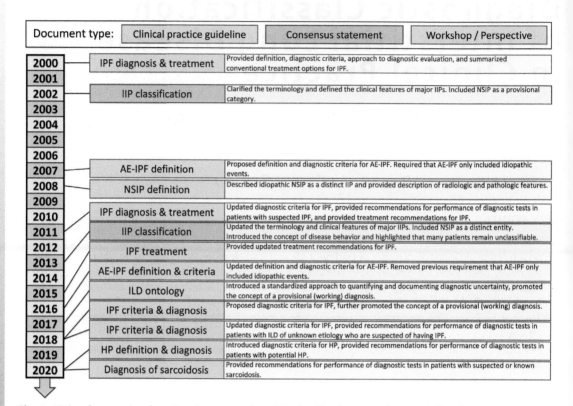

Document type:	Clinical practice guideline	Consensus statement	Workshop / Perspective

Year	Document	Description
2000	IPF diagnosis & treatment	Provided definition, diagnostic criteria, approach to diagnostic evaluation, and summarized conventional treatment options for IPF.
2001		
2002	IIP classification	Clarified the terminology and defined the clinical features of major IIPs. Included NSIP as a provisional category.
2003		
2004		
2005		
2006		
2007	AE-IPF definition	Proposed definition and diagnostic criteria for AE-IPF. Required that AE-IPF only included idiopathic events.
2008	NSIP definition	Described idiopathic NSIP as a distinct IIP and provided description of radiologic and pathologic features.
2009		
2010	IPF diagnosis & treatment	Updated diagnostic criteria for IPF, provided recommendations for performance of diagnostic tests in patients with suspected IPF, and provided treatment recommendations for IPF.
2011	IIP classification	Updated the terminology and clinical features of major IIPs. Included NSIP as a distinct entity. Introduced the concept of disease behavior and highlighted that many patients remain unclassifiable.
2012	IPF treatment	Provided updated treatment recommendations for IPF.
2013		
2014	AE-IPF definition & criteria	Updated definition and diagnostic criteria for AE-IPF. Removed previous requirement that AE-IPF only included idiopathic events.
2015	ILD ontology	Introduced a standardized approach to quantifying and documenting diagnostic uncertainty, promoted the concept of a provisional (working) diagnosis.
2016	IPF criteria & diagnosis	Proposed diagnostic criteria for IPF, further promoted the concept of a provisional (working) diagnosis.
2017	IPF criteria & diagnosis	Updated diagnostic criteria for IPF, provided recommendations for performance of diagnostic tests in patients with ILD of unknown etiology who are suspected of having IPF.
2018	HP definition & diagnosis	Introduced diagnostic criteria for HP, provided recommendations for performance of diagnostic tests in patients with potential HP.
2019		
2020	Diagnosis of sarcoidosis	Provided recommendations for performance of diagnostic tests in patients with suspected or known sarcoidosis.

Fig. 1. Major documents advancing the approach to ILD classification over the past 2 decades.

idiopathic interstitial pneumonias (IIPs),[4] which was refined in the most recent 2013 update to this document.[5] Additional documents have helped establish diagnostic criteria and approaches for many of the most common ILD subtypes.[5–16]

The first major change in ILD classification over the past 2 decades has been movement toward an integrated multidisciplinary approach, specifically based on the conclusions arising from a multidisciplinary discussion (MDD) that includes an ILD clinician, a chest radiologist, and a lung pathologist, as described later in this article. Three major challenges in the diagnosis of ILD provided justification for this evolution. First, individual features are very rarely pathognomonic for a given ILD subtype, indicating the need to incorporate many findings from multiple domains. Second, there is significant interobserver variability in interpretation of these features,[17] particularly among less experienced physicians,[18] and contextualizing specific features within the full constellation of findings helps reduce the impact of outlying results that are more likely to be inaccurate. Third, the potential harms of surgical lung biopsy are increasingly recognized and fewer patients are undergoing this procedure,[19,20] with MDD helpful in this situation to overcome the limitations arising from a less comprehensive diagnostic evaluation.

A second major change has been the increasing emphasis on disease behavior that was clearly described in the 2013 IIP classification document,[5] and since referenced in multiple recent publications. Demonstrating benefit of antifibrotic medications across a variety of ILD subtypes with progressive fibrosis has provided some support for the concept of disease behavior[21,22]; however, it is necessary to consider a disease behavior classification as a complementary tool to the ILD diagnosis. This has led to the current approach that is evolving toward a hybrid of lumping and splitting fibrotic ILDs. Specifically, it may be appropriate to lump groups of patients when considering relatively nonselective or nonspecific treatments (eg, oxygen supplementation, pulmonary rehabilitation), while splitting groups of patients will likely be more informative for detailed studies of disease biology and development of future targeted pharmacotherapies.

Despite recent advances in ILD diagnosis and classification, there remain frequent discrepancies even across experienced groups.[23] These ongoing issues primarily relate to uncertainties and inconsistencies in the interpretation of individual ILD features, as well as how these features are best combined to arrive at a confident diagnosis that then informs optimal management. In the following sections we describe the major building blocks that are integrated to help diagnose patients with ILD, and further describe how MDD should be used to optimize diagnostic accuracy.

DIAGNOSTIC TOOLS ROUTINELY EMPLOYED TO SUPPORT INTERSTITIAL LUNG DISEASE CLASSIFICATION
History and Physical Examination

Despite the overlap of initial symptoms and signs across ILD subtypes and with other diseases,[24] diagnostic accuracy is substantially improved by eliciting a careful and detailed medical history,[25] sometimes supported by a structured questionnaire.[15] Basic demographic characteristics such as age and sex are important initial considerations. For example, autoimmune-related ILDs are more prevalent among young female individuals,[26,27] whereas idiopathic pulmonary fibrosis (IPF) more commonly affects older men and current or former smokers.[26,27] Differences in racial demographics may also exist across ILD subtypes, as Black individuals are diagnosed with ILD at a younger age and less often with IPF compared with White patients.[28] Environmental exposures to avian antigens, mold, and organic dust have been linked to the development of hypersensitivity pneumonitis (HP),[15] and various inorganic exposures are associated with pneumoconioses (eg, silicosis, asbestosis). Multisystem disorders such as connective tissue disease and sarcoidosis can also result in pulmonary involvement with concomitant ILD, with extrapulmonary manifestations frequently predating overt pulmonary manifestations.[16,29] Although these many features are often not universal or pathognomonic, they are often helpful when contextualized with other findings to increase or decrease the likelihood of a given ILD subtype.

Chest Imaging

Chest high-resolution computed tomography (HRCT) is a central component in the diagnostic classification of ILD. HRCT patterns of ILD can be broadly categorized as fibrotic or nonfibrotic. Common patterns of fibrosis include usual interstitial pneumonia (UIP), fibrotic nonspecific interstitial pneumonia (NSIP), and fibrotic HP, with many patients also having a relatively nonspecific or unclassifiable pattern of fibrosis (**Fig. 2**). Distinguishing among these patterns provides critical information for the subclassification of ILD, with consequent impact on management and prognostication.

Imaging features of typical UIP include honeycombing, reticulation, and traction bronchiectasis.[13] Ground glass should be absent or at most inconspicuous, but can be more prominent during an acute illness and can sometimes represent microfibrosis when ground-glass opacification and fine reticulation are present concurrently with tractional changes. A radiologic pattern of UIP is strongly associated with a histopathologic pattern of UIP when findings are primarily distributed in a subpleural and basilar pattern.[13] Fibrotic HP is more varied in its radiological appearance.[15] In addition to coarse reticulation often without a zonal predominance,[30] HP classically has features of small airway disease, such as poorly defined centrilobular nodules, ground-glass opacities, air trapping, and mosaic attenuation.[15,31] The combination of normal lung, lucent lung (suggesting obstructive abnormality), and high-attenuation lung (ground glass) is described as the "3-density pattern," which is considered highly specific for fibrotic HP. A radiologic pattern of fibrotic NSIP typically consists of varying ground-glass attenuation with underlying reticulation and occasionally subpleural sparing, but without prominent honeycombing.[8]

It is essential to distinguish these imaging patterns from the clinical diagnosis, as the radiologic pattern provides only a starting point for accurate classification. For example, identifying a pattern of UIP on HRCT substantially narrows the differential diagnosis and provides important prognostic information, but additional clinical, laboratory, and sometimes histopathological data are still required to differentiate between common causes of a UIP pattern (eg, IPF, connective tissue disease [CTD]-ILD, fibrotic HP). In some patients, additional imaging features may be present that suggest potential causes of a UIP pattern. For example, the radiologic UIP pattern that is, typical of IPF is characterized by a basal and subpleural predominant distribution with the absence of features that might suggest an alternative diagnosis.[25] Conversely, peribronchovascular extension of fibrosis might suggest a diagnosis of fibrotic HP, whereas the presence of exuberant honeycombing (ie, honeycombing that is disproportionately severe compared with other features of fibrosis) raises the likelihood of a CTD-ILD. Although such features are rarely diagnostic in isolation, they inform the clinical-radiological differential diagnosis and together with other features can sometimes impact the decision to pursue more invasive diagnostic tests.

Importantly, the interpretation of chest HRCTs is best performed by thoracic radiologists with expertise in ILD and preferably within the context of an MDD.[18,23] Although not clinically available at this time, complementary imaging techniques

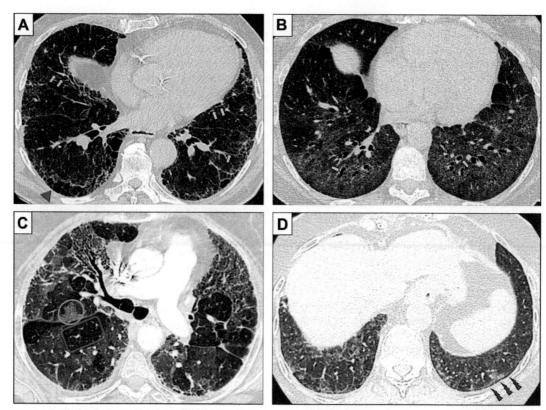

Fig. 2. Representative axial CT images of common ILD patterns. (*A*) A typical UIP pattern characterized by sub-pleural and basal predominant honeycombing (*blue triangle*), reticulation (*red asterisks*), and traction bronchi-ectasis (*yellow arrows*). (*B*) A typical nonspecific interstitial pneumonia (NSIP) pattern with peripheral and lower lung predominant abnormalities, including the classic feature of subpleural sparing that is seen in approx-imately 25% of patients with NSIP and helps distinguish from UIP when present. In this case, the presence of bronchiectasis (*yellow arrows*) indicates the presence of "microfibrosis" that is represented by ground glass on this image. (*C*) A typical pattern of fibrotic HP including the 3-density sign that is indicated by the presence of well-demarcated areas of high attenuation or ground glass (*green circle*), low attention (*blue rectangle*), and normal attenuation. There is diffuse abnormality in both the craniocaudal and axial planes, with presence of reticulation (*red asterisks*) and traction bronchiectasis (*yellow arrows*). (*D*) An indeterminate pattern of fibrosis characterized by mild peripheral reticulation and ground-glass abnormality without any defining feature. The suggestion of well-demarcated subpleural sparing (*red lightning bolts*) is an image processing artifact and does not suggest NSIP.

such as computerized quantitative algorithms may eventually be useful to help eliminate the interob-server variability that currently exists, particularly among nonexperts.[32,33] This approach also holds appeal for its potential to improve precision in assessing ILD severity and estimating prognosis.[32–34]

Pulmonary Function Testing

Although pulmonary function tests are typically un-helpful in distinguishing ILD subtypes, these are a critical component of assessing disease severity and disease behavior.[35,36] Longitudinal monitoring of forced vital capacity (FVC) and diffusing capac-ity of the lung for carbon monoxide (DLCO) is valuable for monitoring therapeutic response, quantifying disease progression, and identifying patients with high mortality risk. Even in patients without a defined ILD, the subtle presence of inter-stitial lung abnormalities on chest HRCT is associ-ated with an increased rate of pulmonary function decline,[37] indicating the importance of monitoring patients with subtle abnormalities on chest imag-ing. In some patients, disease behavior provides useful information that impacts the diagnostic like-lihood. For example, long-term stability decreases the probability of IPF, whereas ongoing rapid worsening may argue against non-IPF etiologies, particularly if a potential offending cause has been removed (eg, a potentially offending medica-tion or environmental exposure).

The most common physiologic pattern in fibrotic ILD is that of a restrictive ventilatory defect showing decreased total lung capacity and FVC, with an increase in the ratio of the forced expiratory volume in the first second to the FVC (FEV1:FVC).[9] This restrictive ventilatory defect is frequently accompanied by a reduction in the DLCO, which is often severely reduced in fibrotic ILD.[38] A minority of patients with fibrotic ILD will have a concurrent obstructive process, most frequently occurring in patients who have a second pulmonary diagnosis such as asthma or chronic obstructive pulmonary disease.[39] In the absence of a second diagnosis, this mixed ventilatory pattern is also observed in pulmonary sarcoidosis,[40,41] HP,[42,43] and rarely in patients with CTD-ILD who can have underlying intrinsic airway disease.[44]

Serologic Analysis

Testing for autoantibodies in patients diagnosed with ILD is crucial to disease classification, approach to management, and determining outcomes.[5] Although it is recommended that antinuclear antibody, anticyclic citrullinated peptide (anti-CCP), and rheumatoid factor (RF) be obtained at baseline evaluation for ILD, additional serologic autoantibodies such as anti-Jo1, PL-7, PL-12, anti-Scl70, SSA/Ro, SSB/La, RNP, and Sm autoantibodies may also be helpful in patients suspected of having an underlying CTD.[5] When a defined CTD is confirmed, the ILD is highly likely to be ascribed to the CTD given the heterogeneous ILD patterns that are possible in patients with CTD; however, there are infrequently alternative causes in this setting, most notably including drug-related ILD that can occur with many of the medications that are used to treat CTD.

Patients with idiopathic interstitial pneumonias may also demonstrate autoimmune features, including the presence of relatively specific autoantibodies, but without meeting criteria for a specific autoimmune disease.[15,45,46] This group of patients has previously been labeled as autoimmune-featured ILD,[47] undifferentiated CTD-related ILD,[48,49] and lung-dominant-CTD.[50] A joint research statement from a multinational task force proposed standardized criteria for interstitial pneumonia with autoimmune features (IPAF),[44] although additional consensus is required to support the clinically utility of this entity.

In patients with newly identified ILD for which a clinical suspicion of HP is being entertained, current guidelines suggest serum-specific immunoglobulin testing that targets potential antigens known to be associated with HP.[15] This serologic evaluation might direct further exploration of potential exposures in the patient's environment and can help secure a specific diagnosis or strengthen diagnostic confidence; however, there is substantial variability in these tests across centers and further research is still required to confirm their clinical utility.

Bronchoalveolar Lavage

Bronchoalveolar lavage (BAL) cellular analysis has a relatively limited role in patients with suspected IPF who have a UIP pattern on HRCT, and current guidelines recommend against performing BAL in this situation unless there is specific concern for infection or malignancy.[9,13] BAL can provide useful information in other situations, but is rarely diagnostic in isolation.[9] Situations in which BAL can be helpful include nonfibrotic and less commonly fibrotic HP (lymphocytosis with/without plasma cells), sarcoidosis (lymphocytosis, increased CD4/CD8 T-cell ratio), cellular NSIP (lymphocytosis), acute interstitial pneumonia (neutrophilic predominance), diffuse alveolar damage (neutrophilic predominance with Type II pneumocytes), lymphangitic carcinoma (malignant cells), eosinophilic pneumonia (eosinophilia), and diffuse alveolar hemorrhage (sequential increasingly bloody lavage).[51]

Lung Biopsy

Surgical lung biopsy (SLB) provides important information that frequently directs management and supports prognostication when performed adequately[52]; however, there is potential for significant complications that prohibits this procedure in many patients with fibrotic ILD.[19,20] Most notably, the 30-day mortality following elective SLB is 1.7%,[19,20] approaching 15% to 20% for patients with a respiratory-related admission to hospital.[19,20] Proceeding with a surgical lung biopsy therefore requires careful consideration of how results might impact management decisions, as well as a detailed discussion with the patient about whether this expected benefit outweighs the potential risks.

The incremental benefit of a biopsy is not justified in patients with clear clinical and radiological features that suggest a specific diagnosis with high confidence. For example, the presence of a typical and often a probable UIP pattern on HRCT obviates the need for lung biopsy to confirm a diagnosis of IPF in the appropriate clinical setting,[25,53] and this procedure is similarly not justified in patients with a clear CTD or a typical HP exposure with consistent imaging patterns.

Video-assisted thoracoscopic surgery (VATS) is almost universally performed when SLB is indicated due to its associated lower morbidity and shorter hospital stay compared with traditional open lung biopsies.[54] Alternative forms of sampling lung tissue (eg, conventional transbronchial biopsy, lung cryobiopsy) have a potential role and may be preferred in some centers for specific patient populations.[55,56]

Multidisciplinary Discussion

MDD is an integral component of the ILD diagnostic process (**Fig. 3**).[5,13] Although geographic variations exist in the specific format and team composition,[57] most centers include a pulmonologist, chest radiologist, thoracic pathologist, and frequently a rheumatologist. The pulmonologist directly caring for the patient presents the clinical information, which is then integrated with additional data and input from other members of the MDD team, culminating in a consensus diagnosis.[57] This approach is now considered the gold standard for classifying patients with ILD.[5]

In community settings in which diagnostic doubt exists or where MDD is not viable, strong consideration should be given to referral of the patient to an ILD center, as this likely improves diagnostic accuracy,[18] and also provides access to clinical trials and lung transplant services.[58,59] Recent data also suggest that performing remote MDD for patients unable to travel to a tertiary center is a feasible option and could permit improved and more rapid access to ILD expertise for community clinicians.[60,61]

CONTEMPORARY APPROACHES TO INTERSTITIAL LUNG DISEASE CLASSIFICATION

Accurate diagnosis of ILD is essential for guiding treatment and estimating prognosis; however, there are multiple overlapping approaches to ILD classification and each has advantages and disadvantages. It is therefore common for patients to simultaneously be classified based on multiple approaches as described later (see **Fig. 3**). An additional complementary approach is to consider diagnostic confidence and the concept of a

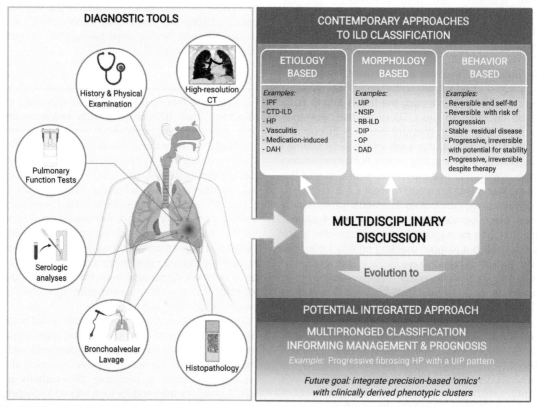

Fig. 3. Schematic depicting the application of diagnostic tools to various approaches for the classification of ILD. DAH, diffuse alveolar hemorrhage; DIP, desquamative interstitial pneumonia; OP, organizing pneumonia; PFT, pulmonary function testing; RB, respiratory bronchiolitis; RF, rheumatoid factor; UIP, usual interstitial pneumonia. Created with BioRender.com.

working diagnosis. An international working group suggested definitions of a confident diagnosis (≥90% confidence and/or meeting guideline criteria), a provisional high-confidence diagnosis (70%–89% confidence), and a provisional low-confidence diagnosis (51%–69% confidence), with unclassifiable ILD defined by the inability to provide a diagnosis that is more likely than not.[12] This approach has been adopted in recent clinical practice guidelines and provides a practical framework that helps support management decisions.[62]

Etiology-Based Classification

The conventional etiology-based classification divides patients by the underlying cause of their ILD.[63] This approach has proven value in ILD management, as the choice of pharmacotherapy has historically varied across ILD subtypes, and the identified cause may be directly treated or mitigated itself. A major limitation of this approach is that it ignores similarities in disease morphology or behavior across distinct ILD subtypes that may have important prognostic and management implications, as well as different phenotypes within ILDs that also carry significance.

Morphology-Based Classification

The morphology-based approach classifies patients based on radiologic and/or histopathologic patterns. Previous consensus documents recognize 6 major idiopathic interstitial pneumonias based on their histopathologic features: UIP, nonspecific interstitial pneumonia, respiratory bronchiolitis, desquamative interstitial pneumonia, organizing pneumonia, and diffuse alveolar damage.[5] Several of these histopathologic patterns correlate strongly with corresponding radiologic patterns. These patterns correspond to 3 major clinical groups: (1) chronic fibrosing idiopathic ILDs (IPF, idiopathic NSIP); (2) smoking-related idiopathic ILDs (respiratory bronchiolitis–ILD, desquamative interstitial pneumonia); and (3) acute/subacute idiopathic ILDs (cryptogenic organizing pneumonia, acute interstitial pneumonia).

The advantage of this approach relates to the prognostic significance of certain morphologic patterns even within a given ILD (eg, UIP typically has a worse prognosis than non-UIP patterns regardless of the clinical diagnosis).[64–67] Recent data have also suggested potential therapeutic implications of different morphologies, with a greater relative benefit of antifibrotic therapy in patients with progressive fibrosis who have a UIP-like pattern on HRCT across a variety of ILD subtypes.[21] However, limitations to a morphologic approach to ILD classification includes the limited

insight into the disease's etiology, potential existence of multiple morphologic patterns within an individual patient, and inconsistent agreement between radiologic and pathologic patterns.

Behavior-Based Classification

The behavior-based classification groups patients by their observed and/or anticipated disease behavior. The utility of this approach lies in the ease with which clinicians can apply it to routine patient care and increasing evidence that some therapies apply to certain phenotypes that span different ILDs.[21] There are a number of features that can be used to help inform separation of patients according to the anticipated disease behavior. For example, predominance of ground glass on chest imaging suggests a greater potential for therapeutic response to immunosuppressive therapy, in contrast to patients with a predominance of fibrosis in which antifibrotic therapy may be the preferred option.[21,65,68] However, this approach remains constrained by its inability to provide additional insight into etiopathogenesis and is less useful for supporting development of targeted therapies.

FUTURE PERSPECTIVES

ILD classification is evolving into a multipronged approach that integrates etiology, morphology, and disease behavior into a framework that attempts to account for the complex pathobiology of fibrosis while informing management decisions and prognostication. For example, the classification of a patient as having "progressive fibrosing HP with a UIP pattern" captures critical components of the approaches mentioned previously and provides greater insight into potential prognosis and therapeutic options compared with simply labeling a patient as "HP" (see **Fig. 3**). Although this multipronged approach to ILD classification remains at a nascent stage, it is likely that future studies will generate additional data to support its refinement and confirm clinical utility.

An important missing component of the preceding approaches to ILD classification is a robust incorporation of disease biology. A biology-based approach to ILD classification would consider etiopathogenic factors such as gene variants and risk polymorphisms,[69] epigenomic modifications by environmental exposures, transcriptomic and proteomic biomarker pathways,[70] and molecular imaging techniques.[71] Together, these would allow better characterization of mechanisms that account for phenotypic and functional alterations of the lung parenchyma, and would facilitate identification of potential therapeutic targets. Technologies based on genomic, epigenomic, and proteomic data have proven invaluable in improving our understanding of many diseases, and these tools are similarly being used to support a greater biological understanding of ILD classification.[72,73]

As we move toward an era of personalized ILD care, these markers will then become useful to identify potential therapeutic targets, effectively stratify patients for clinical trials, and then predict response to emergent pharmacotherapies. High-throughput genomic and transcriptomic analytical techniques have resulted in a high-resolution reference map of the human lungs, which will promote further insights into pulmonary cell-cell interactions.[74] There are also relatively new statistical techniques (eg, cluster analysis) that appear promising for classifying ILDs into discrete phenotypes, providing another strategy to identify novel classification approaches that may have greater biological and clinical relevance.[75] As we harness these new technologies, it is likely that "omics"-focused, cluster-based schema, and machine-learning algorithms will help support development of the next classification approach for patients with ILD.

SUMMARY

Optimizing diagnostic precision in the classification of ILDs in clinical practice hinges on careful and thorough acquisition of data from routinely used tools such as the history and physical examination, chest imaging, pulmonary function testing, serologic analyses, BAL, and histopathologic evaluation of surgical lung biopsy specimens; all integrated within the setting of an MDD. Continued progress in our understanding of the etiology, morphology, and disease behavior of these ILDs with increasing access to more novel "omics"-based biomarkers and statistical algorithms will hopefully facilitate a shift toward a more accurate and meaningful multipronged approach to ILD classification with substantial improvements in its therapeutic and prognostic value.

CLINICS CARE POINTS

- The most important distinction in ILD classification is between IPF and non-IPF ILDs.
- A history, physical examination, autoimmune serologies, and high-resolution chest CT are essential components of evaluation that should be performed in all patients presenting with a new ILD.
- BAL cellular analysis has a role in specific situations.

- Surgical lung biopsy is associated with potential for serious complications and the risk of this procedure should be carefully considered against the potential benefit on a case-by-case basis.
- All available data should be considered within a multidisciplinary discussion, which is considered the gold standard for ILD diagnosis and can provide additional information on the anticipated disease behavior and expected response to therapy.

AUTHOR'S CONTRIBUTIONS

Conception and design, acquisition of data for the work, analysis and interpretation, and drafting the article for important intellectual content: All authors (A. Adegunsoye, C.J. Ryerson).

CONFLICT OF INTEREST DISCLOSURES

A. Adegunsoye is supported by a career development award from the National Heart, Lung, and Blood Institute (K23HL146942), and has received speaking and advisory board fees from Boehringer Ingelheim and grant funding for interstitial lung disease research from the Pulmonary Fibrosis Foundation. C.J. Ryerson is supported by a Health Professional Investigator Award from the Michael Smith Foundation for Health Research.

REFERENCES

1. Liebow A, Carrington CB. The interstitial pneumonias. In: Simon M, Potchen EJ, LeMay M, editors. Frontiers of pulmonary radiology. New York: Grune & Stratton; 1969. p. 102–41.
2. Katzenstein AA, Askin FB. Surgical pathology of non-neoplastic lung disease. Can J Surg 1997; 40(5):394.
3. Müller NL, Coiby TV. Idiopathic interstitial pneumonias: high-resolution CT and histologic findings. Radiographics 1997;17(4):1016–22.
4. American Thoracic Society, European Respiratory Society. American Thoracic Society/European Respiratory Society International Multidisciplinary Consensus Classification of the Idiopathic Interstitial Pneumonias. This joint statement of the American Thoracic Society (ATS), and the European Respiratory Society (ERS) was adopted by the ATS board of directors, June 2001 and by the ERS Executive Committee, June 2001. Am J Respir Crit Care Med 2002;165(2):277–304.
5. Travis WD, Costabel U, Hansell DM, et al. An official American Thoracic Society/European Respiratory Society statement: update of the international multidisciplinary classification of the idiopathic interstitial

pneumonias. Am J Respir Crit Care Med 2013; 188(6):733–48.

6. American Thoracic Society. Idiopathic pulmonary fibrosis: diagnosis and treatment. International consensus statement. American Thoracic Society (ATS), and the European Respiratory Society (ERS). Am J Respir Crit Care Med 2000;161(2 Pt 1):646–64.

7. Collard HR, Moore BB, Flaherty KR, et al. Acute exacerbations of idiopathic pulmonary fibrosis. Am J Respir Crit Care Med 2007;176(7):636–43.

8. Travis WD, Hunninghake G, King TE Jr, et al. Idiopathic nonspecific interstitial pneumonia: report of an American Thoracic Society project. Am J Respir Crit Care Med 2008;177(12):1338–47.

9. Raghu G, Collard HR, Egan JJ, et al. An official ATS/ERS/JRS/ALAT statement: idiopathic pulmonary fibrosis: evidence-based guidelines for diagnosis and management. Am J Respir Crit Care Med 2011;183(6):788–824.

10. Raghu G, Rochwerg B, Zhang Y, et al. An official ATS/ERS/JRS/ALAT clinical practice guideline: treatment of idiopathic pulmonary fibrosis. An update of the 2011 clinical practice guideline. Am J Respir Crit Care Med 2015;192(2):e3–19.

11. Collard HR, Ryerson CJ, Corte TJ, et al. Acute exacerbation of idiopathic pulmonary fibrosis. An international working group report. Am J Respir Crit Care Med 2016;194(3):265–75.

12. Ryerson CJ, Corte TJ, Lee JS, et al. A standardized diagnostic ontology for fibrotic interstitial lung disease. An international working group perspective. Am J Respir Crit Care Med 2017;196(10):1249–54.

13. Raghu G, Remy-Jardin M, Myers JL, et al. Diagnosis of idiopathic pulmonary fibrosis. An official ATS/ERS/JRS/ALAT clinical practice guideline. Am J Respir Crit Care Med 2018;198(5):e44–68.

14. Raghu G, Remy-Jardin M, Myers J, et al. The 2018 diagnosis of idiopathic pulmonary fibrosis guidelines: surgical lung biopsy for radiological pattern of probable usual interstitial pneumonia is not mandatory. Am J Respir Crit Care Med 2019; 200(9):1089–92.

15. Raghu G, Remy-Jardin M, Ryerson CJ, et al. Diagnosis of hypersensitivity pneumonitis in adults. An official ATS/JRS/ALAT clinical practice guideline. Am J Respir Crit Care Med 2020;202(3):e36–69.

16. Crouser ED, Maier LA, Wilson KC, et al. Diagnosis and detection of sarcoidosis. An official American Thoracic Society Clinical Practice Guideline. Am J Respir Crit Care Med 2020;201(8):e26–51.

17. Walsh SL, Calandriello L, Sverzellati N, et al. Interobserver agreement for the ATS/ERS/JRS/ALAT criteria for a UIP pattern on CT. Thorax 2016;71(1):45–51.

18. Flaherty KR, Andrei AC, King TE Jr, et al. Idiopathic interstitial pneumonia: do community and academic physicians agree on diagnosis? Am J Respir Crit Care Med 2007;175(10): 1054–60.

19. Hutchinson JP, Fogarty AW, McKeever TM, et al. In-hospital mortality after surgical lung biopsy for interstitial lung disease in the United States. 2000 to 2011. Am J Respir Crit Care Med 2016;193(10): 1161–7.

20. Hutchinson JP, McKeever TM, Fogarty AW, et al. Surgical lung biopsy for the diagnosis of interstitial lung disease in England: 1997-2008. Eur Respir J 2016; 48(5):1453–61.

21. Flaherty KR, Wells AU, Cottin V, et al. Nintedanib in progressive fibrosing interstitial lung diseases. N Engl J Med 2019;381(18):1718–27.

22. Maher TM, Corte TJ, Fischer A, et al. Pirfenidone in patients with unclassifiable progressive fibrosing interstitial lung disease: a double-blind, randomised, placebo-controlled, phase 2 trial. Lancet Respir Med 2020;8(2):147–57.

23. Walsh SLF, Wells AU, Desai SR, et al. Multicentre evaluation of multidisciplinary team meeting agreement on diagnosis in diffuse parenchymal lung disease: a case-cohort study. Lancet Respir Med 2016;4(7):557–65.

24. Raghu G, Brown KK. Interstitial lung disease: clinical evaluation and keys to an accurate diagnosis. Clin Chest Med 2004;25(3):409–19, v.

25. Lynch DA, Sverzellati N, Travis WD, et al. Diagnostic criteria for idiopathic pulmonary fibrosis: a Fleischner Society white paper. Lancet Respir Med 2018; 6(2):138–53.

26. Han MK, Murray S, Fell CD, et al. Sex differences in physiological progression of idiopathic pulmonary fibrosis. Eur Respir J 2008;31(6):1183–8.

27. Han MK, Arteaga-Solis E, Blenis J, et al. Female sex and gender in lung/sleep health and disease. Increased understanding of basic biological, pathophysiological, and behavioral mechanisms leading to better health for female patients with lung disease. Am J Respir Crit Care Med 2018;198(7): 850–8.

28. Adegunsoye A, Oldham JM, Bellam SK, et al. African-American race and mortality in interstitial lung disease: a multicentre propensity-matched analysis. Eur Respir J 2018;51(6):1800255.

29. Vij R, Strek ME. Diagnosis and treatment of connective tissue disease-associated interstitial lung disease. Chest 2013;143(3):814–24.

30. Salisbury ML, Gross BH, Chughtai A, et al. Development and validation of a radiological diagnosis model for hypersensitivity pneumonitis. Eur Respir J 2018;52(2):1800443.

31. Salisbury ML, Myers JL, Belloli EA, et al. Diagnosis and treatment of fibrotic hypersensitivity pneumonia. where we stand and where we need to go. Am J Respir Crit Care Med 2017;196(6):690–9.

32. Jacob J, Bartholmai BJ, Rajagopalan S, et al. Automated quantitative computed tomography versus visual computed tomography scoring in idiopathic pulmonary fibrosis: validation against pulmonary function. J Thorac Imaging 2016;31(5):304–11.

33. Jacob J, Bartholmai BJ, Rajagopalan S, et al. Predicting outcomes in idiopathic pulmonary fibrosis using automated computed tomographic analysis. Am J Respir Crit Care Med 2018;198(6):767–76.

34. Elicker BM, Kallianos KG, Henry TS. The role of high-resolution computed tomography in the follow-up of diffuse lung disease: number 2 in the Series "Radiology" Edited by Nicola Sverzellati and Sujal Desai. Eur Respir Rev 2017;26(144):170008.

35. Ryerson CJ, Vittinghoff E, Ley B, et al. Predicting survival across chronic interstitial lung disease: the ILD-GAP model. Chest 2014;145(4):723–8.

36. Ley B, Ryerson CJ, Vittinghoff E, et al. A multidimensional index and staging system for idiopathic pulmonary fibrosis. Ann Intern Med 2012;156(10):684–91.

37. Araki T, Putman RK, Hatabu H, et al. Development and progression of interstitial lung abnormalities in the Framingham heart study. Am J Respir Crit Care Med 2016;194(12):1514–22.

38. Robbie H, Daccord C, Chua F, et al. Evaluating disease severity in idiopathic pulmonary fibrosis. Eur Respir Rev 2017;26(145):170051.

39. Cottin V, Nunes H, Brillet PY, et al. Combined pulmonary fibrosis and emphysema: a distinct underrecognised entity. Eur Respir J 2005;26(4):586–93.

40. Calaras D, Munteanu O, Scaletchi V, et al. Ventilatory disturbances in patients with intrathoracic sarcoidosis - a study from a functional and histological perspective. Sarcoidosis Vasc Diffuse Lung Dis 2017;34(1):58–67.

41. Thillai M, Potiphar L, Eberhardt C, et al. Obstructive lung function in sarcoidosis may be missed, especially in older white patients. Eur Respir J 2012; 39(3):775–7.

42. Selman M, Pardo A, King TE Jr. Hypersensitivity pneumonitis: insights in diagnosis and pathobiology. Am J Respir Crit Care Med 2012;186(4):314–24.

43. Tseng HJ, Henry TS, Veeraraghavan S, et al. Pulmonary function tests for the radiologist. Radiographics 2017;37(4):1037–58.

44. Fischer A, Antoniou KM, Brown KK, et al. An official European Respiratory Society/American Thoracic Society research statement: interstitial pneumonia with autoimmune features. Eur Respir J 2015;46(4): 976–87.

45. Adegunsoye A, Oldham JM, Demchuk C, et al. Predictors of survival in coexistent hypersensitivity pneumonitis with autoimmune features. Respir Med 2016;114:53–60.

46. Buendia-Roldan I, Santiago-Ruiz L, Perez-Rubio G, et al. A major genetic determinant of autoimmune diseases is associated with the presence of autoantibodies in hypersensitivity pneumonitis. Eur Respir J 2020;56(2):1901380.

47. Vij R, Noth I, Strek ME. Autoimmune-featured interstitial lung disease: a distinct entity. Chest 2011; 140(5):1292–9.

48. Kinder BW, Collard HR, Koth L, et al. Idiopathic nonspecific interstitial pneumonia: lung manifestation of undifferentiated connective tissue disease? Am J Respir Crit Care Med 2007;176(7):691–7.

49. Corte TJ, Copley SJ, Desai SR, et al. Significance of connective tissue disease features in idiopathic interstitial pneumonia. Eur Respir J 2012;39(3): 661–8.

50. Omote N, Taniguchi H, Kondoh Y, et al. Lung-dominant connective tissue disease: clinical, radiologic, and histologic features. Chest 2015;148(6):1438–46.

51. Meyer KC, Raghu G. Bronchoalveolar lavage for the evaluation of interstitial lung disease: is it clinically useful? Eur Respir J 2011;38(4):761–9.

52. Raj R, Raparia K, Lynch DA, et al. Surgical lung biopsy for interstitial lung diseases. Chest 2017; 151(5):1131–40.

53. Chung JH, Chawla A, Peljto AL, et al. CT scan findings of probable usual interstitial pneumonitis have a high predictive value for histologic usual interstitial pneumonitis. Chest 2015;147(2):450–9.

54. Ambrogi V, Mineo TC. VATS biopsy for undetermined interstitial lung disease under non-general anesthesia: comparison between uniportal approach under intercostal block vs. three-ports in epidural anesthesia. J Thorac Dis 2014;6(7):888–95.

55. Sheth JS, Belperio JA, Fishbein MC, et al. Utility of transbronchial vs surgical lung biopsy in the diagnosis of suspected fibrotic interstitial lung disease. Chest 2017;151(2):389–99.

56. Troy LK, Grainge C, Corte TJ, et al. Diagnostic accuracy of transbronchial lung cryobiopsy for interstitial lung disease diagnosis (COLDICE): a prospective, comparative study. Lancet Respir Med 2020;8(2): 171–81.

57. Jo HE, Corte TJ, Moodley Y, et al. Evaluating the interstitial lung disease multidisciplinary meeting: a survey of expert centres. BMC Pulm Med 2016;16:22.

58. Oldham JM, Noth I. Idiopathic pulmonary fibrosis: early detection and referral. Respir Med 2014; 108(6):819–29.

59. Lamas DJ, Kawut SM, Bagiella E, et al. Delayed access and survival in idiopathic pulmonary fibrosis: a cohort study. Am J Respir Crit Care Med 2011; 184(7):842–7.

60. Valenzi E, Kass DJ. Diagnosis from Afar: is remote multidisciplinary discussion appropriate for interstitial lung disease care? Ann Am Thorac Soc 2019; 16(4):434–6.

61. Grewal JS, Morisset J, Fisher JH, et al. Role of a regional multidisciplinary conference in the

diagnosis of interstitial lung disease. Ann Am Thorac Soc 2019;16(4):455–62.

62. Walsh SLF, Lederer DJ, Ryerson CJ, et al. Diagnostic likelihood thresholds that define a working diagnosis of idiopathic pulmonary fibrosis. Am J Respir Crit Care Med 2019;200(9):1146–53.

63. Ryerson CJ, Collard HR. Update on the diagnosis and classification of ILD. Curr Opin Pulm Med 2013;19(5):453–9.

64. Ley B, Collard HR, King TE Jr. Clinical course and prediction of survival in idiopathic pulmonary fibrosis. Am J Respir Crit Care Med 2011;183(4):431–40.

65. Adegunsoye A, Oldham JM, Bellam SK, et al. Computed tomography honeycombing identifies a progressive fibrotic phenotype with increased mortality across diverse interstitial lung diseases. Ann Am Thorac Soc 2019;16(5):580–8.

66. Solomon JJ, Chung JH, Cosgrove GP, et al. Predictors of mortality in rheumatoid arthritis-associated interstitial lung disease. Eur Respir J 2016;47(2): 588–96.

67. Oldham JM, Adegunsoye A, Valenzi E, et al. Characterisation of patients with interstitial pneumonia with autoimmune features. Eur Respir J 2016;47(6):1767–75.

68. Wijsenbeek M, Cottin V. Spectrum of fibrotic lung diseases. N Engl J Med 2020;383(10):958–68.

69. Allen RJ, Guillen-Guio B, Oldham JM, et al. Genome-wide association study of susceptibility to idiopathic pulmonary fibrosis. Am J Respir Crit Care Med 2020;201(5):564–74.

70. Inoue Y, Kaner RJ, Guiot J, et al. Diagnostic and prognostic biomarkers for chronic fibrosing interstitial lung diseases with a progressive phenotype. Chest 2020;158(2):646–59.

71. Weatherley ND, Eaden JA, Stewart NJ, et al. Experimental and quantitative imaging techniques in interstitial lung disease. Thorax 2019;74(6):611–9.

72. Herazo-Maya JD, Kaminski N. Personalized medicine: applying 'omics' to lung fibrosis. Biomark Med 2012;6(4):529–40.

73. Adegunsoye A, Vij R, Noth I. Integrating genomics into management of fibrotic interstitial lung disease. Chest 2019;155(5):1026–40.

74. Schiller HB, Montoro DT, Simon LM, et al. The human lung cell atlas: a high-resolution reference map of the human lung in health and disease. Am J Respir Cell Mol Biol 2019;61(1):31–41.

75. Adegunsoye A, Oldham JM, Chung JH, et al. Phenotypic clusters predict outcomes in a longitudinal interstitial lung disease cohort. Chest 2018;153(2): 349–60.

Rethinking Idiopathic Pulmonary Fibrosis

Justin M. Oldham, MD, MS[a],*, Carlo Vancheri, MD, PhD[b]

KEYWORDS

- Idiopathic pulmonary fibrosis • Usual interstitial pneumonia • Interstitial lung disease
- Idiopathic interstitial pneumonia

KEY POINTS

- Idiopathic pulmonary fibrosis (IPF) is a chronic fibrosing interstitial lung disease of unknown etiology that may result from several sources of alveolar injury in genetically predisposed individuals.
- IPF can be diagnosed by high-resolution computed tomography in a majority of cases. These include patients with the classic pattern of usual interstitial pneumonia (UIP) and those with probable UIP.
- IPF is best treated with therapies targeting fibrotic pathways and no longer should be treated with immunosuppressive therapies.

INTRODUCTION

Decades of research and patient-physician interactions have proved idiopathic pulmonary fibrosis (IPF) to be a devastating disease for those affected by the disease and their caretakers and loved ones. Although the cause of IPF remains elusive, understanding of the disease has evolved considerably since being characterized in the 1960s. Once called fibrosing alveolitis, it is now known that IPF results in minimal alveolar inflammation. Previously diagnosed by surgical lung biopsy (SLB) in a substantial number of patients, now only a small minority undergo this invasive and morbid diagnostic modality. Once treated with medications aimed at suppression of the immune system, this approach now is understood to be harmful in patients with IPF. These course corrections have required a constant rethinking of IPF on a molecular level, clinical level, and everywhere in-between. This review highlights key areas in which understanding of IPF recently has evolved over the past several decades, including paradigms of disease pathogenesis, diagnosis, and treatment.

RETHINKING IDIOPATHIC PULMONARY FIBROSIS PATHOGENESIS

Limited to case series that described variable histologic features through 1960s, modern-day IPF was coined, *diffuse fibrosing alveolitis*, in 1964 and thought to represent an inflammatory parenchymal process affecting primarily the alveoli.[1,2] Later studies, acknowledging the unclear etiology of this process, referred to it as *cryptogenic fibrosing alveolitis*[3] and IPF.[4] In 1969, Liebow and Carrington[5] described a spectrum of histologic features in patients with idiopathic interstitial pneumonia, including IPF, and hypothesized that such histologic stratification may provide useful prognostic information. The next 30 years supported this hypothesis, because 1 particular histologic subtype, usual interstitial pneumonia (UIP), portended a worse prognosis compared with other patterns.[5–9] Poor survival in patients with UIP, along with minimal alveolar inflammation observed in this histologic subtype, solidified IPF as the preferred name for this condition, with UIP a requisite finding to diagnose IPF.[10,11]

[a] Department of Internal Medicine, Division of Pulmonary, Critical Care and Sleep Medicine, University of California, Davis, 4150 V Street Suite 3400, Sacramento, CA 95817, USA; [b] Department of Clinical and Experimental Medicine, University of Catania, Regional Referral Center for Rare Lung Diseases, University-Hospital "Policlinico -Vittorio Emanuele", Catania, Italy
* Corresponding author.
E-mail address: joldham@ucdavis.edu

Clin Chest Med 42 (2021) 263–273
https://doi.org/10.1016/j.ccm.2021.03.005

Although alveolar inflammation initially was thought to drive fibrosis formation,[12,13] IPF now is thought to result from repetitive alveolar injury followed by abnormal wound healing, characterized by cellular senescence, fibroblast activation and delayed apoptosis, and eventually extracellular matrix remodeling (**Fig. 1**).[14–16] Why this cascade of events occurs in only a small number of individuals remains unclear, but a host of risk factors appear to influence susceptibility. Well-documented risk factors are rare and common gene variants, increasing age, cigarette smoking, chronic infection/colonization, microaspiration, and environmental and occupational exposures.[17–22] That most patients at the time of diagnosis are long removed from these exposures suggests that IPF is a long evolving process, with many years of quiescent disease prior to symptom onset.

Genetic risk factors play an important role in IPF pathogenesis. Through linkage analysis, Seibold and colleagues[23] identified a common variant in the promoter region of *MUC5B* on the short arm of chromosome 11. *MUC5B* encodes mucin-5B, a protein that contributes to mucin production, and is critical for airway homeostasis and host defense.[23,24] The *MUC5B* promoter polymorphism, which has a frequency of approximately 10% in the general population, is highly enriched in patients with IPF, with a frequency of 30% to 40%.[25,26] Another well-characterized genetic phenomenon linked to IPF susceptibility is telomere length. Telomeres are composed of a repeating sequence of nucleotides and serve as protective caps at the end of each chromosome.[27] Although gene variants are static, telomere maintenance is a dynamic process that can result in critically short telomere length in the setting of deleterious telomerase gene mutations, increasing age, and repetitive toxic exposures.[28,29] This critical telomere shortening may provide the conditions for initiation of the fibrotic cascade characteristic of IPF.[14]

Two notable and potentially modifiable risk factors are chronic bacterial colonization and recurrent microaspiration. Studies of the microbiome have begun to characterize the complex interaction between the human body and colonizing bacteria.[17,30–32] Using bronchoalveolar lavage (BAL) fluid, investigators have shown that bacterial burden and presence of specific bacterial species in the lower airway, including streptococcus and staphylococcus, are associated with worse outcomes in IPF.[17,30] Whether direct alveolar injury results from these colonizers remains unclear, but differential expression of genes involved in immune signaling has been demonstrated in the presence of some species.[32] Another potentially modifiable risk factor, enduring and controversial, is microaspiration. A large number of studies have demonstrated that gastroesophageal reflux disease (GERD) and hiatal hernia occur in a large proportion of patients with IPF,[33–36] leading some investigators to hypothesize that GERD followed by microaspiration may lead to alveolar injury characteristic of IPF.[37] Other investigators have pointed out, however, that GERD is an expected physiologic phenomena stemming from increasingly negative intrathoracic pressure in the setting of fibrosis-associated pulmonary restriction.[38]

Together, these findings show IPF to be a complex disease resulting from numerous potential sources of alveolar injury in genetically predisposed individuals. Identifying those genetically predisposed individuals remains a challenge, because the utility of genetic testing remains largely undefined. At present, this testing can provide useful information in high-risk individuals, including those with familial forms of IPF and multisystem findings suggestive of a telomerase mutation.[39,40] Several clinical trials targeting potentially modifiable risk factors recently have been completed, which provide additional useful insight into these risk factors. Additionally, hard work by investigators around the world has improved understanding of the molecular pathways underpinning IPF, resulting in a rapid expansion of antifibrotic compounds, some of which now are entering the final phases of development (discussed later).

RETHINKING IDIOPATHIC PULMONARY FIBROSIS DIAGNOSIS

Prior to the widespread availability and use of high-resolution computed tomography (HRCT), most studies characterizing IPF relied heavily on histologically confirmed cases of UIP. SLB played a prominent role in the 2000 IPF diagnosis and treatment guidelines, which recommended that SLB be performed "in patients with suspected IPF and without contraindications to surgery,"[41] despite the observation that very few patients during that time actually underwent SLB as part of their diagnostic work-up for IPF[42] and several studies showing a strong correlation between histologic UIP and its radiologic corollary by the same name,[43–46] characterized by lower lobe predominant peripheral reticulation with honeycombing with or without traction bronchiectasis (**Fig. 2**).[10,47] The 2011 IPF diagnostic guidelines codified this by effectively allowing a confident diagnosis of IPF to be made in those with UIP on

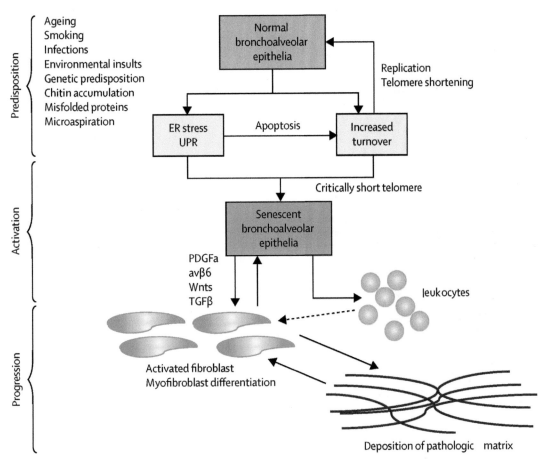

Fig. 1. Three-stage description of the pathogenesis of IPF. In the predisposition stage, recurrent environmental insults lead, in genetically predisposed individuals, to increased turnover of alveolar type II cells, ER stress–mediated activation of UPR, apoptosis, and progressive telomere attrition. In the activation stage, accumulation of a lifetime insults leads to pathologic alterations of the lung epithelium, such as senescence reprogramming, and release of profibrotic mediators (eg, TGFβ, Wnts, and PDGFβ) by the alveolar epithelium. These mediators, either directly or indirectly via leukocytes, activate fibroblasts to deposit pathologic matrix. In the progression stage, the pathologic matrix promotes additional differentiation of fibroblasts to myofibroblasts, which deposit more matrix and further activate fibroblasts in a feed-forward loop of lung remodeling. ER, endoplasmic reticulum; PDGF, platelet-derived growth factor; TGF, transforming growth factor; UPR, unfolded protein response. (*From* Wolters PJ, Blackwell TS, Eickelberg O, et al. Time for a change: is idiopathic pulmonary fibrosis still idiopathic and only fibrotic? Lancet Respir Med. 2018;6(2):154-160. Reprinted with permission from Elsevier.)

HRCT alone, which accounted for nearly half of patients.[48] These guidelines still called for SLB to be performed in patients displaying patterns on HRCT other than UIP when possible.

A 2017 Fleischner Society white paper on the diagnosis of IPF challenged the diagnostic construct established by the 2011 IPF consensus guidelines.[47] Citing studies showing a high correlation between histologic UIP and the radiologic probable UIP,[49] a pattern characterized by lower lobe predominant peripheral reticulation and traction bronchiectasis or bronchiolectasis without honeycombing (see **Fig. 2**), the Fleischner Society recommended that a confident diagnosis of IPF be made in patients with UIP and probable UIP on HRCT once other potential causes of interstitial lung disease (ILD) had been excluded. This recommendation mirrored common practice within the ILD community, where SLB remained a diagnostic procedure reserved for patients for whom IPF was not strongly suspected. Clinical trials also supported this approach, because IPF patients with probable UIP demonstrated a rate of lung function decline similar to that in patients with definite UIP.[50] The 2018 IPF diagnostic guidelines offered a more ambiguous message as a conditional recommendation for SLB remained in patients with probable UIP.[10] The 2018 IPF guidelines later

UIP on HRCT (with honeycombing)

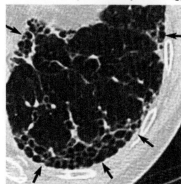

Probable UIP on HRCT (traction bronchiectasis and bronchiolectasis without honeycombing)

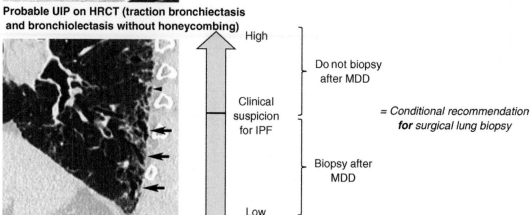

= Strong recommendation *against* surgical lung biopsy

= Conditional recommendation *for* surgical lung biopsy

Fig. 2. Consideration of SLB to determine histologic features in patients with HRCT patterns of UIP and probable UIP. (*Top*) UIP magnified view of the left lower lobe (transverse computed tomography section) showing typical characteristics of honeycombing, consisting of clustered cystic airspaces with well-defined walls and variable diameters, seen in single or multiple layers (*arrows*). (*Bottom*) Probable UIP magnified sagittal view (reconstructed) of the right lower lobe illustrating the presence of a reticular pattern with subpleural, peripheral, and basal predominance of traction bronchiolectasis that appears as tubular (*arrows*) or cystic (*arrowhead*) structures. Images reprinted from.[10] (*Reprinted from* Raghu G, Remy-Jardin M, Myers J, Richeldi L, Wilson KC. The 2018 Diagnosis of Idiopathic Pulmonary Fibrosis Guidelines: Surgical Lung Biopsy for Radiological Pattern of Probable Usual Interstitial Pneumonia Is Not Mandatory. Am J Respir Crit Care Med. 2019;200(9):1089-1092; with permission of the American Thoracic Society. Copyright © 2020 American Thoracic Society. All rights reserved.)

clarified that their conditional recommendation meant that patients with a high clinical suspicion of IPF after multidisciplinary discussion (MDD) need not undergo SLB, whereas this diagnostic modality should be considered in those with a lower pretest probability of IPF after MDD (see **Fig. 2**).[51]

Although bronchoscopy and BAL may assist in the diagnosis of ILDs, such as chronic hypersensitivity pneumonitis, the role of bronchoscopy in diagnosing IPF remains limited. The 2018 IPF diagnostic guidelines provide a conditional recommendation for BAL and cellular analysis in patients with suspected IPF and patterns other than UIP on HRCT, because this may help differentiate IPF from alternate ILDS. No recommendation for or against the use of transbronchial biopsy (TBB)

was provided due to paucity of data on the subject. Given the patchy nature of IPF, however, TBBs often fail to provide a sample of sufficient size to appreciate the temporal heterogeneity and architectural distortion characteristic of UIP.

Although histologic utility remains limited with TBBs, recent advances in genomic technology may prove TBBs to be useful in the diagnostic work-up of IPF. Using SLB histology as the gold standard, investigators used machine learning methods to identify gene transcripts associated with UIP on SLB. An aggregated transcriptomic signature and categorical classifier then was derived using these data. Validation of this classifier in an independent cohort demonstrated sensitivity of 76% and specificity of 88%. Given the high prevalence of UIP in these cohorts, this translated to positive and negative predictive values of 81% and 85%, respectively.[52] These data suggest that this classifier may serve as a reliable confirmatory test for patients unable or unwilling to undergo SLB but do not provide sufficient sensitivity for use as a screening tool. The role of this genomic classifier in the work-up of IPF remains undefined but is a reasonable consideration for patients with an indeterminate pattern on HRCT.

Transbronchial lung cryobiopsy (TBLC) may serve as an alternative to SLB in selected patients, because the sample size provided by this intervention is significantly larger than traditional transbronchial biopsies and allows for a histologic diagnosis to be made in a majority of cases.[53] A recent prospective investigation of TBLC in Australia demonstrated greater than 70% agreement between TBLC and SLB and 95% concordance in patients, with a high confidence diagnosis of IPF after MDD.[54] Risks of bleeding and pneumothorax remain a major concern with this diagnostic modality and need to be weighed against the benefit of a confident ILD diagnosis.

For those in whom SLB is deemed appropriate and necessary, video-assisted thoracoscopic surgery (VATS) has become the preferred method for obtaining lung tissue in patients with suspected IPF and other ILDs. This stems from data suggesting that a VATS approach results in reduced operative time and hospital stay compared with an open approach.[55] Irrespective of approach, perioperative mortality ranges 2% to 5% for elective cases,[42,56,57] underscoring the importance of patient education and individualized risk/benefit assessment. An awake thoracoscopic approach with regional nerve blocks also has been studied and shown to be safe and effective in small, single-center studies.[58,59] This approach, which may mitigate risks associated with general anesthesia and mechanical ventilation, provides an intriguing alternative to traditional VATS approach and is worthy of additional investigation.

For patients ultimately diagnosed with ILD, IPF, or otherwise, arriving at the diagnosis through MDD has become a hallmark of ILD centers of excellence. The 2018 IPF diagnostic guidelines provided a conditional recommendation that patients with suspected IPF undergo MDD.[10] This recommendation reflects prior research showing that MDD increases diagnostic confidence, shows good agreement in IPF diagnosis by specialists around the world, and significantly increases the percentage of cases that receive a diagnosis.[60–62] Although IPF severity, comorbidities, and travel distance may preclude ILD center evaluation and MDD for some patients, ILD center evaluation should be made available for otherwise able and interested patients. Virtual MDD represents a potential alternative for patients unable to undergo in-person ILD center evaluation. This approach recently was studied in Canada and showed virtual MDD to change ILD diagnosis in approximately half of external referrals and change in therapy in more than 60%.[63]

RETHINKING IDIOPATHIC PULMONARY FIBROSIS TREATMENT

The paradigm of IPF being an inflammatory-driven process persisted for decades and resulted in the regular administration of corticosteroids and other immunosuppressant therapies, such as cyclophosphamide[64] and azathioprine.[65] This approach was supported by the 2000 IPF treatment guidelines, which recommended combination therapy with corticosteroids and azathioprine in those with early disease.[41] Other immunomodulatory therapies were assessed over the next decade but failed to show benefit.[66–69] Then, in 2011, the PANTHER trial revealed that a higher proportion of deaths and hospitalizations occurred in patients treated with combination prednisone, azathioprine, and N-acetylcysteine, effectively ending the era of immunosuppression for the treatment of IPF.[70] Although immune dysregulation appears to contribute to IPF pathogenesis, PANTHER and other trials assessing immunosuppressive therapies suggest this phenomenon occurs downstream from alveolar injury and supports, rather than drives, profibrotic signaling (see **Fig. 1**).

Concurrent to immunosuppressant clinical trials were those assessing the efficacy of therapies with antifibrotic properties, including pirfenidone and nintedanib. After promising phase II results, these therapies were studied in large phase III clinical trials and showed each therapy to effectively slow lung function decline in patients with IPF,[71–73] resulting in their approval for the treatment of IPF in many countries around the world. Post hoc analyses of the pirfenidone and nintedanib clinical trial datasets also suggested that these therapies reduced the risk of acute exacerbation, hospitalization, and death.[71,74–76] A growing number of investigations reinforce these findings, suggesting a survival benefit in those treated with antifibrotic therapy.[77–80] Although the 2015 IPF treatment guidelines provided a conditional recommendation for the use of antifibrotic in IPF, subsequent investigations suggest efficacy of these drugs irrespective of age, lung function, need for supplemental oxygen, or duration of disease.[81] Side effects remain a major concern for each drug but are tolerable or can be managed effectively in most patients in whom they develop.

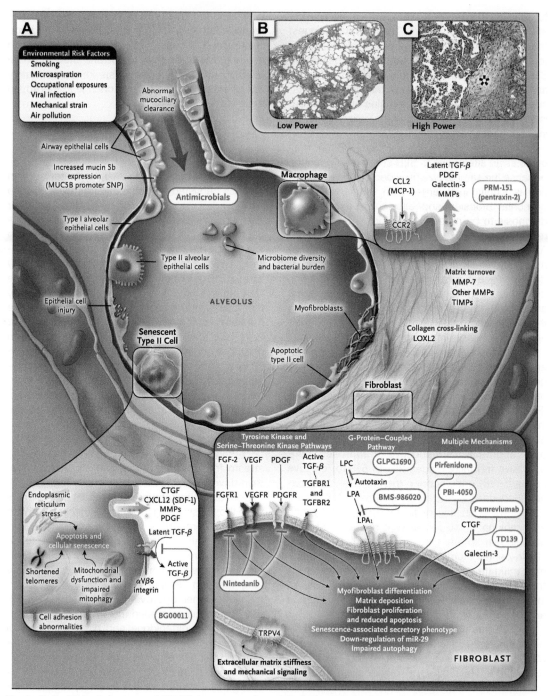

Fig. 3. Pathobiologic features of IPF. (*A*) A conceptual model of the pathobiology of IPF, which is characterized by recurrent epithelial cell injury, senescent alveolar epithelial cells, profibrotic mediators leading to matrix deposition by myofibroblasts, microbiome changes, and host defense abnormalities. Potential therapeutic interventions are shown in green. Histologic features of UIP are shown in (*B*) at low magnification and (*C*) at high magnification (hematoxylin-eosin). The photomicrographs show a marked patchy fibrosis in a peripheral, lobular (paraseptal) distribution. Fibroblastic foci (*asterisk*) typically are a prominent (but nonspecific) feature. Absent are features that would suggest an alternative ILD, such as granulomas, hyaline membranes, organizing pneumonia, or marked inflammation. AEC, alveolar epithelial cell; CCL2, chemokine (C-C motif) ligand 2; CCR2, chemokine (C-C motif) receptor 2; CTGF, connective-tissue growth factor; CXCL12, C-X-C motif chemokine ligand 12; FGF-2, fibroblast growth factor 2; FGFR1, fibroblast growth factor receptor 1; LOXL2, lysyl oxidase–like 2; LPA,

Phase III trials of newer antifibrotic therapies now are being planned or are under way, each with an independent mechanism of action (**Fig. 3**). Ziritaxestat (GLP1690) is an autotaxin inhibitor taken orally once daily. Pamrevlumab is a monoclonal antibody inhibitor of connective tissue growth factor that is administered via intravenous infusion every 3 weeks. PRM-151 is a recombinant human pentraxin-2 protein that inhibits monocyte differentiation into profibrotic fibrocytes administered via intravenous infusion every 4 weeks. Each of these therapies demonstrated good safety profiles in phase II trials[82–84] and is being assessed for efficacy in phase III trials. The phase III trials for ziritaxestat (GLPG1690) (NCT 03711162/ 03733444) allows background therapy with pirfenidone or nintedanib, as will the PRM-151 trial, which currently is in planning stages. Background therapy currently is not allowed in those enrolling in the phase III pamrevlumab trial (NCT03955146).

Targeting of modifiable IPF risk factors also has been pursued. Studies of the microbiome showing increased mortality in patients with high bacterial burden[17] and streptococcus and staphylococcus species[30] prompted 2 studies assessing whether potential modulation of the microbial composition of the lower airways may affect disease progression in IPF. The CleanUp study in the United States and EME-TIPAC study in the United Kingdom each assessed the impact of add-on co-trimoxazole to standard of care compared with standard of care as it related to death and hospitalization.[85,86] Results for these trials are due in the near future. Both studies collected biospecimens, which will allow for further assessment of these results in relation to relevant biomarkers and microbial landscape.

Given prior studies implicating microaspiration as a potential cause of alveolar injury in IPF, the phase II WRAP-IPF trial assessed whether Nissen fundoplication modulated disease progression in patients with IPF and pathologic GERD.[87] Although the trial did not show a difference in the primary endpoint of change in forced vital capacity over 24 weeks, there was a suggestion of hospitalization-free survival benefit in those undergoing this procedure. Until these findings can be validated in a larger trial, the potential benefits of this surgery need to be weighed against the risks associated with any surgical intervention on a case-by-case basis.[88] Antacid therapy also has been proposed for the treatment of IPF given the high prevalence of GERD in this population, although retrospective data have been mixed.[89,90] A small trial assessing the efficacy of omeprazole for the treatment of IPF-related cough showed worsened lung function in those treated with omeprazole.[91] As such, although antacid therapy certainly should be considered for the treatment of symptomatic GERD in IPF, the role of such therapy as an adjunct IPF therapy remains unclear.

The first precision medicine study in IPF also is set to begin enrolling soon. The PRECISIONS trial (NCT04300920) will prospectively test a prior observation that patients enrolled in the PANTHER trial[92] with a common gene variant in the *TOLLIP* gene displayed better progression-free survival when treated with *N*-acetylcysteine.[93] PRECISIONS will focus on patients with both variant alleles of rs3750920 in *TOLLIP*, which represent approximately 25% of patients with IPF. This trial will allow background therapy with pirfenidone or nintedanib and will collect large-scale genomic data to allow for further characterization of genomic, transcriptomic and proteomic factors influencing IPF progression, and treatment response.

CHALLENGES AHEAD

Although the past decade has seen great optimism emerge in the field of IPF, much work remains to better identify and treat these patients. A survey conducted in 2007 showed that more than 50% of respondents with IPF reported waiting more than a year from the time of symptom onset to diagnosis.[94] A similar survey conducted a decade later showed little change in this experience.[95] Efforts to characterize the factors underpinning diagnostic delays are under way, but screening of high-risk groups, including those undergoing chest CT for lung cancer screening and other indications with shared IPF risk factors, is a reasonable starting point. Interstitial lung abnormalities likely represent early IPF in a significant number of cases,[96] so reliable interstitial lung

lysophosphatidic acid; LPA$_1$, lysophosphatidic acid receptor type 1; LPC, lysophosphatidylcholine; MCP-1, monocyte chemoattractant protein 1; MMP, matrix metalloproteinase; PDGF, platelet-derived growth factor; PDGFR, platelet-derived growth factor receptor; SDF-1, stromal-cell–derived factor 1; TGF-β, transforming growth factor β; TGFBR1 TGF-β receptor type 1; TIMP, tissue inhibitor of metalloproteinases; TRPV4, transient receptor potential cation channel subfamily V member 4; VEGF, vascular endothelial growth factor; VEGFR, vascular endothelial growth factor receptor. (*From* Lederer DJ, Martinez FJ. Idiopathic Pulmonary Fibrosis. *N Engl J Med*. 2018;378(19):1811-1823. Copyright © 2020 Massachusetts Medical Society. Reprinted with permission from Massachusetts Medical Society.)

abnormalities reporting by radiologists followed by referral of such patients to an ILD center of excellence should be prioritized.[97]

Although early diagnosis provides the best opportunity for early intervention in IPF, intervention still is required to impact disease course. Despite emerging data supporting the benefit of antifibrotic therapy in IPF and other ILDs, a large proportion of patients with IPF remains untreated. This may reflect the conditional recommendation for antifibrotic use by the 2015 IPF treatment guidelines, but several physician-level factors leading to the recommendation against treatment are concerning. Age, sex, disease duration, and severity do not appear to impact antifibrotic efficacy. Moreover, the idea of stable IPF is a fallacy discredited by innumerable studies. IPF by definition is a progressive disease. Understanding of disease pathogenesis reaffirms this, as does the authors' experience caring for and studying patients with IPF. With increasingly less-invasive procedures needed to diagnose IPF, the goal as a community should be near universal treatment in those who want it along with tireless investment in making effective therapies available for patients.

CLINICS CARE POINTS

- Initially thought to be an inflammatory interstitial lung disease, idiopathic pulmonary fibrosis is now known to be driven by aberrant wound repair and pronounced extracellular matrix formation in response to alveolar injury.

- Previously requiring a definite UIP pattern for diagnosis, IPF can now be diagnosed in patients with a probable UIP pattern on high-resolution computed tomography in the appropriate clinical context.

- While suppression of the immune system is now known to harm patients with IPF, therapies targeting pathways involved in fibrogenesis have proven effective in slowing IPF progression.

DISCLOSURE

J.M. Oldham reports consulting fees from Genentech and Boehringer Ingelheim unrelated to this work. C. Vancheri reports consulting fees from Roche and Boehringer Ingelheim unrelated to this work. National Heart Lung and Blood Institute (K23HL138190) for Dr. Oldham. The NHLBI had no role in the conceptualization or writing of this review.

REFERENCES

1. Scadding JG. Fibrosing alveolitis. Br Med J 1964; 2(5410):686.
2. Livingstone JL, Lewis JG, Reid L, et al. Diffuse interstitial pulmonary fibrosis.a clinical, radiological, and pathological study based on 45 patients. Q J Med 1964;33:71–103.
3. Stack BH, Choo-Kang YF, Heard BE. The prognosis of cryptogenic fibrosing alveolitis. Thorax 1972; 27(5):535–42.
4. Crystal RG, Fulmer JD, Roberts WC, et al. Idiopathic pulmonary fibrosis. Clinical, histologic, radiographic, physiologic, scintigraphic, cytologic, and biochemical aspects. Ann Intern Med 1976;85(6): 769–88.
5. Liebow A, Carrington CB. The interstitial pneumonias, frontiers of pulmonary radiology. New York: Grune and Stratton; 1969.
6. Katzenstein AL, Myers JL. Idiopathic pulmonary fibrosis: clinical relevance of pathologic classification. Am J Respir Crit Care Med 1998;157(4 Pt 1): 1301–15.
7. Bjoraker JA, Ryu JH, Edwin MK, et al. Prognostic significance of histopathologic subsets in idiopathic pulmonary fibrosis. Am J Respir Crit Care Med 1998; 157(1):199–203.
8. Panos RJ, Mortenson RL, Niccoli SA, et al. Clinical deterioration in patients with idiopathic pulmonary fibrosis: causes and assessment. Am J Med 1990; 88(4):396–404.
9. Flaherty KR, Toews GB, Travis WD, et al. Clinical significance of histological classification of idiopathic interstitial pneumonia. Eur Respir J 2002;19(2): 275–83.
10. Raghu G, Remy-Jardin M, Myers JL, et al. Diagnosis of idiopathic pulmonary fibrosis. an official ATS/ERS/ JRS/ALAT clinical practice guideline. Am J Respir Crit Care Med 2018;198(5):e44–68.
11. Noble PW, Homer RJ. Back to the future: historical perspective on the pathogenesis of idiopathic pulmonary fibrosis. Am J Respir Cell Mol Biol 2005; 33(2):113–20.
12. Crystal RG, Bitterman PB, Rennard SI, et al. Interstitial lung diseases of unknown cause. Disorders characterized by chronic inflammation of the lower respiratory tract. N Engl J Med 1984;310(4):235–44.
13. Crystal RG, Bitterman PB, Rennard SI, et al. Interstitial lung diseases of unknown cause. Disorders characterized by chronic inflammation of the lower respiratory tract (first of two parts). N Engl J Med 1984;310(3):154–66.
14. Wolters PJ, Blackwell TS, Eickelberg O, et al. Time for a change: is idiopathic pulmonary fibrosis still

idiopathic and only fibrotic? Lancet Respir Med 2018;6(2):154–60.

15. Lederer DJ, Martinez FJ. Idiopathic pulmonary fibrosis. N Engl J Med 2018;378(19):1811–23.

16. Blackwell TS, Tager AM, Borok Z, et al. Future directions in idiopathic pulmonary fibrosis research. An NHLBI workshop report. Am J Respir Crit Care Med 2014;189(2):214–22.

17. Molyneaux PL, Cox MJ, Willis-Owen SA, et al. The role of bacteria in the pathogenesis and progression of idiopathic pulmonary fibrosis. Am J Respir Crit Care Med 2014;190(8):906–13.

18. Baumgartner KB, Samet JM, Stidley CA, et al. Cigarette smoking: a risk factor for idiopathic pulmonary fibrosis. Am J Respir Crit Care Med 1997;155(1):242–8.

19. Raghu G, Weycker D, Edelsberg J, et al. Incidence and prevalence of idiopathic pulmonary fibrosis. Am J Respir Crit Care Med 2006;174(7):810–6.

20. Taskar VS, Coultas DB. Is idiopathic pulmonary fibrosis an environmental disease? Proc Am Thorac Soc 2006;3(4):293–8.

21. Puglisi S, Torrisi SE, Giuliano R, et al. What we know about the pathogenesis of idiopathic pulmonary fibrosis. Semin Respir Crit Care Med 2016;37(3):358–67.

22. Kropski JA, Blackwell TS, Loyd JE. The genetic basis of idiopathic pulmonary fibrosis. Eur Respir J 2015;45(6):1717–27.

23. Seibold MA, Wise AL, Speer MC, et al. A common MUC5B promoter polymorphism and pulmonary fibrosis. N Engl J Med 2011;364(16):1503–12.

24. Roy MG, Livraghi-Butrico A, Fletcher AA, et al. Muc5b is required for airway defence. Nature 2014;505(7483):412–6.

25. Fingerlin TE, Murphy E, Zhang W, et al. Genome-wide association study identifies multiple susceptibility loci for pulmonary fibrosis. Nat Genet 2013;45(6):613–20.

26. Noth I, Zhang Y, Ma SF, et al. Genetic variants associated with idiopathic pulmonary fibrosis susceptibility and mortality: a genome-wide association study. Lancet Respir Med 2013;1(4):309–17.

27. Armanios M, Blackburn EH. The telomere syndromes. Nat Rev Genet 2012;13(10):693–704.

28. Harley CB, Futcher AB, Greider CW. Telomeres shorten during ageing of human fibroblasts. Nature 1990;345(6274):458–60.

29. Allsopp RC, Vaziri H, Patterson C, et al. Telomere length predicts replicative capacity of human fibroblasts. Proc Natl Acad Sci U S A 1992;89(21):10114–8.

30. Han MK, Zhou Y, Murray S, et al. Lung microbiome and disease progression in idiopathic pulmonary fibrosis: an analysis of the COMET study. Lancet Respir Med 2014;2(7):548–56.

31. Huang Y, Ma SF, Espindola MS, et al. Microbes are associated with host innate immune response in idiopathic pulmonary fibrosis. Am J Respir Crit Care Med 2017;196(2):208–19.

32. Molyneaux PL, Willis-Owen SAG, Cox MJ, et al. Host-microbial interactions in idiopathic pulmonary fibrosis. Am J Respir Crit Care Med 2017;195(12):1640–50.

33. Raghu G. The role of gastroesophageal reflux in idiopathic pulmonary fibrosis. Am J Med 2003;115(Suppl 3A):60S–4S.

34. Tobin RW, Pope CE 2nd, Pellegrini CA, et al. Increased prevalence of gastroesophageal reflux in patients with idiopathic pulmonary fibrosis. Am J Respir Crit Care Med 1998;158(6):1804–8.

35. Raghu G, Freudenberger TD, Yang S, et al. High prevalence of abnormal acid gastro-oesophageal reflux in idiopathic pulmonary fibrosis. Eur Respir J 2006;27(1):136–42.

36. Noth I, Zangan SM, Soares RV, et al. Prevalence of hiatal hernia by blinded multidetector CT in patients with idiopathic pulmonary fibrosis. Eur Respir J 2012;39(2):344–51.

37. Lee JS, Collard HR, Raghu G, et al. Does chronic microaspiration cause idiopathic pulmonary fibrosis? Am J Med 2010;123(4):304–11.

38. Ghisa M, Marinelli C, Savarino V, et al. Idiopathic pulmonary fibrosis and GERD: links and risks. Ther Clin Risk Manag 2019;15:1081–93.

39. Diaz de Leon A, Cronkhite JT, Yilmaz C, et al. Subclinical lung disease, macrocytosis, and premature graying in kindreds with telomerase (TERT) mutations. Chest 2011;140(3):753–63.

40. Parry EM, Alder JK, Qi X, et al. Syndrome complex of bone marrow failure and pulmonary fibrosis predicts germline defects in telomerase. Blood 2011;117(21):5607–11.

41. American Thoracic Society. Idiopathic pulmonary fibrosis: diagnosis and treatment. International consensus statement. American Thoracic Society (ATS), and the European Respiratory Society (ERS). Am J Respir Crit Care Med 2000;161(2 Pt 1):646–64.

42. Hutchinson JP, McKeever TM, Fogarty AW, et al. Surgical lung biopsy for the diagnosis of interstitial lung disease in England: 1997-2008. Eur Respir J 2016;48(5):1453–61.

43. Flaherty KR, Thwaite EL, Kazerooni EA, et al. Radiological versus histological diagnosis in UIP and NSIP: survival implications. Thorax 2003;58(2):143–8.

44. Hunninghake GW, Zimmerman MB, Schwartz DA, et al. Utility of a lung biopsy for the diagnosis of idiopathic pulmonary fibrosis. Am J Respir Crit Care Med 2001;164(2):193–6.

45. Swensen SJ, Aughenbaugh GL, Myers JL. Diffuse lung disease: diagnostic accuracy of CT in patients undergoing surgical biopsy of the lung. Radiology 1997;205(1):229–34.

46. Raghu G, Mageto YN, Lockhart D, et al. The accuracy of the clinical diagnosis of new-onset idiopathic

pulmonary fibrosis and other interstitial lung disease: a prospective study. Chest 1999;116(5):1168–74.

47. Lynch DA, Sverzellati N, Travis WD, et al. Diagnostic criteria for idiopathic pulmonary fibrosis: a Fleischner Society white paper. Lancet Respir Med 2018;6(2):138–53.

48. Raghu G, Collard HR, Egan JJ, et al. An official ATS/ERS/JRS/ALAT statement: idiopathic pulmonary fibrosis: evidence-based guidelines for diagnosis and management. Am J Respir Crit Care Med 2011;183(6):788–824.

49. Raghu G, Lynch D, Godwin JD, et al. Diagnosis of idiopathic pulmonary fibrosis with high-resolution CT in patients with little or no radiological evidence of honeycombing: secondary analysis of a randomised, controlled trial. Lancet Respir Med 2014;2(4):277–84.

50. Raghu G, Wells AU, Nicholson AG, et al. Effect of nintedanib in subgroups of idiopathic pulmonary fibrosis by diagnostic criteria. Am J Respir Crit Care Med 2017;195(1):78–85.

51. Raghu G, Remy-Jardin M, Myers J, et al. The 2018 diagnosis of idiopathic pulmonary fibrosis guidelines: surgical lung biopsy for radiological pattern of probable usual interstitial pneumonia is not mandatory. Am J Respir Crit Care Med 2019;200(9):1089–92.

52. Raghu G, Flaherty KR, Lederer DJ, et al. Use of a molecular classifier to identify usual interstitial pneumonia in conventional transbronchial lung biopsy samples: a prospective validation study. Lancet Respir Med 2019;7(6):487–96.

53. Tomassetti S, Wells AU, Costabel U, et al. Bronchoscopic lung cryobiopsy increases diagnostic confidence in the multidisciplinary diagnosis of idiopathic pulmonary fibrosis. Am J Respir Crit Care Med 2016;193(7):745–52.

54. Troy LK, Grainge C, Corte TJ, et al. Diagnostic accuracy of transbronchial lung cryobiopsy for interstitial lung disease diagnosis (COLDICE): a prospective, comparative study. Lancet Respir Med 2020;8(2):171–81.

55. Mouroux J, Clary-Meinesz C, Padovani B, et al. Efficacy and safety of videothoracoscopic lung biopsy in the diagnosis of interstitial lung disease. Eur J Cardiothorac Surg 1997;11(1):22–4, 25–26.

56. Kreider ME, Hansen-Flaschen J, Ahmad NN, et al. Complications of video-assisted thoracoscopic lung biopsy in patients with interstitial lung disease. Ann Thorac Surg 2007;83(3):1140–4.

57. Hutchinson JP, Fogarty AW, McKeever TM, et al. In-hospital mortality after surgical lung biopsy for interstitial lung disease in the United States. 2000 to 2011. Am J Respir Crit Care Med 2016;193(10):1161–7.

58. Pompeo E, Rogliani P, Cristino B, et al. Awake thoracoscopic biopsy of interstitial lung disease. Ann Thorac Surg 2013;95(2):445–52.

59. Jeon CS, Yoon DW, Moon SM, et al. Non-intubated video-assisted thoracoscopic lung biopsy for interstitial lung disease: a single-center experience. J Thorac Dis 2018;10(6):3262–8.

60. Flaherty KR, King TE Jr, Raghu G, et al. Idiopathic interstitial pneumonia: what is the effect of a multidisciplinary approach to diagnosis? Am J Respir Crit Care Med 2004;170(8):904–10.

61. De Sadeleer LJ, Meert C, Yserbyt J, et al. Diagnostic ability of a dynamic multidisciplinary discussion in interstitial lung diseases: a retrospective observational study of 938 cases. Chest 2018;153(6):1416–23.

62. Walsh SLF, Wells AU, Desai SR, et al. Multicentre evaluation of multidisciplinary team meeting agreement on diagnosis in diffuse parenchymal lung disease: a case-cohort study. Lancet Respir Med 2016;4(7):557–65.

63. Grewal JS, Morisset J, Fisher JH, et al. Role of a regional multidisciplinary conference in the diagnosis of interstitial lung disease. Ann Am Thorac Soc 2019;16(4):455–62.

64. Kolb M, Kirschner J, Riedel W, et al. Cyclophosphamide pulse therapy in idiopathic pulmonary fibrosis. Eur Respir J 1998;12(6):1409–14.

65. Raghu G, Depaso WJ, Cain K, et al. Azathioprine combined with prednisone in the treatment of idiopathic pulmonary fibrosis: a prospective double-blind, randomized, placebo-controlled clinical trial. Am Rev Respir Dis 1991;144(2):291–6.

66. King TE Jr, Albera C, Bradford WZ, et al. Effect of interferon gamma-1b on survival in patients with idiopathic pulmonary fibrosis (INSPIRE): a multicentre, randomised, placebo-controlled trial. Lancet 2009;374(9685):222–8.

67. Raghu G, Brown KK, Bradford WZ, et al. A placebo-controlled trial of interferon gamma-1b in patients with idiopathic pulmonary fibrosis. N Engl J Med 2004;350(2):125–33.

68. Raghu G, Brown KK, Costabel U, et al. Treatment of idiopathic pulmonary fibrosis with etanercept: an exploratory, placebo-controlled trial. Am J Respir Crit Care Med 2008;178(9):948–55.

69. Tzouvelekis A, Bouros E, Oikonomou A, et al. Effect and safety of mycophenolate mofetil in idiopathic pulmonary fibrosis. Pulm Med 2011;2011:849035.

70. Idiopathic Pulmonary Fibrosis Clinical Research Network, Raghu G, Anstrom KJ, et al. Prednisone, azathioprine, and N-acetylcysteine for pulmonary fibrosis. N Engl J Med 2012;366(21):1968–77.

71. King TE Jr, Bradford WZ, Castro-Bernardini S, et al. A phase 3 trial of pirfenidone in patients with idiopathic pulmonary fibrosis. N Engl J Med 2014;370(22):2083–92.

72. Noble PW, Albera C, Bradford WZ, et al. Pirfenidone in patients with idiopathic pulmonary fibrosis (CAPACITY): two randomised trials. Lancet 2011;377(9779):1760–9.

73. Richeldi L, du Bois RM, Raghu G, et al. Efficacy and safety of nintedanib in idiopathic pulmonary fibrosis. N Engl J Med 2014;370(22):2071–82.

74. Collard HR, Richeldi L, Kim DS, et al. Acute exacerbations in the INPULSIS trials of nintedanib in idiopathic pulmonary fibrosis. Eur Respir J 2017;49(5):1601339.

75. Lancaster L, Crestani B, Hernandez P, et al. Safety and survival data in patients with idiopathic pulmonary fibrosis treated with nintedanib: pooled data from six clinical trials. BMJ Open Respir Res 2019;6(1):e000397.

76. Ley B, Swigris J, Day BM, et al. Pirfenidone reduces respiratory-related hospitalizations in idiopathic pulmonary fibrosis. Am J Respir Crit Care Med 2017;196(6):756–61.

77. Adegunsoye A, Alqalyoobi S, Linderholm A, et al. Circulating plasma biomarkers of survival in antifibrotic-treated patients with idiopathic pulmonary fibrosis. Chest 2020;158(4):1526–34.

78. Dempsey TM, Sangaralingham LR, Yao X, et al. Clinical effectiveness of antifibrotic medications for idiopathic pulmonary fibrosis. Am J Respir Crit Care Med 2019;200(2):168–74.

79. Tran T, Sterclova M, Mogulkoc N, et al. The European MultiPartner IPF registry (EMPIRE): validating long-term prognostic factors in idiopathic pulmonary fibrosis. Respir Res 2020;21(1):11.

80. Guenther A, Krauss E, Tello S, et al. The European IPF registry (eurIPFreg): baseline characteristics and survival of patients with idiopathic pulmonary fibrosis. Respir Res 2018;19(1):141.

81. Maher TM, Strek ME. Antifibrotic therapy for idiopathic pulmonary fibrosis: time to treat. Respir Res 2019;20(1):205.

82. Raghu G, van den Blink B, Hamblin MJ, et al. Effect of recombinant human pentraxin 2 vs placebo on change in forced vital capacity in patients with idiopathic pulmonary fibrosis: a randomized clinical trial. JAMA 2018;319(22):2299–307.

83. Richeldi L, Fernandez Perez ER, Costabel U, et al. Pamrevlumab, an anti-connective tissue growth factor therapy, for idiopathic pulmonary fibrosis (PRAISE): a phase 2, randomised, double-blind, placebo-controlled trial. Lancet Respir Med 2020;8(1):25–33.

84. Maher TM, van der Aar EM, Van de Steen O, et al. Safety, tolerability, pharmacokinetics, and pharmacodynamics of GLPG1690, a novel autotaxin inhibitor, to treat idiopathic pulmonary fibrosis (FLORA): a phase 2a randomised placebo-controlled trial. Lancet Respir Med 2018;6(8):627–35.

85. Anstrom KJ, Noth I, Flaherty KR, et al. Design and rationale of a multi-center, pragmatic, open-label randomized trial of antimicrobial therapy - the study of clinical efficacy of antimicrobial therapy strategy using pragmatic design in Idiopathic Pulmonary Fibrosis (CleanUP-IPF) clinical trial. Respir Res 2020;21(1):68.

86. Hammond M, Clark AB, Cahn AP, et al. The efficacy and mechanism evaluation of treating idiopathic pulmonary fibrosis with the addition of Co-trimoxazole (EME-TIPAC): study protocol for a randomised controlled trial. Trials 2018;19(1):89.

87. Raghu G, Pellegrini CA, Yow E, et al. Laparoscopic anti-reflux surgery for the treatment of idiopathic pulmonary fibrosis (WRAP-IPF): a multicentre, randomised, controlled phase 2 trial. Lancet Respir Med 2018;6(9):707–14.

88. Johannson KA, Strambu I, Ravaglia C, et al. Antacid therapy in idiopathic pulmonary fibrosis: more questions than answers? Lancet Respir Med 2017;5(7):591–8.

89. Kreuter M, Wuyts W, Renzoni E, et al. Antacid therapy and disease outcomes in idiopathic pulmonary fibrosis: a pooled analysis. Lancet Respir Med 2016;4(5):381–9.

90. Lee JS, Collard HR, Anstrom KJ, et al. Anti-acid treatment and disease progression in idiopathic pulmonary fibrosis: an analysis of data from three randomised controlled trials. Lancet Respir Med 2013;1(5):369–76.

91. Dutta P, Funston W, Mossop H, et al. Randomised, double-blind, placebo-controlled pilot trial of omeprazole in idiopathic pulmonary fibrosis. Thorax 2019;74(4):346–53.

92. Idiopathic Pulmonary Fibrosis Clinical Research N, Martinez FJ, de Andrade JA, et al. Randomized trial of acetylcysteine in idiopathic pulmonary fibrosis. N Engl J Med 2014;370(22):2093–101.

93. Oldham JM, Ma SF, Martinez FJ, et al. TOLLIP, MUC5B, and the response to N-acetylcysteine among individuals with idiopathic pulmonary fibrosis. Am J Respir Crit Care Med 2015;192(12):1475–82.

94. Collard HR, Tino G, Noble PW, et al. Patient experiences with pulmonary fibrosis. Respir Med 2007;101(6):1350–4.

95. Cosgrove GP, Bianchi P, Danese S, et al. Barriers to timely diagnosis of interstitial lung disease in the real world: the INTENSITY survey. BMC Pulm Med 2018;18(1):9.

96. Putman RK, Gudmundsson G, Axelsson GT, et al. Imaging patterns are associated with interstitial lung abnormality progression and mortality. Am J Respir Crit Care Med 2019;200(2):175–83.

97. Oldham JM, Adegunsoye A, Khera S, et al. Underreporting of interstitial lung abnormalities on lung cancer screening computed tomography. Ann Am Thorac Soc 2018;15(6):764–6.

Management of Idiopathic Pulmonary Fibrosis

Margaret L. Salisbury, MD[a],*, Marlies S. Wijsenbeek, MD, PhD[b]

KEYWORDS

- Pharmacotherapy • Idiopathic pulmonary fibrosis • Palliative care

KEY POINTS

- Pulmonary fibrosis results from recurrent injury to the lung epithelium, with fibroblast accumulation, myofibroblast activation, and deposition of matrix.
- Progress in the past 2 decades has led to use of 2 medications to slow loss of lung function in patients with pulmonary fibrosis.
- Use of currently available pharmacotherapies can be limited by side effects, and neither has a consistent effect on patient symptoms or function.
- Several promising new pharmacotherapies under development target the innate immune response to epithelial injury or reduce fibroblast/myofibroblast activities by targeting epithelial-mesenchymal transition and transforming growth factor beta effects.
- Comprehensive management of pulmonary fibrosis hinges on shared decision making about pharmacotherapy, with early identification and management of symptoms and comorbidities.

INTRODUCTION

Management of idiopathic pulmonary fibrosis (IPF) has rapidly evolved in the past decade, with 2 disease-modifying pharmacologic therapies now widely available. Despite this landmark progress, available treatments are not curative, and prognosis remains poor. Care in IPF aims to make patients live as long and as well as possible, based on their individual preferences and values.[1] Therefore, a multidimensional approach to treatment is needed, with choices about use of pharmacologic treatments and nonpharmacologic treatments, attention to patient and caregiver education, management of comorbidities and symptoms, consideration of lung transplant, and end-of life care most optimally delivered simultaneously and from the onset of disease. This article provides an overview of literature guiding the use of available disease-modifying therapy, summarizes evidence for promising pharmacologic treatments in

the final stages of development, and discusses the role of nonpharmacologic therapies, each with attention to improving the well-being of patients affected by IPF.

PATIENT AND CAREGIVER EDUCATION: APPLICATIONS TO DISEASE MANAGEMENT

Receiving a diagnosis of IPF may be a breathtaking experience for patients and their families. Identifying patients' needs is crucial throughout the disease course, and starts at the time pulmonary fibrosis is recognized.[2] Patient and caregivers report a high need for information on what to expect from the disease and how their future will look.[3] Appropriate education of patient and caregivers is the first step toward implementing each component in a comprehensive care scheme for IPF (**Fig. 1**). It is important that patients receive information not only on pharmacologic treatments but also on preventive and supportive measures,

---

a Department of Medicine, Division of Allergy, Pulmonary and Critical Care, Vanderbilt University Medical Center, 1161 21st Avenue South, T-1209A Medical Center North, Nashville, TN 37232, USA; b Department of Respiratory Medicine, Centre for Interstitial Lung Diseases and Sarcoidosis, Erasmus Medical Center, University Medical Centre Rotterdam, Dr. Molewaterplein 40, Rotterdam 3015, GD, the Netherlands
* Corresponding author.
E-mail address: Margaret.Salisbury@vumc.org

Clin Chest Med 42 (2021) 275–285
https://doi.org/10.1016/j.ccm.2021.03.004

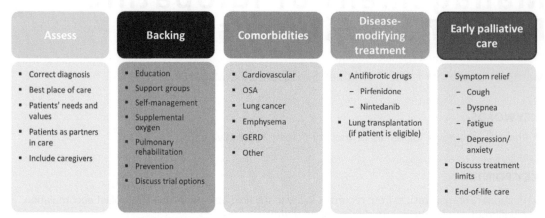

Fig. 1. Comprehensive management of IPF starts with education about each component. GERD, gastroesophageal reflux disease; OSA, obstructive sleep apnea. (*Adapted from*: van Manen MJ, Geelhoed JJ, Tak NC, Wijsenbeek MS. Optimizing quality of life in patients with idiopathic pulmonary fibrosis. *Ther Adv Respir Dis.* 2017;11(3):157-169; with permission.)

options for participation in clinical trials, patient support groups, and advanced care planning.[3,4] Pacing information and being attentive to discrepancies between patients and their caregivers may improve education.[3,4] More insights into their disease and management options may empower patients to become partners in care decisions, enhancing quality and customization of care.

DISEASE-MODIFYING THERAPY FOR IDIOPATHIC PULMONARY FIBROSIS
Current Pharmacologic Therapy

Following completion of large, randomized, placebo-controlled trials (RCT), monotherapy with either nintedanib or pirfenidone has been widely adopted in practice and is conditionally recommended for use in patients with IPF.[5] A large body of literature now guides their use in clinical practice.

Nintedanib is an intracellular, competitive inhibitor of multiple tyrosine kinases (fibroblast growth factor receptor, platelet-derived growth factor receptor, colony stimulating factor receptor (CSFR), FLT3, vascular endothelial growth factor [VEGF] receptor), with effects including inhibition of intracellular signaling of fibroblasts.[6–8] Two concurrent phase 3 trials enrolled more than 1000 patients, randomized 3:2 to receive nintedanib 150 mg orally twice daily or placebo, for 52 weeks. The primary efficacy end point was change in forced vital capacity (FVC) between baseline and week 52. Treatment with nintedanib resulted in approximately 50% slower decline in FVC relative to placebo, with an absolute between-group difference of approximately 100 mL.[7] Pooled data from phase 2 and 3 RCTs showed that nintedanib also prolongs

time to first acute disease exacerbation and preserves quality of life by 1 measure.[9] Pirfenidone has a pleiotropic effect, including regulation of transforming growth factor beta (TGF-β) and tumor necrosis factor alpha (TNF-alpha) to inhibit fibroblast proliferation and collagen synthesis.[10,11] The concurrent phase 3 CAPACITY [Clinical Studies Assessing Pirfenidone in Idiopathic Pulmonary Fibrosis: Research of Efficacy and Safety Outcomes] trials randomized more than 700 subjects either in a 2:1:2 ratio to oral pirfenidone 2403 mg/d, 1197 mg/d, or placebo, or in a 1:1 ratio to pirfenidone 2403 mg/d or placebo for 72 weeks.[10] The primary end point, change in FVC percentage predicted, was met in only 1 of the trials. Subsequently, the ASCEND [Assessment of Pirfenidone to Confirm Efficacy and Safety in Idiopathic Pulmonary Fibrosis] trial randomized 555 subjects 1:1 to oral pirfenidone 2403 mg/d or placebo for 52 weeks. The primary end point, proportion with FVC decline greater than 10% or death at 52 weeks, significantly favored pirfenidone (16.5% vs 31.8%).[11] Pooled data from all 3 RCTs showed a reduction in all-cause (3.5% vs 6.7%) and IPF-related (1.1% vs 3.5%) deaths in pirfenidone-treated compared with placebo-treated subjects.[11] Pirfenidone also seems to reduce respiratory-related, but not all-cause or non–respiratory-related, hospitalizations.[12] Pirfenidone is titrated to goal dose over a 2-week period at initiation, with dosage divided to 3 times daily and administered with food.[10,11] Several phase 2 trials evaluated the safety and pharmacology of combined therapy with pirfenidone and nintedanib, showing a modest increase in adverse events and medication discontinuation.[13,14] Efficacy data on the potential for additive benefit of combination therapy do not exist.

Adverse events were common among clinical trial participants, and patient education about common side effects is crucial before medication initiation. Side effects most attributable to nintedanib in phase 3 trials most often occurred in the first 3 months of dosing, and included diarrhea (up to 63% in nintedanib vs 18% in placebo) and nausea (26% vs 7%), with gastrointestinal disorders leading to drug discontinuation in up to 8.4% of nintedanib-treated subjects.[7] Increased liver enzyme levels (3 times normal or higher) were observed in approximately 5% of nintedanib-treated and fewer than 1% of placebo-treated subjects.[7] Diarrhea can often be managed with hydration and antidiarrheal medications; experts have suggested that scheduled dosing may be more effective than as-needed dosing of antidiarrheal medications.[15] Dose reduction to 100 mg twice daily can facilitate medication tolerance in practice, when other measures fail.[7,15] In the phase 3 RCTs, nintedanib-treated subjects experienced a numerically higher number of adverse cardiac events; however, pooled analysis of phase 2 and 3 data showed similar rates regardless of treatment.[7,16] Adverse events most attributable to pirfenidone in phase 3 trials most often occurred within the first 6 months of dosing, and included nausea (up to 36% vs 17%), rash (32% vs 12%), dyspepsia (19% vs 7%), and vomiting (14% vs 4%).[10,11,17] Taking pirfenidone during or just after a meal can mitigate gastrointestinal side effects.[18,19] For mild or moderate side effects of pirfenidone, experts suggest the use of a protocolized approach to dosing, consisting first of dose reduction, temporary withholding if dose reduction fails, followed by slow escalation back to the target dose with side effect resolution.[18] Given the side effect profile of each medication, monitoring of laboratory parameters for hepatic toxicity is advised.

Despite insight on selection of patients for treatment and timing of drug initiation increasing over recent years, up to 40% of patients are not treated with antifibrotic drugs near the time of diagnosis.[20,21] Several secondary data analyses of RCTs have not identified differential treatment effects of antifibrotic drugs based on several key demographics, comorbidities, or disease severity measures (ie, age, baseline FVC, smoking history),[22–24] although patients with more severe disease may derive a greater benefit in terms of symptoms stabilization.[25–27] Several open-label and real-world registry analyses suggest that patients with IPF treated with antifibrotic drugs have more severe disease compared with those not treated.[28–31] Consistent with this finding, surveyed physicians are less likely to favor treatment in patients with good quality of life or less severe disease.[20,32] Subjects transitioning from placebo to pirfenidone as part of the RECAP [An Open-Label Study of the Long-Term Safety of Pirfenidone in Patients with Idiopathic Pulmonary Fibrosis] open-label extension seem to have experienced irreversible loss of lung function during the placebo treatment period.[33] Taken together, these data suggest that offering treatment to all patients with IPF at the time of diagnosis is a reasonable approach, allowing shared decision making on choice of drug and when to start. In patients with more severe disease, pharmacotherapy should be offered along with a clear discussion of benefit/adverse event ratio, because several analyses suggest that patients with more severe disease are more likely to discontinue treatment and/or experience adverse events.[17,21,24,34]

Pharmacotherapy Pipeline: the Future of Disease-modifying Therapy

Although the pathobiology of human IPF is incompletely elucidated, it is generally accepted that recurrent injury to the lung epithelium leads, through several key pathways, to aberrant scar formation with fibroblast accumulation, myofibroblast activation, and deposition of matrix.[35,36] The innate immune response to epithelial injury may play a key role in fibrosis.[37–40] Fibroblasts and myofibroblasts in scar tissue resulting from epithelial injury can be derived from alveolar epithelial cells following epithelial-mesenchymal transition, a process in which the cytokine TGF-β plays a key role.[36,41] More pharmacotherapies for IPF are currently under development than ever before, with many targeting the previously mentioned fibrosis mechanisms directly, and others aiming to reduce lung injury. With current competition for centers and patients in the expanding clinical trials field, clinicians and patients should be well informed to guide their decisions on trial participation. This article summarizes potential future IPF treatments that have completed phase 2 randomized trials (**Table 1**), with a focus on mechanism of action.

Although untargeted immunosuppression is harmful to patients with IPF,[42] treatments targeting an aberrant innate immune response are under development. Monocyte-derived alveolar macrophages may play a key role in pulmonary fibrosis.[38] Pentraxin 2 (PRM-151), a recombinant amyloid P, inhibits monocyte differentiation into

Table 1
Disease-modifying pharmacotherapy pipeline for idiopathic pulmonary fibrosis: phase 2 clinical trial results

Treatment	Mechanism of Action	Weeks	Doses, Route	N	Efficacy	Notes
GLPG1690[55]	Autotaxin inhibitor, reduces LPA; LPA modulates fibroblast responses via LPA_1 receptor	12	600 mg PO daily Placebo	17 6	FVC + 25 mL (95% CI, −75, 124) FVC, −70 mL (95% CI, −208, 68)	Similar MOA: BMS-986020 (halted for safety), BMS-986278 (phase 2 planned), PBI-4050 (open-label phase 2 complete)
Pamrevlumab (FG-3019)[59]	mAb against CTGF; CTGF modulates actions of TGF-β, VEGF, and integrins	48	30 mg/kg IV q3 wk Placebo	50 53	FVC, −2.9% FVC, −7.2% difference 4.3% (95% CI, 0.4, 8.3)	No safety concerns re. antihuman antibodies. Similar MOA: BG00011 (halted for safety concerns), omipalisib (phase 1 complete)
Pentraxin 2 (PRM-151)[45]	Recombinant amyloid P, inhibits monocyte to fibrocyte and proinflammatory macrophage differentiation, inhibits TGF-β1 production	24	10 mg/kg IV q4 wk Placebo	77 37	FVC, −2.5% FVC, −4.8% difference 2.3% (90% CI, 1.1, 3.5)	Allowed background therapy with approved drugs for IPF. Antidrug antibodies developed in n = 7 treated subjects. Similar MOA: TD139 (phase 2a complete and 2b underway)
Cotrimoxazole[68]	Reduce lung bacterial burden, a hypothesized lung epithelial injury	52	960 mg PO BID Placebo	—	FVC, −188 mL FVC, −196 mL	Intention-to-treat analysis included only those with end-study FVC measurement; N per group was not clearly stated. Per-protocol analysis: cotrimoxazole reduced all-cause mortality (3 out of 53 vs 14 out of 65 in placebo)
Antireflux[71]	Reduce reflux of acid and other gastric contents, a hypothesized lung epithelial injury	48	Laparoscopic antireflux surgery No surgery (unblinded)	27 20	FVC, −50 mL (95% CI, −150, 50) FVC, −130 mL (95% CI, −230, −20)	Powered to detect a 200-mL FVC difference in FVC at 48 wk. AE, respiratory hospitalization, and death (n = 1 vs n = 4) were numerically less common in the surgery group. 29% had dysphagia and 14% had abdominal distention after surgery

Abbreviations: AE, adverse event; BID, twice a day; CI, confidence interval; CTGF, connective tissue growth factor; IV, intravenously; LPA, lysophosphatidic acid; mAb, monoclonal antibody; MOA, Mechanism of action; PO, by mouth; q, every.

profibrotic fibrocytes and proinflammatory macrophages, and inhibits TGF-β1 production.[43–46] In a phase II trial, pentraxin 2 significantly slowed decline in FVC (the primary end point) and 6-minute walk distance compared with placebo.[45] A similar proportion of drug-treated (7%) and placebo-treated (10%) subjects experienced serious adverse events, with antidrug antibodies detected in some subjects.[44,45]

Acetylcysteine is a glutathione (antioxidant) precursor with hypothesized antifibrotic properties. Although not efficacious in unselected IPF patients in a large phase 3 trial,[47] post hoc analysis suggested that patients with the toll interacting protein (TOLLIP) TT genotype may selectively benefit; another trial will soon assess efficacy in this group (https://clinicaltrials.gov/ct2/show/NCT04300920).[48] TOLLIP is an inhibitory adaptor protein within the toll-like receptor pathway of innate immunity.[39,48] Of note, phase 2 trials of acetylcysteine added to pirfenidone suggested harm (larger decrease in FVC) in acetylcysteine-treated compared with placebo-treated subjects.[49,50]

Linking innate immune components and TGF-β, the molecule galectin-3 is a β-galactoside–binding lectin expressed in fibrotic lung and macrophages of patients with IPF, and may play a role in TGF-β1 signaling.[51,52] TD139, an anti–galectin-3 small molecule, showed an acceptable safety profile, with target engagement shown by reduction in galectin-3 expression on alveolar macrophages in TD139-treated patients.[53] A larger phase 2 efficacy study is underway (https://www.clinicaltrials.gov/ct2/show/NCT03832946). Several therapeutics targeting the adaptive immune response are in early-phase (2 or earlier) development, including ofatumumab (VAY736), a monoclonal antibody (mAb) against the B cell–activating factor (cytokine) BlyS (https://clinicaltrials.gov/ct2/show/NCT03287414), and rituximab, a B cell–depleting agent (https://www.clinicaltrials.gov/ct2/show/NCT01969409). Development of several anti–IL-13 agents has been halted for lack of efficacy in phase 2 studies.[54]

Lysophosphatidic acid (LPA), produced by the enzyme autotaxin, is increased in bronchoalveolar lavage fluid and exhaled breath concentrate of patients with IPF. LPA may act through the LPA$_1$ receptor to modulate fibroblast responses.[55,56] A 12-week phase II trial of GLPG1690 (an autotaxin inhibitor) randomized 23 subjects, finding an acceptable safety profile, with change in FVC numerically favoring GLPG1690.[55] Target engagement was shown based on reduction in plasma concentration of LPA C18:2.[55] Phase 3 trials are ongoing (https://www.clinicaltrials.gov/ct2/show/NCT03733444).

Of note, the LPA$_1$ receptor antagonist BMS-986020 slowed FVC decline in a 26-week phase 2 trial; the study was terminated because of hepatotoxicity attributed to the study drug.[57] A phase 2 trial using an alternative formulation (BMS-986278) is planned (https://clinicaltrials.gov/ct2/show/NCT04308681). Another agent, PBI-4050, a 3-pentylbenzeneacetic acid salt with GPR40 and GPR84 activity (regulates macrophages, fibroblasts, and epithelial cells to inhibit fibroblast to myofibroblast differentiation), completed an open-label phase 2 single-arm study.[58]

Connective tissue growth factor (CTGF) is a glycoprotein secreted by fibroblasts, myofibroblasts, and endothelial cells. Through interactions with regulatory modulators (TGF-β, VEGF, and integrins), CTGF modulates cellular responses (eg, secretion of extracellular matrix) central to tissue repair and fibrosis. Pamrevlumab (FG-3019) is a human recombinant mAB that neutralizes CTGF. In a 48-week phase 2 trial enrolling 103 subjects, Pamrevlumab-treated subjects experienced a smaller decrease in FVC and smaller increase in quantitatively measured volume of lung with fibrosis.[59] Serious adverse events were observed in numerically more pamrevlumab-treated (12%, 24%) than placebo-treated (8%, 15%) subjects.[59,60] Phase 3 RCTs are underway (https://clinicaltrials.gov/ct2/show/NCT04419558). Of note, a phase 2 trial of an mAb against integrin αvβ6 (BG00011), a driver of TGF-β activation and fibrosis, was halted for safety concerns.[61] Omipalisib, an inhibitor of PI3Ks/mTOR signaling, attenuated fibroblast proliferation and TGF-β–induced collagen synthesis, completed a phase I placebo-controlled dose escalation study, which showed target engagement including inhibition of phosphatidylinositol 3,4,5 trisphosphate, phosphorylated Akt, and reduced 18F-fluorodeoxyglucose uptake on PET–computed tomography scan.[62]

Several treatments aim to reduce sources of recurrent lung epithelial injury. The lung microbiome may play a role in fibrosis pathobiology, possibly through innate immune mechanisms.[63,64] IPF is associated with an increased lung bacterial load, and patients with higher bacterial load are at increased risk of disease progression.[63–67] Several studies have tested antibiotics intended to reduce the lung bacterial burden. A phase 2 trial showed no benefit of cotrimoxazole compared with placebo on 12-month change in FVC in the intention-to-treat population, although a per-protocol analysis suggested a reduction in all-cause mortality.[68] A subsequent phase 3 trial (open-label trimethoprim-sulfamethoxazole or doxycycline vs placebo) has finished and results are pending (https://clinicaltrials.gov/ct2/show/NCT02759120). Gastroesophageal reflux (GER) is another hypothesized source of lung injury.

Retrospective analyses of the benefit of proton pump inhibitor treatment showed mixed evidence of efficacy.[69,70] A phase 2 trial of surgical GER management (via Nissen fundoplication) numerically favored surgery to reduce FVC decline.[71] Current expert guidelines conditionally recommend antacid treatment of symptomatic GER in patients with IPF, although without RCT-based efficacy data.[5,72]

Lung Transplant

At present, lung transplant is the only cure for IPF, although only a minority of patients are eligible. Anticipation of disease progression remains challenging[26,73,74]; coupled with unexpected events (infections, acute exacerbation), early referral to a transplant center is recommended. Theoretically both pirfenidone and nintedanib could affect wound healing, but case series identified no perioperative complications among patients treated with antifibrotics at the time of transplant.[75,76]

SUPPORTIVE MEASURES AND MANAGING COMORBIDITIES

In addition to disease-modifying therapy, a primary focus should be on improving patient self-management, improving physical functioning, and alleviating symptoms (see **Fig. 1**). Early palliative care directed at common symptoms should start at the time of diagnosis and continue through the disease course.[77]

Patient education about self-management could prove disease modifying. With cigarette smoking a common risk factor for pulmonary fibrosis, all patients should be asked about ongoing use and advised about cessation.[78] Vaccination against influenza and pneumococcal pneumonia may prevent pulmonary complications and resultant acute disease progression.[79] Likewise, mechanical ventilation could be a risk factor for lung injury, although elective surgery can be safe in carefully-selected patients.[80]

Dyspnea is present in most patients with IPF and not always related to the level of hypoxemia. Addressing the multidimensional aspects of dyspnea by approaches such as pulmonary rehabilitation or a multidisciplinary breathlessness service have been successful.[81,82] Targeting several common symptoms, exercise as part of a structured pulmonary rehabilitation program improves exercise tolerance (measured by 6-minute walk distance), dyspnea, and quality of life.[81] Although often reserved for patients with more significant limitations, those with milder disease may benefit the most.[83] Durability of benefits is limited, especially in patients with advanced disease,

underlining the importance of early referral for pulmonary rehabilitation.[83,84]

Supplemental oxygen is commonly prescribed for patients with IPF. With little quality evidence on efficacy or appropriate timing of prescription, clinical practices vary. A recent Delphi study yielded expert consensus that oxygen should be recommended for patients with resting hypoxemia, and in cases of exertional desaturation to less than 85% to 89%.[5,85] Data from incompletely blinded RCTs suggest that ambulatory oxygen administration to patients with exertional hypoxia improves quality of life,[86] subjective symptoms, and endurance.[87] A sham-controlled triple-blind RCT of ambulatory oxygen is ongoing.[88]

Although opioids alleviate dyspnea in nonmalignant pulmonary diseases, physicians hesitate to use them for IPF because of potential adverse effects and limited evidence of benefit.[89] Low-dose diamorphine showed dyspnea alleviation,[90] whereas morphine drops administered for 1 week had no effect on dyspnea.[91] Retrospective studies of terminally ill patients have suggested relief of breathlessness in most patients.[92,93] None of the studies reported increased risk of respiratory depression, hospitalization, or mortality,[89] but constipation and nausea occurred.

Cough is reported by up to 80% of patients with IPF, affecting physical, psychological, and social well-being.[94] Exclusion of comorbidities that may contribute to cough (eg, reflux, rhinosinusitis, asthma, GER, and obstructive sleep apnea) is an important first step.[71,72,94] With no therapy known to benefit IPF-related cough specifically, a trial-and-error approach similar to treatment of other causes of chronic cough is commonly used.[95] It is hoped that several new treatments for chronic cough, including speech therapy and medications acting both in the peripheral and central nervous systems, will also be tested in IPF.[96]

Although IPF is restricted to the lungs, its impact extends beyond. Fatigue and anxiety occur in many patients with IPF, often with multifactorial origins.[1,97] Frailty and comorbidities such as cardiovascular disease, pulmonary hypertension, sleep apnea, GER disease, emphysema, lung cancer, diabetes, and weight loss are frequently present, and their interactions with IPF are not completely elucidated.[98,99] Optimization of these comorbidities should be pursued, but in reality may be challenging.

Despite progress in pharmacologic treatment and supportive measures, IPF remains a deadly disease. Discussing advanced care planning and end-of-life considerations is an integral part of management, even though often difficult for patients and clinicians. Conversations should be tailored to patient needs, and collaboration with palliative care providers can be useful.[1,2] The use of decisions aids and participation in multidisciplinary advanced care programs may avoid futile medical interventions and promote a dignified death.[97,100]

SUMMARY

IPF continues to be a challenging diagnosis for patients and clinicians, with limited treatment options. Despite this, significant steps toward improved therapies have been made recently, including better knowledge of the practical use of currently available pharmacotherapies and several promising drugs targeting myriad components of disease pathways currently under investigation. Concurrent implementation of supportive treatments directed at symptoms is also key to improving quality of life for patients living with IPF.

CLINICS CARE POINTS

- Two medications tested in phase 3 randomized, placebo-controlled trials slow the loss of lung function in patients with IPF. Patient and caregiver education about recognition and management of common side effects (e.g., gastrointestinal distress, skin rash, others) can facilitate use.

- Several promising pharmacotherapies under development target the innate immune response to epithelial injury or reduce fibroblast/myofibroblast activities by targeting epithelial-mesenchymal transition and transforming growth factor beta effects; clinical trials options should be discussed with patients as part of routine care.

- Early attention to management of symptoms and comorbidities can improve patient quality of life. For example, chronic cough may improve after instituting treatments directed at underlying causes other than pulmonary fibrosis, such as gastroesophageal reflux disease, rhinitis with post-nasal drainage, or chronic bronchitis due to smoking-related lung disease (i.e., COPD/emphysema).

DISCLOSURE

Dr M.L. Salisbury reports grants from National Institutes of Health; personal fees from Boehringer Ingelheim Pharmaceuticals, Inc; Orinove, Inc; and Roche. Dr M.S. Wijsenbeek reports no personal fees or grants, but her institution received grants and fees from Boehringer Ingelheim and Hoffman-La Roche and fees from Respivant, Galapagos, Savara, and Novartis.

REFERENCES

1. Wijsenbeek MS, Holland AE, Swigris JJ, et al. Comprehensive supportive care for patients with fibrosing interstitial lung disease. Am J Respir Crit Care Med 2019;200(2):152–9.
2. Kreuter M, Bendstrup E, Russell AM, et al. Palliative care in interstitial lung disease: living well. Lancet Respir Med 2017;5(12):968–80.
3. Ramadurai D, Corder S, Churney T, et al. Idiopathic pulmonary fibrosis: educational needs of healthcare providers, patients, and caregivers. Chron Respir Dis 2019;16. 1479973119858961.
4. Overgaard D, Kaldan G, Marsaa K, et al. The lived experience with idiopathic pulmonary fibrosis: a qualitative study. Eur Respir J 2016;47(5):1472–80.
5. Raghu G, Rochwerg B, Zhang Y, et al. An Official ATS/ERS/JRS/ALAT clinical practice guideline: treatment of idiopathic pulmonary fibrosis. an update of the 2011 clinical practice guideline. Am J Respir Crit Care Med 2015;192(2):e3–19.
6. Chaudhary NI, Roth GJ, Hilberg F, et al. Inhibition of PDGF, VEGF and FGF signalling attenuates fibrosis. Eur Respir J 2007;29(5):976–85.
7. Richeldi L, du Bois RM, Raghu G, et al. Efficacy and safety of nintedanib in idiopathic pulmonary fibrosis. N Engl J Med 2014;370(22):2071–82.
8. Wollin L, Maillet I, Quesniaux V, et al. Antifibrotic and anti-inflammatory activity of the tyrosine kinase inhibitor nintedanib in experimental models of lung fibrosis. J Pharmacol Exp Ther 2014;349(2):209–20.
9. Richeldi L, Cottin V, du Bois RM, et al. Nintedanib in patients with idiopathic pulmonary fibrosis: combined evidence from the TOMORROW and INPULSIS((R)) trials. Respir Med 2016;113:74–9.
10. Noble PW, Albera C, Bradford WZ, et al. Pirfenidone in patients with idiopathic pulmonary fibrosis (CAPACITY): two randomised trials. Lancet 2011;377(9779):1760–9.
11. King TE Jr, Bradford WZ, Castro-Bernardini S, et al. A phase 3 trial of pirfenidone in patients with idiopathic pulmonary fibrosis. N Engl J Med 2014;370(22):2083–92.
12. Ley B, Swigris J, Day BM, et al. Pirfenidone reduces respiratory-related hospitalizations in idiopathic pulmonary fibrosis. Am J Respir Crit Care Med 2017;196(6):756–61.
13. Flaherty KR, Fell CD, Huggins JT, et al. Safety of nintedanib added to pirfenidone treatment for idiopathic pulmonary fibrosis. Eur Respir J 2018;52(2):1800230.
14. Vancheri C, Kreuter M, Richeldi L, et al. Nintedanib with add-on pirfenidone in idiopathic pulmonary

fibrosis. results of the INJOURNEY trial. Am J Respir Crit Care Med 2018;197(3):356–63.

15. Bendstrup E, Wuyts W, Alfaro T, et al. Nintedanib in idiopathic pulmonary fibrosis: practical management recommendations for potential adverse events. Respiration 2019;97(2):173–84.

16. Noth I, Wijsenbeek M, Kolb M, et al. Cardiovascular safety of nintedanib in subgroups by cardiovascular risk at baseline in the TOMORROW and INPULSIS trials. Eur Respir J 2019;54(3).

17. Nathan SD, Lancaster LH, Albera C, et al. Dose modification and dose intensity during treatment with pirfenidone: analysis of pooled data from three multinational phase III trials. BMJ Open Respir Res 2018;5(1):e000323.

18. Costabel U, Bendstrup E, Cottin V, et al. Pirfenidone in idiopathic pulmonary fibrosis: expert panel discussion on the management of drug-related adverse events. Adv Ther 2014;31(4):375–91.

19. Lancaster LH, de Andrade JA, Zibrak JD, et al. Pirfenidone safety and adverse event management in idiopathic pulmonary fibrosis. Eur Respir Rev 2017;26(146):170057.

20. Maher TM, Molina-Molina M, Russell AM, et al. Unmet needs in the treatment of idiopathic pulmonary fibrosis-insights from patient chart review in five European countries. BMC Pulm Med 2017;17(1):124.

21. Salisbury ML, Conoscenti CS, Culver DA, et al. Antifibrotic drug use in patients with IPF: data from the IPF-PRO registry. Ann Am Thorac Soc 2020;17(11):1413–23.

22. Costabel U, Inoue Y, Richeldi L, et al. Efficacy of nintedanib in idiopathic pulmonary fibrosis across prespecified subgroups in INPULSIS. Am J Respir Crit Care Med 2016;193(2):178–85.

23. Cottin V, Azuma A, Raghu G, et al. Therapeutic effects of nintedanib are not influenced by emphysema in the INPULSIS trials. Eur Respir J 2019;53(4):1801655.

24. Costabel U, Albera C, Glassberg MK, et al. Effect of pirfenidone in patients with more advanced idiopathic pulmonary fibrosis. Respir Res 2019;20(1):55.

25. Glassberg MK, Wijsenbeek MS, Gilberg F, et al. Effect of pirfenidone on breathlessness in patients with idiopathic pulmonary fibrosis. Eur Respir J 2019;54(3):1900399.

26. Ley B, Ryerson CJ, Vittinghoff E, et al. A multidimensional index and staging system for idiopathic pulmonary fibrosis. Ann Intern Med 2012;156(10):684–91.

27. Kreuter M, Wuyts WA, Wijsenbeek M, et al. Health-related quality of life and symptoms in patients with IPF treated with nintedanib: analyses of patient-reported outcomes from the INPULSIS(R) trials. Respir Res 2020;21(1):36.

28. Behr J, Kreuter M, Hoeper MM, et al. Management of patients with idiopathic pulmonary fibrosis in clinical practice: the INSIGHTS-IPF registry. Eur Respir J 2015;46(1):186–96.

29. Jo HE, Glaspole I, Grainge C, et al. Baseline characteristics of idiopathic pulmonary fibrosis: analysis from the Australian Idiopathic Pulmonary Fibrosis Registry. Eur Respir J 2017;49(2):1601592.

30. Pesonen I, Carlson L, Murgia N, et al. Delay and inequalities in the treatment of idiopathic pulmonary fibrosis: the case of two Nordic countries. Multidiscip Respir Med 2018;13:14.

31. Holtze CH, Freiheit EA, Limb SL, et al. Patient and site characteristics associated with pirfenidone and nintedanib use in the United States; an analysis of idiopathic pulmonary fibrosis patients enrolled in the Pulmonary Fibrosis Foundation Patient Registry. Respir Res 2020;21(1):48.

32. Maher TM, Swigris JJ, Kreuter M, et al. Identifying barriers to idiopathic pulmonary fibrosis treatment: a survey of patient and physician views. Respiration 2018;96(6):514–24.

33. Maher TM, Lancaster LH, Jouneau S, et al. Pirfenidone treatment in individuals with idiopathic pulmonary fibrosis: impact of timing of treatment initiation. Ann Am Thorac Soc 2019;16(7):927–30.

34. Fletcher SV, Jones MG, Renzoni EA, et al. Safety and tolerability of nintedanib for the treatment of idiopathic pulmonary fibrosis in routine UK clinical practice. ERJ Open Res 2018;4(4).

35. Lederer DJ, Martinez FJ. Idiopathic pulmonary fibrosis. N Engl J Med 2018;378(19):1811–23.

36. Selman M, Pardo A. Revealing the pathogenic and aging-related mechanisms of the enigmatic idiopathic pulmonary fibrosis. an integral model. Am J Respir Crit Care Med 2014;189(10):1161–72.

37. Fingerlin TE, Murphy E, Zhang W, et al. Genome-wide association study identifies multiple susceptibility loci for pulmonary fibrosis. Nat Genet 2013;45(6):613–20.

38. Misharin AV, Morales-Nebreda L, Reyfman PA, et al. Monocyte-derived alveolar macrophages drive lung fibrosis and persist in the lung over the life span. J Exp Med 2017;214(8):2387–404.

39. Noth I, Zhang Y, Ma SF, et al. Genetic variants associated with idiopathic pulmonary fibrosis susceptibility and mortality: a genome-wide association study. Lancet Respir Med 2013;1(4):309–17.

40. Peljto AL, Zhang Y, Fingerlin TE, et al. Association between the MUC5B promoter polymorphism and survival in patients with idiopathic pulmonary fibrosis. JAMA 2013;309(21):2232–9.

41. Willis BC, Borok Z. TGF-beta-induced EMT: mechanisms and implications for fibrotic lung disease. Am J Physiol Lung Cell Mol Physiol 2007;293(3):L525–34.

42. Raghu G, Anstrom KJ, King TE Jr, et al. Prednisone, azathioprine, and N-acetylcysteine for

pulmonary fibrosis. N Engl J Med 2012;366(21): 1968–77.

43. Dillingh MR, van den Blink B, Moerland M, et al. Recombinant human serum amyloid P in healthy volunteers and patients with pulmonary fibrosis. Pulm Pharmacol Ther 2013;26(6):672–6.

44. Raghu G, van den Blink B, Hamblin MJ, et al. Long-term treatment with recombinant human pentraxin 2 protein in patients with idiopathic pulmonary fibrosis: an open-label extension study. Lancet Respir Med 2019;7(8):657–64.

45. Raghu G, van den Blink B, Hamblin MJ, et al. Effect of recombinant human pentraxin 2 vs placebo on change in forced vital capacity in patients with idiopathic pulmonary fibrosis: a randomized clinical trial. JAMA 2018;319(22):2299–307.

46. van den Blink B, Dillingh MR, Ginns LC, et al. Recombinant human pentraxin-2 therapy in patients with idiopathic pulmonary fibrosis: safety, pharmacokinetics and exploratory efficacy. Eur Respir J 2016;47(3):889–97.

47. Martinez FJ, de Andrade JA, Anstrom KJ, et al. Randomized trial of acetylcysteine in idiopathic pulmonary fibrosis. N Engl J Med 2014;370(22): 2093–101.

48. Oldham JM, Ma SF, Martinez FJ, et al. TOLLIP, MUC5B, and the response to N-acetylcysteine among individuals with idiopathic pulmonary fibrosis. Am J Respir Crit Care Med 2015;192(12): 1475–82.

49. Behr J, Bendstrup E, Crestani B, et al. Safety and tolerability of acetylcysteine and pirfenidone combination therapy in idiopathic pulmonary fibrosis: a randomised, double-blind, placebo-controlled, phase 2 trial. Lancet Respir Med 2016;4(6):445–53.

50. Sakamoto S, Kataoka K, Kondo Y, et al. Pirfenidone plus inhaled N-acetylcysteine for idiopathic pulmonary fibrosis: a randomised trial. Eur Respir J 2020; 57(1):2000348.

51. Ho JE, Gao W, Levy D, et al. Galectin-3 is associated with restrictive lung disease and interstitial lung abnormalities. Am J Respir Crit Care Med 2016;194(1):77–83.

52. Mackinnon AC, Gibbons MA, Farnworth SL, et al. Regulation of transforming growth factor-beta1-driven lung fibrosis by galectin-3. Am J Respir Crit Care Med 2012;185(5):537–46.

53. Mackinnon A, Nicol L, Walker J, et al. TD139, A Novel Inhaled Galectin-3 Inhibitor for the Treatment of Idiopathic Pulmonary Fibrosis (IPF). Results from the First in (IPF) Patients Study. American Journal of Respiratory and Critical Care Medicine 2020; 201:A7560.

54. Wijsenbeek MS, Kool M, Cottin V. Targeting interleukin-13 in idiopathic pulmonary fibrosis: from promising path to dead end. Eur Respir J 2018;52(6):1802111.

55. Maher TM, van der Aar EM, Van de Steen O, et al. Safety, tolerability, pharmacokinetics, and pharmacodynamics of GLPG1690, a novel autotaxin inhibitor, to treat idiopathic pulmonary fibrosis (FLORA): a phase 2a randomised placebo-controlled trial. Lancet Respir Med 2018;6(8):627–35.

56. Tager AM, LaCamera P, Shea BS, et al. The lyso-phosphatidic acid receptor LPA1 links pulmonary fibrosis to lung injury by mediating fibroblast recruitment and vascular leak. Nat Med 2008; 14(1):45–54.

57. Palmer SM, Snyder L, Todd JL, et al. Randomized, double-blind, placebo-controlled, phase 2 trial of BMS-986020, a lysophosphatidic acid receptor antagonist for the treatment of idiopathic pulmonary fibrosis. Chest 2018;154(5):1061–9.

58. Khalil N, Manganas H, Ryerson CJ, et al. Phase 2 clinical trial of PBI-4050 in patients with idiopathic pulmonary fibrosis. Eur Respir J 2019;53(3): 1800663.

59. Richeldi L, Fernandez Perez ER, Costabel U, et al. Pamrevlumab, an anti-connective tissue growth factor therapy, for idiopathic pulmonary fibrosis (PRAISE): a phase 2, randomised, double-blind, placebo-controlled trial. Lancet Respir Med 2019; 8(1):25–33.

60. Raghu G, Scholand MB, de Andrade J, et al. FG-3019 anti-connective tissue growth factor monoclonal antibody: results of an open-label clinical trial in idiopathic pulmonary fibrosis. Eur Respir J 2016;47(5):1481–91.

61. Mouded M, Culver DA, Hamblin MJ, et al. Randomized, Double-Blind, Placebo-Controlled, Multiple Dose, Dose-Escalation Study of BG00011 (Formerly STX-100) in Patients with Idiopathic Pulmonary Fibrosis (IPF). In: D14. ILD: CLINICAL RESEARCH.A7785-A7785.

62. Lukey PT, Harrison SA, Yang S, et al. A randomised, placebo-controlled study of omipalisib (PI3K/mTOR) in idiopathic pulmonary fibrosis. Eur Respir J 2019;53(3):1801992.

63. Huang Y, Ma SF, Espindola MS, et al. Microbes are associated with host innate immune response in idiopathic pulmonary fibrosis. Am J Respir Crit Care Med 2017;196(2):208–19.

64. Molyneaux PL, Willis-Owen SAG, Cox MJ, et al. Host-microbial interactions in idiopathic pulmonary fibrosis. Am J Respir Crit Care Med 2017;195(12): 1640–50.

65. Han MK, Zhou Y, Murray S, et al. Lung microbiome and disease progression in idiopathic pulmonary fibrosis: an analysis of the COMET study. Lancet Respir Med 2014;2(7):548–56.

66. Molyneaux PL, Cox MJ, Willis-Owen SA, et al. The role of bacteria in the pathogenesis and progression of idiopathic pulmonary fibrosis. Am J Respir Crit Care Med 2014;190(8):906–13.

67. O'Dwyer DN, Ashley SL, Gurczynski SJ, et al. Lung microbiota contribute to pulmonary inflammation and disease progression in pulmonary fibrosis. Am J Respir Crit Care Med 2019;199(9):1127–38.

68. Shulgina L, Cahn AP, Chilvers ER, et al. Treating idiopathic pulmonary fibrosis with the addition of co-trimoxazole: a randomised controlled trial. Thorax 2013;68(2):155–62.

69. Kreuter M, Wuyts W, Renzoni E, et al. Antacid therapy and disease outcomes in idiopathic pulmonary fibrosis: a pooled analysis. Lancet Respir Med 2016;4(5):381–9.

70. Lee JS, Ryu JH, Elicker BM, et al. Gastroesophageal reflux therapy is associated with longer survival in patients with idiopathic pulmonary fibrosis. Am J Respir Crit Care Med 2011;184(12):1390–4.

71. Raghu G, Pellegrini CA, Yow E, et al. Laparoscopic anti-reflux surgery for the treatment of idiopathic pulmonary fibrosis (WRAP-IPF): a multicentre, randomised, controlled phase 2 trial. Lancet Respir Med 2018;6(9):707–14.

72. Dutta P, Funston W, Mossop H, et al. Randomised, double-blind, placebo-controlled pilot trial of omeprazole in idiopathic pulmonary fibrosis. Thorax 2019;74(4):346–53.

73. Salisbury ML, Lynch DA, van Beek EJ, et al. Idiopathic pulmonary fibrosis: the association between the adaptive multiple features method and fibrosis outcomes. Am J Respir Crit Care Med 2017;195(7):921–9.

74. Salisbury ML, Xia M, Zhou Y, et al. Idiopathic pulmonary fibrosis: gender-age-physiology index stage for predicting future lung function decline. Chest 2016;149(2):491–8.

75. Delanote I, Wuyts WA, Yserbyt J, et al. Safety and efficacy of bridging to lung transplantation with antifibrotic drugs in idiopathic pulmonary fibrosis: a case series. BMC Pulm Med 2016;16(1):156.

76. Leuschner G, Stocker F, Veit T, et al. Outcome of lung transplantation in idiopathic pulmonary fibrosis with previous anti-fibrotic therapy. J Heart Lung Transplant 2017. https://doi.org/10.1016/j.healun.2017.07.002.

77. Glaspole IN, Chapman SA, Cooper WA, et al. Health-related quality of life in idiopathic pulmonary fibrosis: data from the Australian IPF Registry. Respirology 2017;22(5):950–6.

78. Baumgartner KB, Samet JM, Stidley CA, et al. Cigarette smoking: a risk factor for idiopathic pulmonary fibrosis. Am J Respir Crit Care Med 1997;155(1):242–8.

79. Knippenberg S, Ueberberg B, Maus R, et al. Streptococcus pneumoniae triggers progression of pulmonary fibrosis through pneumolysin. Thorax 2015;70(7):636–46.

80. Patel NM, Kulkarni T, Dilling D, et al. Interstitial, diffuse lung disease network steering C. Preoperative evaluation of patients with interstitial lung disease. Chest 2019;156(5):826–33.

81. Dowman LM, McDonald CF, Hill CJ, et al. The evidence of benefits of exercise training in interstitial lung disease: a randomised controlled trial. Thorax 2017;72(7):610–9.

82. Higginson IJ, Bausewein C, Reilly CC, et al. An integrated palliative and respiratory care service for patients with advanced disease and refractory breathlessness: a randomised controlled trial. Lancet Respir Med 2014;2(12):979–87.

83. Jarosch I, Schneeberger T, Gloeckl R, et al. Short-term effects of comprehensive pulmonary rehabilitation and its maintenance in patients with idiopathic pulmonary fibrosis: a randomized controlled trial. J Clin Med 2020;9(5):1567.

84. Wallaert B, Duthoit L, Drumez E, et al. Long-term evaluation of home-based pulmonary rehabilitation in patients with fibrotic idiopathic interstitial pneumonias. ERJ Open Res 2019;5(2). 00045-2019.

85. Lim RK, Humphreys C, Morisset J, et al. Oxygen in patients with fibrotic interstitial lung disease: an international Delphi survey. Eur Respir J 2019;54(2):1900421.

86. Visca D, Mori L, Tsipouri V, et al. Effect of ambulatory oxygen on quality of life for patients with fibrotic lung disease (AmbOx): a prospective, open-label, mixed-method, crossover randomised controlled trial. Lancet Respir Med 2018;6(10):759–70.

87. Arizono S, Furukawa T, Taniguchi H, et al. Supplemental oxygen improves exercise capacity in IPF patients with exertional desaturation. Respirology 2020;25(11):1152–9.

88. Khor YH, Holland AE, Goh NSL, et al. Ambulatory oxygen in fibrotic interstitial lung disease: a pilot, randomized, triple-blinded, sham-controlled trial. Chest 2020;158(1):234–44.

89. Bajwah S, Davies JM, Tanash H, et al. Safety of benzodiazepines and opioids in interstitial lung disease: a national prospective study. Eur Respir J 2018;52(6):1801278.

90. Allen S, Raut S, Woollard J, et al. Low dose diamorphine reduces breathlessness without causing a fall in oxygen saturation in elderly patients with end-stage idiopathic pulmonary fibrosis. Palliat Med 2005;19(2):128–30.

91. Kronborg-White S, Andersen CU, Kohberg C, et al. Palliation of chronic breathlessness with morphine in patients with fibrotic interstitial lung disease - a randomised placebo-controlled trial. Respir Res 2020;21(1):195.

92. Matsuda Y, Maeda I, Tachibana K, et al. Low-dose morphine for dyspnea in terminally ill patients with

idiopathic interstitial pneumonias. J Palliat Med 2017;20(8):879–83.

93. Takeyasu M, Miyamoto A, Kato D, et al. Continuous intravenous morphine infusion for severe dyspnea in terminally ill interstitial pneumonia patients. Intern Med 2016;55(7):725–9.

94. van Manen MJG, Wijsenbeek MS. Cough, an unresolved problem in interstitial lung diseases. Curr Opin Support Palliat Care 2019;13(3):143–51.

95. Birring SS, Kavanagh JE, Irwin RS, et al. Treatment of interstitial lung disease associated cough: CHEST guideline and expert panel report. Chest 2018;154(4):904–17.

96. Smith JA, Badri H. Cough: new pharmacology. J Allergy Clin Immunol Pract 2019;7(6):1731–8.

97. Bajwah S, Ross JR, Wells AU, et al. Palliative care for patients with advanced fibrotic lung disease: a randomised controlled phase II and feasibility trial of a community case conference intervention. Thorax 2015;70(9):830–9.

98. Caminati A, Lonati C, Cassandro R, et al. Comorbidities in idiopathic pulmonary fibrosis: an underestimated issue. Eur Respir Rev 2019;28(153): 190044.

99. Sheth JS, Xia M, Murray S, et al. Frailty and geriatric conditions in older patients with idiopathic pulmonary fibrosis. Respir Med 2019;148:6–12.

100. Kalluri M, Claveria F, Ainsley E, et al. Beyond idiopathic pulmonary fibrosis diagnosis: multidisciplinary care with an early integrated palliative approach is associated with a decrease in acute care utilization and hospital deaths. J Pain Symptom Manage 2018;55(2):420–6.

Clinical Trials for Idiopathic Pulmonary Fibrosis and the Role of Health Systems

Erica Farrand, MD[a],*, Andrew H. Limper, MD[b]

KEYWORDS

- Learning health care systems • Digital innovation • Alternative trials • Adaptive trials
- Real world data

KEY POINTS

- Evolution in the scope of clinical trial questions and trial design have increased the breadth and depth of clinical trials in idiopathic pulmonary fibrosis (IPF). Unfortunately mounting clinical questions have outpaced the generation of evidence.
- Health systems are positioned to be a central stakeholder in future IPF clinical research by making strategic investments in health information technology and infrastructure to support adaptive study designs and cultivating broad stakeholder engagement.

INTRODUCTION

The history of clinical trials in idiopathic pulmonary fibrosis (IPF), although short, is distinguished by immense growth. Since the first randomized controlled trial (RCT) in IPF was published in 1991, there are have been more than 200 interventional studies conducted globally, with more than 300 related publications.[1] Over this period, the field has engaged in intensive discovery about the natural history, diagnosis, and management of IPF.[2] We have witnessed an evolution in the scope of clinical trial questions, expanded the number of IPF research partners, and refined trial design for this rare disease.[3–7] However, pressure to improve clinical trial efficiency, shorten trial duration, identify novel endpoints, and increase stakeholder engagement highlights the continued logistical and ethical challenges faced by IPF clinical trialists.[8,9] Collectively, these challenges serve as major catalysts for continued evolution and innovation in IPF clinical research.

Despite major strides in the understanding of IPF, mounting clinical questions have outpaced the generation of evidence, resulting in a rapidly expanding knowledge-evidence gap (a discrepancy between what is known and what should be known). The RCT, the gold-standard design for interventional studies, is considered the most reliable evidence of the efficacy of interventions. By reducing bias and enabling rigorous examination of the cause-and-effect relationship between an intervention and outcome, traditional RCTs are the backbone of evidence-based medicine. However, there are fundamental limitations to RCTs with respect to feasibility and generalizability. RCTs are time-intensive and cost-intensive and have limited external validity, particularly the ability to apply findings to other contexts.[10,11] Furthermore, RCTs are poorly suited for answering questions related to when and for whom an intervention works (ie, real-world efficacy) or why an intervention strategy is effective. As a result, a research pipeline that depends heavily on RCTs is unable to address the

[a] 505 Parnassus Avenue, Room M1083, Box 0111, San Francisco, CA 94117, USA; [b] Mayo Clinic, Gonda 18 South, Rochester, MN 55905, USA
* Corresponding author.
E-mail address: erica.farrand@ucsf.edu
Twitter: @ericafarrandMD (E.F.)

Clin Chest Med 42 (2021) 287–294
https://doi.org/10.1016/j.ccm.2021.03.006
0272-5231/21/© 2021 Elsevier Inc. All rights reserved.

complex and evolving questions faced by stakeholders. Although this phenomenon is pervasive throughout medicine, it is felt acutely in rare diseases such as IPF, for which the clinical research pipeline is further limited. Without enough patients to make research cost-effective, rare diseases are challenging to study using traditional paradigms, as it can be difficult to reach recruitment targets or observe sufficient events during the study period. When RCTs are conducted, the carefully selected patient populations and highly regulated study conditions challenge the generalizability of the evidence or the ability to implement findings into routine clinical practice. These challenges result in failed translation of existing high-quality evidence into actual practice (evidence-practice gaps).[12] Consequently, many IPF management decisions rely heavily on expert opinion, manifesting as significant practice variation and little understanding of the impact on outcomes.[13–15] Absent a transformative broadening of how we conduct IPF clinical research, these knowledge-evidence-practice gaps will persist and undermine our ability to make timely and accurate diagnoses or deliver high-quality, safe, and effective care.

Historically, clinical research and more specifically clinical trials have existed as a separate domain within health systems. Traditionally, health systems have supported clinical trials by serving as trial sites, responsible for enrolling participants, completing study visits, conducting procedures, reporting outcomes, and surveillance. The operational challenges of site recruitment, start-up costs, and patient enrollment are well appreciated, with an estimated 10% to 20% of clinical trial sites never enrolling a single patient.[16] Furthermore, the overwhelming majority of evidence generated from clinical trials remains within the silo of academic discourse, with limited feedback to the patients to whom health systems are responsible.[17]

For over a decade, the National Academy of Medicine, Agency for Healthcare Research and Quality, and others have advocated to expand our pathways for evidence generation by embedding clinical research within health care delivery.[18–23] Presently, health systems operate in a context that demands continuous improvements as defined by quality measures, cost, and patient outcomes. Meeting this demand has required health systems to make strategic investments to facilitate collaboration between research enterprises and care delivery teams. These collaborations enable research that provides faster insights into health problems and directly informs health care delivery.[24] Arguably the most profound health system investment has been in digital technologies. A revolution in digital health networks, data management and computational power, has enabled health systems to reimagine the role of the electronic health record (EHR) as a powerful tool to advance both clinical care and clinical research.[25–27] This fundamental restructuring and reimagining have shifted health systems from facilitators of clinical research to central stakeholders in the full spectrum of clinical research activities, including clinical trials.

In this article, the authors specifically consider the role of health systems in IPF clinical research. Reflecting on the history of clinical trials in IPF and presenting lessons learned from past experience, the authors describe current knowledge-evidence and evidence-practice gaps. Next, they then consider the changing landscape of health care and what it means for the future of IPF research. Finally, they identify specific investments health systems can make to support continued advancement of IPF clinical trials. The authors intend for this discussion to provide a roadmap for the field to explore the future role of health systems in IPF clinical trials, grounded in historical experience.

NATURE OF THE PROBLEM
Idiopathic Pulmonary Fibrosis Clinical Trial Design

In 1991, results from one of the first randomized double-blind trials in IPF were published.[1] This study, which compared the therapeutic benefit of prednisone plus placebo versus prednisone plus azathioprine, enrolled 27 patients over 5 years from 2 study sites and followed participants over a 12-month period. The issues of trial execution in IPF that have challenged the field for 30 years are well exemplified in this study. First and foremost, clinical trials in IPF are challenged by the low number of patients enrolled in any given center. A limited number of centers with IPF expertise and a limited number of patients per center make it challenging to reach target sample sizes. Multicentered and multinational studies are commonly used solutions to meet enrollment targets. However, this approach introduces the added complexities of multiple institutional review boards, lack of workflow standardization, and increased funding requirements.

Second, clinical trials with long study periods are costly and can influence participant recruitment and retention. Most clinical trials in IPF have leveraged a study length of 1 year or less, providing sufficient time to observe the outcome or outcomes while minimizing loss to follow-up and cost. However, limited follow-up can potentially underestimate the long-term impact of interventions.[28] Choices about study population and clinical trial endpoints are heavily influenced by the selected study period. Enrolling patients earlier in the disease course is thought to optimize a drug's likelihood of success. However, patients with early IPF are likely to have lower mortalities, lower risk of acute exacerbation, and therefore, require longer follow-up, especially when clinical endpoints are used. All-cause mortality has been identified as the most important clinical endpoint for patients with IPF. However, the number of patients and study duration needed to adequately power time-to-event studies using clinical endpoints are often prohibitive. As a result, traditional phase 2 and 3 trials in IPF have used surrogate endpoints related to lung function (change in forced vital capacity [FVC]) or functional assessments (6-minute walk distance) instead of clinical endpoints.[29,30]

Arguably, the most important limitation of traditional IPF RCTs is the inability to generalize the results to real-world populations. IPF clinical trial populations are biased toward enrolling patients with less severe disease, more typical disease presentations, and fewer comorbidities. In contrast, real-world populations often present with advanced disease, as defined by percent predicted FVC or carbon monoxide diffusing capacity. Real-world IPF patients experience significant variability in time to diagnosis and clinical course, have a high burden of comorbid conditions and concomitant medication use, and report lower health-related quality of life than patients in clinical trials.[31–36] Finally, as with clinical trials in general, racial and ethnic minorities and older adults are underrepresented or excluded from clinical trials in general, and similar trends are observed in IPF studies.[37] Although strict patient inclusion and exclusion criteria are important to reducing bias and confounding factors in RCTs, they are used at the expense of external validity and at times generalizability.

Over the last 3 decades, we have witnessed clinical trial design in IPF continue to grapple with these foundational issues of study design and rely on varied approaches, most notably multicenter studies, limited follow-up, use of surrogate outcomes, and modification of inclusion and exclusion criteria to address challenges inherent to RCTs in rare diseases. Evolution in the structural design of clinical trials has undoubtedly contributed to the landmark RCTs of the last decade, CAPACITY, PANTHER-IPF, ASCEND, INPULSIS, and most recently INBUILD.[38–42] These large RCTs demonstrate the potential for evolution in IPF clinical trial design and the ability to answer important questions in the field. However, we cannot successfully address the knowledge-evidence-practice gaps by relying on RCTs alone.

Expanding the IPF research pipeline requires a transformative broadening in how we conduct clinical research. Clinical trials in heterogenous populations using real-world data sources can complement traditional RCTs by providing insight into the efficacy of interventions in diverse, real-world clinical settings. Conducting such trials require reimagining how we define study populations, collect data, deliver interventions, and structure follow-up. Innovation in IPF trial design is exemplified by CleanUP IPF (#NCT02759120), the first pragmatic clinical trial in the field.[43] Pragmatic trials evaluate the effectiveness of interventions in real-world conditions. CleanUP IPF specifically evaluates the effectiveness of a commonly available antimicrobial intervention strategy in reducing mortality and respiratory-related hospitalizations.[44] The study design differs from traditional clinical trials in several key ways.

1. *Large and generalizable study population:* The study uses a limited set of inclusion and exclusion criteria enabling increased recruitment per center and overall enrollment of a study cohort representative of the broader IPF population. Participants are recruited following routine usual practice visits at enrollment sites, inclusive of both community-based and tertiary care institutions. This pragmatic design feature allowed for a target enrollment of 500 participants at a fraction of the cost required for traditional trials.

2. *Intervention delivery strongly aligned with real-world practices:* Participants are randomized in a 1:1 ratio to usual care versus usual care plus receipt of a prescription drug voucher for oral antimicrobial therapy. The intervention provides access to the study medication rather than direct administration, thereby more closely mimicking real-world conditions. Timing of the intervention can occur at any point during the chronic phase of the disease, encompassing practice variability into the study design.

3. *EHR leveraged to support longitudinal data collection:* Scheduled follow-up for CleanUP IPF is strongly influenced by routine clinical care and designed to minimize the number of research-specific visits and optimize use of data generated in routine practice. Sites are encouraged to use real-world data sources, most notably the EHR, to collect longitudinal data. This approach improves the cost-effectiveness and feasibility of an extended follow-up period of up to 42 months.

CleanUP IPF demonstrates how pragmatic trials can solve some of the inherent challenges of traditional RCTs by making studies more cost-effective and efficient and the results applicable to a broader target population. As discussed later, strategic investment in digital technologies can further advance clinical trial design. EHR data can be used to evaluate pretrial feasibility, streamline patient recruitment, automate data collection, and enable longitudinal follow-up. Continued innovation in clinical trial design can significantly expand the IPF research pipeline.

Idiopathic Pulmonary Fibrosis Clinical Trial Scope

Although we have witnessed an evolution in the design of IPF clinical trials, the parallel expansion in their scope beyond pharmacologic therapy has been much slower. Early research priorities in IPF centered on understanding the natural history, pathobiology, and clinical significance of IPF. Unsurprisingly, early clinical trials in the field responded to the pressing need for disease-specific treatment by focusing on the safety and efficacy of pharmacologic interventions. Although most of these studies failed to meet their primary outcomes, they informed the successes of the ASCEND and INPULSIS trials and ultimately Food and Drug Administration approval of 2 medications for the treatment of IPF, pirfenidone and nintedanib.[40,41] Both of these drugs modulate disease progression, but neither medication addresses the severe symptom burden, uncertain disease course, related comorbidities, and education needs that collectively erode quality of life for patients and their caregivers. International clinical practice guidelines reflect the complexity of IPF management and specify 5 strategies to improve health-related quality of life in IPF: (1) defined clinical follow-up, (2) supplemental oxygen, (3) pulmonary rehabilitation, (4) evaluation of comorbidities, and (5) consideration for pharmacologic management with nintedanib or pirfenidone.[13,14] Notably, only one of the 5 recommendations directly relate to pharmacologic management. However, in the last 5 years, more than 75% of published clinical trials in IPF have focused on pharmacologic interventions. This persistent bias in clinical trial scope limits the ability of clinical research to meet the broad and complex needs of IPF stakeholders, most notably patients, caregivers, and clinicians.

The limited scope of IPF clinical trials also contributes to evidence-practice gaps. This phenomenon is well illustrated by the story of immunosuppression in IPF. In 2012, the pivotal RCT PANTHER-IPF demonstrated that a combination of prednisone, azathioprine, and N-acetylcysteine, then the cornerstone of IPF management,

was associated with increased risk of death and hospitalization.[39] Eight years later, prednisone is still commonly prescribed to IPF patients, and current guidelines include a weak recommendation for its use in acute exacerbations of the disease.[14,33,45] Evidence-practice gaps extend beyond pharmacologic management. A 2016 retrospective single-cohort study by Kulkarni and colleagues[46] evaluated the association between a bundled delivery approach to guideline-based care and transplant-free survival in 284 patients with IPF. The study demonstrated that higher adherence to structured management practices (as defined by the 2015 ATS/ERS/JRS/ALAT consensus guidelines) was associated with improved transplant-free survival.[13] Unfortunately, only 12% of IPF patients received at least 4 of the 5 components of guideline-based care, and lower adherence was associated with a significantly higher risk of death or lung transplant (hazard ratio [HR], 2.234; 95% confidence interval [CI], 1.18–4.24) as compared with patients with comprehensive adherence (P value = .014). The implications of this work are profound. In IPF, a disease with high morbidity and mortality, with limited clinical practice guidelines, the overwhelming majority of patients are still not receiving comprehensive evidence-based care.

Fortunately, clinicians, health systems, and policymakers increasingly recognize the importance of patient-centered approaches to care and support an expanded scope of IPF research. For example, patient registry studies have been instrumental in evaluating nonpharmacologic management strategies designed to improve quality of life and symptoms in IPF.[3,47] Innovation in clinical trial design provides another pathway for studying a wide range of new and expanded use interventions not supported by the existing pharmacoeconomic model. In IPF, these interventions include supplemental oxygen use, pulmonary rehabilitation, patient and provider education tools, and targeted referrals to lung transplantation or palliative care, in addition to pharmacologic therapies. Both clinical trial design innovation and an expanded scope of IPF research are needed to generate the next era of IPF evidence and translate that evidence into clinical practice.

THE ROLE OF HEALTH SYSTEMS IN CLINICAL RESEARCH

A review of IPF research highlights the immense progress the field has made as well as the depth and breadth of the unmet need. The limitations of traditional RCTs, combined with resource constraints, increased emphasis on patient-centered research, and rapid proliferation of technology have catalyzed the changing landscape of clinical research. Health systems constantly generate real-world data through patient encounters and actively consume real-world evidence to improve value-based care delivery models. Likewise, health systems are uniquely positioned to align science, incentives, and informatics in order to continuously generate knowledge as a result of the delivery experience. Health systems are now uniformly recognized as central stakeholders in clinical research activities, with an unmistakable role to shape the future of clinical research through strategic investments. This transformative prospect extends across medical fields, but the implications for rare diseases, such as IPF, are notable. Limited volume, breadth, and depth of data in IPF have contributed to significant unmet medical need. Innovation in clinical research platforms that merge innovative data sources, flexible study designs, and novel analytics have the potential to decrease time to diagnosis, identify variations in IPF phenotypes, enhance understanding of the longitudinal disease course, and accelerate treatment pathways.

Health systems are well positioned to catalyze the future of clinical research and improve the understanding of health and health care delivery. However, there are important limitations to realizing this vision. Many, but not all health care systems, enjoy the benefits of unified EHR systems, including ready transfer of computed tomographic and lung function data. Fortunately, major EHR platforms are rapidly evolving to better interface, which will continue to address this concern over time. There may also be financial barriers that can limit clinical research in some settings. Health systems often contain central larger academic centers surrounded by smaller clinical practices. The resources supporting research and the financial drivers of these differing practices vary, with sufficient resources not always available to support research in smaller clinical settings. Trial designs with greater reliance on routine clinical visits, data readily available in the EHR and automated transfer of relevant data, are essential to overcoming these obstacles. Finally, there may also be cultural challenges with certain providers or practices reluctant to share outcomes and quality measures, or to practice in a fashion that supports clinical trials. Ongoing communication with greater transparency and collaboration is needed to meet and overcome these challenges.

THE FUTURE OF CLINICAL TRIALS IN IDIOPATHIC PULMONARY FIBROSIS

Equipped with a historical appreciation of IPF clinical trials, an understanding of the existing knowledge-evidence-practice gaps, and an awareness of the role of health systems in clinical research, we are well positioned to reimagine the future of clinical trials in IPF. Following are 3 specific investments health systems can make to support the next phase of IPF clinical trials.

1. *Investment in health information technology.* There is no larger or more comprehensive data source in IPF than the EHR. EHR-based clinical research can accelerate the pace and expand the scope of research discovery in IPF. Although EHR data have been successfully leveraged to support retrospective analyses,[48–50] thoughtful investment in EHR-based tools has the potential to transform EHR systems from passive data sources to powerful tools for prospective research. EHR-based tools can be leveraged to conduct landscape analyses of current clinical practice and identify areas of practice heterogeneity, outcome variability, and evidence-practice gaps, which can then be used to formulate clinically impactful research questions. EHR tools can support pretrial feasibility and planning by assessing the impact of inclusion and exclusion criteria on IPF study populations and estimating clinical event rates (eg, respiratory hospitalizations, acute exacerbations, mortality) using center-specific historical data. Such information would enable more intentional study design and informed decision making by health systems about trial participation. In the active phase, EHR tools can improve patient identification, recruitment, and enrollment by prescreening populations, providing automatic alerts to providers about study eligibility, and engaging with patients directly about research opportunities. The EHR platform can be used for allocation assignment, to deliver interventions (eg, decision support), and collect monitoring and outcome data through automatic data extractions. In addition, EHR tools can be used to support multipurpose use of trial data, including the development of IPF-specific dashboards, integration of patient-generated data (eg, surveys, wearables, and home monitoring devices), and facilitation of point-of-care communication and decision support. There is immense potential in EHR-based clinical research to lower the cost, enhance the feasibility, and expand the IPF research pipeline. Realizing this potential requires significant health system investment and broader commitment from EHR vendors.

2. *Adoption of alternative and adaptive study designs.* Alternative clinical trial designs include

pragmatic randomized clinical trials, large simple trials, and comparative effectiveness studies, which use health system–embedded research models and real-world data to generate evidence on the relative effectiveness of treatment strategies in routine clinical practice.[51] These alternative trial designs can balance the explanatory data generated from traditional RCTs and provide critical evidence needed to guide physicians, health systems, and policymakers in choosing the optimal treatment for patients.

Adaptive trial design methods aim to improve the flexibility of clinical trials by allowing modifications to be made to the trial or statistical procedures based on interim data analyses without undermining the validity and integrity of the trial.[52] Adaptive designs are often more informative and efficient than trials with fixed study design, as they make better use of resources, often require fewer participants, avoid underpowered trials, and are better equipped to estimate treatment effects. In rare diseases, adaptive design methods can be used to shorten the development time and increase the probability of successful clinical developments. For example, in IPF, an adaptive trial could be used to compare multiple pharmacologic interventions, including medication combinations (eg, nintedanib or pirfenidone plus a new compound). Experimental arms could be added and removed from the study based on a predefined algorithm (removing underperforming interventions). Efficient evaluation of both the clinical benefits and the harm of new interventions and the comparative effectiveness of different treatment strategies would create more opportunities to identify optimal management in IPF.

The next generation of IPF clinical trials will require design modifications to account for existing therapies, an increasing number of potential therapeutic targets, and competing stakeholder priorities. Adoption of alternative and adaptive study designs will enable health systems to respond to the evolving complexities of IPF clinical trials in a timely manner.

3. *Broad Stakeholder Engagement.* The last 30 years of IPF clinical research have marked significant growth in the field. Thanks to considerable effort and collaboration, we now have 2 pharmacologic therapies that slow disease progression. This would not have been accomplished without a broad coalition of stakeholders, including patients, caregivers, clinicians, scientists, foundations, advocacy organizations, industry, regulatory agencies, and the National Heart, Lung, and Blood Institute. Continued active engagement by each of these stakeholders is important if we are to assure that diversified and comprehensive priorities are established for the next phase of clinical trials. Coordination among stakeholders will be important to facilitate consistency in study design templates, consensus around common data elements, standardized workflows, and improved visibility and collaboration across clinical trial sites. Finally, stakeholder engagement has proven invaluable in other disease contexts for clinical trial execution, including navigating regulatory requirements with centralized review processes and streamlining clinical trial administration.

SUMMARY

We are in the midst of transformative innovation in health care delivery and clinical trials in IPF. Health systems are uniquely positioned at the crossroad of these shifting paradigms, equipped with the resources to expand the research pipeline in IPF through visionary leadership and targeted investments. The authors hope that by prioritizing development of health information technology, supporting a broader range of clinical trial designs, and cultivating broad stakeholder engagement, health systems will generate data to address knowledge-evidence-practice gaps in IPF. This will continue to improve the ability to deliver high-quality, safe, and effective care.

DISCLOSURE

The authors have nothing to disclose.

ACKNOWLEDGMENTS

E. Farrand receives support from the Pulmonary Fibrosis Foundation Scholar, CHEST, and the Nina Ireland Program for Lung Health. A.H. Limper is supported in part by the Three Lakes Foundation and funds from the Mayo Foundation. Erica also receives funding from the National Heart, Lung, and Blood Institute.

REFERENCES

1. Raghu G, Depaso WJ, Cain K, et al. Azathioprine combined with prednisone in the treatment of idiopathic pulmonary fibrosis: a prospective double-blind, randomized, placebo-controlled clinical trial. Am Rev Respir Dis 1991;144(2):291–6.
2. Valenzuela C, Torrisi SE, Kahn N, et al. Ongoing challenges in pulmonary fibrosis and insights from

the nintedanib clinical programme. Respir Res 2020; 21(1):7.

3. Russell AM, Sprangers MA, Wibberley S, et al. The need for patient-centred clinical research in idiopathic pulmonary fibrosis. BMC Med 2015;13:240.

4. Pulmonary Fibrosis Foundation. Partnership grants: increased power through partnership 2019. Available at: https://www.pulmonaryfibrosis.org/medical-community/partnership-grants. Accessed August 3, 2020.

5. Cision PR Newswire. NIH Awards major grant in pulmonary fibrosis research - new study to pave way for precision medicine. 2019. Available at: https://www.prnewswire.com/news-releases/nih-awards-major-grant-in-pulmonary-fibrosis-research-300950527.html. Accessed August 6, 2020.

6. Kaner RJ, Bajwa EK, El-Amine M, et al. Design of idiopathic pulmonary fibrosis clinical trials in the era of approved therapies. Am J Respir Crit Care Med 2019;200(2):133–9.

7. Johannson KA, Vittinghoff E, Morisset J, et al. Home monitoring improves endpoint efficiency in idiopathic pulmonary fibrosis. Eur Respir J 2017;50(1):1602406.

8. Spagnolo P, Maher TM. Clinical trial research in focus: why do so many clinical trials fail in IPF? Lancet Respir Med 2017;5(5):372–4.

9. Somogyi V, Chaudhuri N, Torrisi SE, et al. The therapy of idiopathic pulmonary fibrosis: what is next? Eur Respir Rev 2019;28(153):190021.

10. Sanson-Fisher RW, Bonevski B, Green LW, et al. Limitations of the randomized controlled trial in evaluating population-based health interventions. Am J Prev Med 2007;33(2):155–61.

11. Getz KA, Campo RA. New benchmarks characterizing growth in protocol design complexity. Ther Innov Regul Sci 2018;52(1):22–8.

12. Moor CC, Wijsenbeek MS, Balestro E, et al. Gaps in care of patients living with pulmonary fibrosis: a joint patient and expert statement on the results of a Europe-wide survey. ERJ Open Res 2019;5(4). 00124-2019.

13. Raghu G, Collard HR, Egan JJ, et al. An official ATS/ERS/JRS/ALAT statement: idiopathic pulmonary fibrosis: evidence-based guidelines for diagnosis and management. Am J Respir Crit Care Med 2011;183(6):788–824.

14. Raghu G, Rochwerg B, Zhang Y, et al. An official ATS/ERS/JRS/ALAT clinical practice guideline: treatment of idiopathic pulmonary fibrosis. An update of the 2011 clinical practice guideline. Am J Respir Crit Care Med 2015;192(2):e3–19.

15. Behr J, Kreuter M, Hoeper MM, et al. Management of patients with idiopathic pulmonary fibrosis in clinical practice: the INSIGHTS-IPF registry. Eur Respir J 2015;46(1):186–96.

16. Fogel DB. Factors associated with clinical trials that fail and opportunities for improving the likelihood of success: a review. Contemp Clin Trials Commun 2018;11:156–64.

17. Rees CA, Pica N, Monuteaux MC, et al. Noncompletion and nonpublication of trials studying rare diseases: a cross-sectional analysis. Plos Med 2019; 16(11):e1002966.

18. Institute of Medicine. Large simple trials and knowledge generation in a learning health system: workshop summary. Washington, DC: The National Academies Press; 2013.

19. Institute of Medicine. Sharing clinical research data: workshop summary. Washington, DC: The National Academies Press; 2013.

20. The National Academies of Sciences Engineering Medicine. Advancing the discipline of regulatory science for medical product development: an update on progress and a forward-looking agenda: workshop summary. Washington, DC: The National Academies Press; 2016.

21. Forrest CB, Chesley FD Jr, Tregear ML, et al. Development of the learning health system researcher core competencies. Health Serv Res 2017;53(4): 2615–32.

22. Bindman AB. The agency for healthcare research and quality and the development of a learning health care system. JAMA Intern Med 2017;177(7):909–10.

23. Califf RM, Robb MA, Bindman AB, et al. Transforming evidence generation to support health and health care decisions. N Engl J Med 2016;375(24): 2395–400.

24. Karin Johnson CG, Anau J, Greene S, et al. Integrating research into health care systems: executives' views 2015. Available at: https://nam.edu/wp-content/uploads/2015/06/IntegratingResearchintoHealthcareSystems1.pdf. Accessed July 1, 2021.

25. Evans RS. Electronic health records: then, now, and in the future. Yearb Med Inform 2016;(Suppl 1):S48–61.

26. The National Academies of Sciences Engineering Medicine. Real-world evidence generation and evaluation of therapeutics: proceedings of a workshop. Washington, DC: The National Academies Press; 2017.

27. Miksad RA, Abernethy AP. Harnessing the power of real-world evidence (RWE): a checklist to ensure regulatory-grade data quality. Clin Pharmacol Ther 2018;103(2):202–5.

28. Llewellyn-Bennett R, Bowman L, Bulbulia R. Post-trial follow-up methodology in large randomized controlled trials: a systematic review protocol. Syst Rev 2016;5(1):214.

29. Nathan SD, Meyer KC. IPF clinical trial design and endpoints. Curr Opin Pulm Med 2014;20(5):463–71.

30. Ley B. Clarity on endpoints for clinical trials in idiopathic pulmonary fibrosis. Ann Am Thorac Soc 2017;14(9):1383–4.

31. Cosgrove GP, Bianchi P, Danese S, et al. Barriers to timely diagnosis of interstitial lung disease in the real

world: the INTENSITY survey. BMC Pulm Med 2018; 18(1):9.

32. Kreuter M, Swigris J, Pittrow D, et al. Health related quality of life in patients with idiopathic pulmonary fibrosis in clinical practice: insights-IPF registry. Respir Res 2017;18(1):139.

33. Farrand E, Iribarren C, Vittinghoff E, et al. Impact of idiopathic pulmonary fibrosis on longitudinal healthcare utilization in a community-based cohort of patients. Chest 2020;159(1):219–27.

34. Collard HR, Chen SY, Yeh WS, et al. Health care utilization and costs of idiopathic pulmonary fibrosis in U.S. Medicare beneficiaries aged 65 years and older. Ann Am Thorac Soc 2015;12(7):981–7.

35. Wu N, Yu YF, Chuang CC, et al. Healthcare resource utilization among patients diagnosed with idiopathic pulmonary fibrosis in the United States. J Med Econ 2015;18(4):249–57.

36. Raimundo K, Chang E, Broder MS, et al. Clinical and economic burden of idiopathic pulmonary fibrosis: a retrospective cohort study. BMC Pulm Med 2016;16: 2.

37. Courtright K. POINT: do randomized controlled trials ignore needed patient populations? Yes Chest 2016; 149(5):1128–30.

38. Noble PW, Albera C, Bradford WZ, et al. Pirfenidone in patients with idiopathic pulmonary fibrosis (CAPACITY): two randomised trials. Lancet 2011; 377(9779):1760–9.

39. Idiopathic Pulmonary Fibrosis Clinical Research Network. Prednisone, azathioprine, and N-acetyl-cysteine for pulmonary fibrosis. N Engl J Med 2012;366(21):1968–77.

40. King TE Jr, Bradford WZ, Castro-Bernardini S, et al. A phase 3 trial of pirfenidone in patients with idiopathic pulmonary fibrosis. N Engl J Med 2014; 370(22):2083–92.

41. Richeldi L, du Bois RM, Raghu G, et al. Efficacy and safety of nintedanib in idiopathic pulmonary fibrosis. N Engl J Med 2014;370(22):2071–82.

42. Flaherty KR, Wells AU, Cottin V, et al. Nintedanib in progressive fibrosing interstitial lung diseases. N Engl J Med 2019;381(18):1718–27.

43. ClinicalTrials.gov. CleanUP IPF for the Pulmonary Trials Cooperative. 2017.

44. Anstrom KJ, Noth I, Flaherty KR, et al. Design and rationale of a multi-center, pragmatic, open-label randomized trial of antimicrobial therapy - the study of clinical efficacy of antimicrobial therapy strategy using pragmatic design in Idiopathic Pulmonary Fibrosis (CleanUP-IPF) clinical trial. Respir Res 2020;21(1):68.

45. Wijsenbeek M, Kreuter M, Olson A, et al. Progressive fibrosing interstitial lung diseases: current practice in diagnosis and management. Curr Med Res Opin 2019;35(11):2015–24.

46. Kulkarni T, Willoughby J, Acosta Lara Mdel P, et al. A bundled care approach to patients with idiopathic pulmonary fibrosis improves transplant-free survival. Respir Med 2016;115:33–8.

47. Wuyts WA, Wijsenbeek M, Bondue B, et al. Idiopathic pulmonary fibrosis: best practice in monitoring and managing a relentless fibrotic disease. Respiration 2020;99(1):73–82.

48. Brunnemer E, Wälscher J, Tenenbaum S, et al. Real-world experience with nintedanib in patients with idiopathic pulmonary fibrosis. Respiration 2018; 95(5):301–9.

49. Farrand E, Vittinghoff E, Ley B, et al. Corticosteroid use is not associated with improved outcomes in acute exacerbation of IPF. Respirology 2019;25(6): 629–35.

50. Pastre J, Khandhar S, Barnett S, et al. Surgical lung biopsy for interstitial lung disease: safety and feasibility at a tertiary referral center. Ann Am Thorac Soc 2021;18(3):460–7.

51. Zuidgeest MGP, Goetz I, Groenwold RHH, et al. Series: pragmatic trials and real world evidence: paper 1. Introduction. J Clin Epidemiol 2017;88:7–13.

52. Pallmann P, Bedding AW, Choodari-Oskooei B, et al. Adaptive designs in clinical trials: why use them, and how to run and report them. BMC Med 2018; 16(1):29.

Management of Connective Tissue Disease-Associated Interstitial Lung Disease

Leticia Kawano-Dourado, MD[a,b,c],*, Joyce S. Lee, MD[d]

KEYWORDS

- Connective tissue disease • Interstitial lung disease • Pulmonary fibrosis
- Autoimmune lung disease

KEY POINTS

- The current paradigm for treatment is to manage connective tissue disease (CTD)–interstitial lung diseases (ILDs) based on the underlying CTD. Nevertheless, CTD-ILD management guided by the underlying ILD pattern may also be necessary (eg, organizing pneumonia pattern).
- Immunosuppressants are the mainstem of therapy for CTD-ILDs, whereas antifibrotics seem to be beneficial in some scenarios.
- Management of associated comorbidities, evaluation for oxygen needs, lung transplant, and novel therapies, including clinical trial participation, are also important aspects of patient care.

INTRODUCTION

The term connective tissue disease (CTD) encompasses multiple entities, whose common characteristic is the immune-mediated injury of collagen affecting many organs, including the lungs. Interstitial lung disease (ILD) is a common manifestation of these systemic autoimmune disorders and confers a significant impact on morbidity and mortality, making their diagnosis and treatment a priority.[1] CTD-ILD is not a single diagnosis but rather a group of conditions characterized by a diverse cause of CTDs and a variety of patterns of interstitial pneumonia.[2]

The presence of ILD negatively affects prognosis among patients with an underlying CTD.[3–5]

Factors that negatively affect prognosis in these patients include reduced forced vital capacity (FVC) or signs of fibrosis on the high-resolution computed tomography (HRCT) of the chest.[4,5] ILD is the leading cause of death in systemic sclerosis (SSc), and in rheumatoid arthritis (RA) it is the second leading cause of death.[3]

The current paradigm for treatment is to manage the CTD-ILDs based on the underlying CTD. This approach is mostly based on experience rather than evidence.[6] However, more recently, some indirect and direct evidence is emerging that may support this strategy, including the association of articular disease activity in RA with incident RA-ILD[7] and data from a randomized controlled trial

[a] HCor Research Institute, Hospital do Coracao, Rua Abilio Soares, 250, 12o andar, Sao Paulo, Sao Paulo 04005-909, Brazil; [b] Pulmonary Division, Heart Institute (InCor), Medical School, University of Sao Paulo, Sao Paulo, Brazil; [c] INSERM UMR 1152, University of Paris, Paris, France; [d] Department of Medicine, Division of Pulmonary Sciences and Critical Care Medicine, University of Colorado Denver – Anschutz Medical Campus, 12631 East 17th Avenue, C-323, Academic Office 1, Room 7223, Aurora, CO 80045, USA
* Corresponding author. HCor Research Institute, Hospital do Coracao, Rua Abilio Soares, 250, 12o andar, Sao Paulo, Sao Paulo 04005-909, Brazil.
E-mail address: ldourado@hcor.com.br
Twitter: @leticiakawano (L.K.-D.)

in early SSc with mild ILD showing that patients allocated to the placebo arm continued to have FVC decline compared with patients allocated to tocilizumab (an anti–interleukin [IL]-6).[8] CTD-ILD management guided by the ILD pattern may also be necessary, as in situations where an organizing pneumonia (OP) pattern predominates, regardless of the background CTD, corticosteroids are the treatment of choice. The significance of distinguishing between other interstitial pneumonia patterns (eg, usual interstitial pneumonia [UIP] versus nonspecific interstitial pneumonia [NSIP]) as it relates to pharmacologic management, in the context of an underlying CTD, is less clear.

This article reviews the initial approach to management of CTD-ILDs in general, followed by a discussion of immunosuppressive treatment stratified by underlying CTD, and concludes with other pharmacologic and nonpharmacologic considerations in the management of CTD-ILD.

INITIAL APPROACH

The first and foremost decision in managing CTD-ILDs is to determine which cases should receive therapy targeting ILD, and which cases should only be monitored (**Fig. 1**).[9] There is little direct evidence to be used as guidance; therefore, expert opinion and some indirect evidence are what inform these management decisions at this time.[6,9]

Pharmacologic treatment should be considered in all patients with severe, active, and/or progressive disease. Determining disease severity and activity can be difficult, but a combination of clinical symptoms, pulmonary function tests (PFTs), and chest imaging can be used.[10] It is also important to consider contraindications to therapy, including comorbid conditions and drug interactions.[2,10] The initial approach to CTD-ILDs is further detailed in **Fig. 1**.

Disease severity can be defined by the extent of ILD involvement on HRCT of the chest[11,12] and also by the characteristics of the alterations: subpleural alterations and the presence of traction bronchiectasis and honeycomb are associated with an increased risk of progression.[13,14] The presence of crackles on lung auscultation is a surrogate marker of fibrosis, and therefore a marker of disease severity.[15] Physiology is another determinant of disease severity: the presence of FVC or diffusing capacity of lung for carbon monoxide (DL_{CO}) impairment are markers of disease severity.[16–19] On longitudinal evaluation, evidence of decline in FVC and/or DL_{CO} is associated with worse outcome, and, for that reason, should also be taken as an indication for treatment of the CTD-ILD[4] (see **Fig. 1**).

Differential Diagnosis

The cause of ILD developing in the context of a CTD is usually straightforward: a CTD-ILD. However, in some scenarios, there is the need for a differential diagnosis, especially when the clinical/radiological presentation is not typical or if the onset is acute/subacute (**Fig. 2**). The most common differential diagnoses of CTD-ILD are[20–22]:

- Drug toxicity
- Infection
- Hypersensitivity pneumonitis
- Associated sarcoidosis
- Idiopathic pulmonary fibrosis (IPF)

The need for bronchoalveolar lavage (BAL) evaluation and or histology is especially important when the pretest probability of infection is sufficiently high. Less invasive techniques often fail to yield the diagnosis (see **Fig. 2**). Nevertheless, BAL technique and protocols for processing and analyzing BAL fluid are critically important for the BAL to provide useful information and should be followed.[23]

IMMUNOSUPPRESSIVE TREATMENT STRATIFIED BY CONNECTIVE TISSUE DISEASE
Systemic Sclerosis-Associated Interstitial Lung Disease

SSc-ILD is the CTD-ILD with the best body of evidence supporting specific pharmacologic treatment recommendations.[8,24–27]

Corticosteroids are usually part of the treatment regimen of CTD-ILDs in general, especially if an OP pattern is present. However, in SSc-ILD, caution should be exercised when using corticosteroids: medium to high dosages (≥ 15 mg/d of prednisone or equivalent) are associated with scleroderma renal crisis, which is characterized by acute renal failure usually accompanied by malignant hypertension.[28,29] In addition, given the higher prevalence of pulmonary hypertension (PH) in SSc compared with other CTD-ILDs, the presence or worsening of symptoms and/or low DL_{CO} should prompt an evaluation for PH.[30]

Cytotoxic disease-modifying antirheumatic drugs

Based on data from the Scleroderma Lung Study I and II, cyclophosphamide (CYC), up to 2 mg/kg/d, and mycophenolate mofetil (MMF), 3000 mg/d in divided doses, are the cytotoxic disease-modifying antirheumatic drugs (DMARDs) of choice to treat SSc-ILD.[25,26] Given MMF's better safety profile and comparable efficacy with oral CYC, MMF is preferred to CYC.[26] It should be taken with food because this may decrease

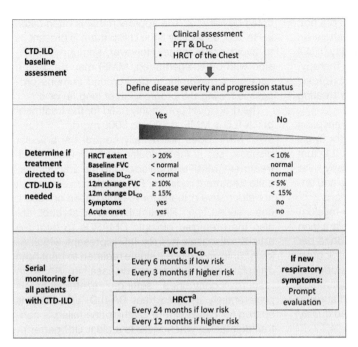

Fig. 1. Suggested algorithm for assessment and management of patients with CTD-ILD. Define disease severity and, if possible, progression status at baseline. Next, depending on markers of severity and/or progression, treatment directed to the CTD-ILD may be needed. Irrespective of treatment, all patients with CTD-ILD need longitudinal follow-up. Frequency of the follow-up depends on the severity of the CTD-ILD and on the risk of progression. [a]The interval time of follow-up with HRCT varies from center to center. 12 m, 12 months; DL_{CO}, diffusing capacity of lung for carbon monoxide; PFT, pulmonary function test.

gastrointestinal side effects of nausea, vomiting, and/or diarrhea. For patients with significant gastrointestinal dysmotility, monthly intravenous pulses of CYC 500 to 750 mg/m^2 may be considered. A Delphi consensus treatment algorithm advocated first-line treatment of SSc-ILD with MMF. Second-line treatments included CYC or rituximab as induction therapy, followed by MMF as maintenance therapy.[31]

Biologic disease-modifying antirheumatic drugs

A phase III clinical trial data has shown that the treatment of early diffuse cutaneous SSc led to stabilization of FVC% in the tocilizumab (anti–IL-6) group compared with the placebo group over 48 weeks.[8] The mean FVC% was 82.1% ± 14.8% at baseline and around 65% of subjects had SSc-ILD at baseline.[8] These data favor treating patients with subclinical ILD with high-risk features (early diffuse cutaneous SSc).[8] Another biologic DMARD that has gained interest in response to promising effects on both ILD and skin thickening is rituximab (RTX). A small randomized controlled trial of RTX versus monthly pulse CYC for early diffuse cutaneous SSc-ILD found that the RTX group had improved FVC% at the end of 6 months (RTX group improved from

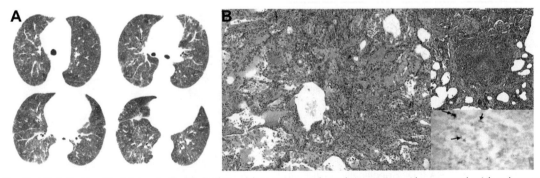

Fig. 2. (A) Patient with RA treated with hydroxychloroquine and prednisone 5 mg/d presented with subacute onset of dyspnea, fever, and interstitial opacities. Sputum and bronchoalveolar lavage were used in order to identify infection, but were nondiagnostic. (B) A surgical lung biopsy was performed revealing extensive OP represented by multiple buds of granulation tissue (*left*). Intra-alveolar edema with fibrin deposition is also seen (*left*), necrotizing granulomas (*upper right*), and mycobacteria (*arrows*) were identified in areas of necrosis through Ziehl-Neelsen stain (*lower right*). (magnification B (left) 100x, [upper right] 200x, [lower right] 1000x). (*Courtesy of* University of São Paulo, ILD clinic, São Paulo; with permission.)

61.3% to 67.5%, whereas the CYC group did not: 59.3% to 58.1%). The efficacy and safety shown in this trial suggested that RTX 1000 mg at day 0 (D0) and D15 may be considered as a first-line therapy, or as an add-on to nonresponders to cytotoxic DMARDs.[32] The long-term role of RTX in treating SSc-ILD warrants further study.

Autologous hematopoietic stem cell transplant represents an emerging treatment option for those patients with early diffuse cutaneous SSc-ILD that is severe and refractory to standard therapy, and who are likely to benefit from the procedure and unlikely to develop posttransplant complications.[30,31] Three key trials (ASSIST [Autologous non-myeloablative haemopoietic stem-cell transplantation compared with pulse cyclophosphamide once per month for systemic sclerosis], ASTIS [Autologous Stem cell Transplantation International Scleroderma trial], and SCOT [Scleroderma: Cyclophosphamide or Transplantation]) have shown improved survival compared with CYC, in addition to improved quality of life, skin thickening, and FVC.[33–36]

Despite this evidence, there remain areas of uncertainty in SSc-ILD treatment, such as whether subclinical SSc-ILD should be treated. One single-center study suggested that immunosuppression should be considered for subclinical SSc-ILD if patients have high-risk features: (1) early diffuse cutaneous SSc phenotype, (2) positive for anti-SCL70, and/or (3) an increased C-reactive protein level ($\geq$10 mg/L), which confers a higher risk of disease progression. Given the uncertainty surrounding treatment of early disease, the risk-benefit considerations should be discussed with the patient and decided on an individual basis.[30,37]

Rheumatoid Arthritis–Associated Interstitial Lung Disease

To date, there have been no randomized controlled trials published on the treatment of RA-ILD. Treatment recommendations are mostly based on expert opinion supported by case series and retrospective observational studies.[38]

It is important to recognize that RA-ILD significantly differs from other CTD-ILDs. RA-ILD is the only CTD-ILD where the UIP pattern predominates (**Fig. 3**).[39] The UIP pattern is the hallmark of IPF,[40] and similarities observed between IPF and RA-ILD have introduced uncertainty regarding how to appropriately treat RA-ILD. Specifically, in IPF, it has been shown that combined immunosuppression with azathioprine and steroids is harmful.[41] It remains unknown whether the harmful signal observed in IPF can be extrapolated to RA-ILD, and whether it is a drug-specific or class-specific effect or whether immunosuppression, in general,

could be harmful. The approach that is often taken in RA-ILD, especially if the UIP pattern is present, is to avoid azathioprine. However, immunosuppression with other agents (eg, MMF) may be used if necessary, assuming a background immune process is fueling the progression of lung fibrosis.

The drug most commonly used for the treatment of RA-ILD is MMF at 2000 to 3000 mg/d.[42–46] However, MMF does not usually control the articular disease, so, if the articular disease also needs treatment, MMF is often added to the articular disease treatment regimen. Rituximab and abatacept are alternative options for RA-ILD based on recent case series.[47–49] Rituximab and abatacept are also the preferred biologic DMARDs to treat RA articular disease when RA-ILD is present, which allows clinicians to use a single regimen to treat both articular and pulmonary disease in RA.[50] In resource-constrained settings, azathioprine is preferentially used to treat RA-ILD, and MMF is spared for cases where azathioprine failed/is contraindicated or when there is a clear UIP pattern.

Methotrexate lung toxicity

Methotrexate (MTX) is the anchor drug for the treatment of RA articular disease and has been suspected to be a contributing cause of RA-ILD.[51,52] MTX-associated acute hypersensitivity pneumonitis is the most frequently reported within the first year of MTX use and seems to be dose independent, suggesting an idiosyncratic hypersensitivity reaction rather than a dose-related toxic lung injury. It is reported in 0.25% to 0.43% of MTX-treated patients or probably less. In many studies, the case definitions used have been weighted toward a diagnosis of MTX pneumonitis

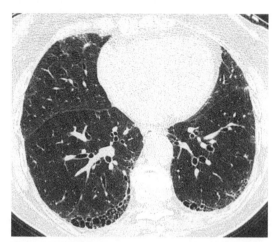

Fig. 3. UIP pattern in a patient with RA. Note the subpleural distribution of the honeycomb and traction bronchiectasis. (*Courtesy of* University of São Paulo, ILD clinic, São Paulo; with permission.)

and have not always adequately ruled out other causes.[51,53,54] A recent large multinational study has shown that MTX use was inversely associated with RA-ILD incidence.[55]

Interstitial Lung Disease in Polymyositis and Dermatomyositis

ILD is one of the most common systemic complications of polymyositis (PM) and dermatomyositis (DM).[56] Specific autoantibodies confer distinct clinical phenotypes. Notably, the antiaminoacyl–transfer RNA (ARS) antibodies and antimelanoma differentiation factor 5 (MDA5), are both associated with a high prevalence of ILD, and the presence of MDA5 is associated with worse prognosis.[57,58]

The management of PM/DM-associated ILD varies considerably. The immunosuppressive agents used are supported by case series or retrospective reviews and there are only a few prospective or randomized studies.[56] Corticosteroids are the mainstay of therapy, and, depending on the disease severity, may be given as pulse (methylprednisolone 500–1000 mg/d for 3 days), whereas more stable patients are treated with 0.75 to 1 mg/kg/d of prednisone.[59–61] When patients do not respond to corticosteroids or when disease activity is not controlled on corticosteroid taper, a second immunosuppressant is added.[61–64] It is common practice to add an additional immunosuppressive agent with initial corticosteroid treatment.[56]

Many immunosuppressive agents have been used for the treatment of PM/DM-ILD, such as azathioprine, MMF, cyclophosphamide, calcineurin inhibitors, rituximab, and intravenous immunoglobulin.[43,59,62,64–69] More recently, tofacitinib, a Janus kinase inhibitor, was reported as a potential treatment of ILD associated with the presence of MDA5, usually presenting as clinically amyopathic dermatomyositis (CADM).[70]

The choice of which immunosuppressive agent to add to conventional corticosteroid therapy depends on the severity of ILD presentation along with other comorbidities for each patient. Patients presenting with mild to moderate ILD should be treated with steroids and azathioprine or MMF. Those with improvement or stabilization undergo steroid tapering with maintenance of the steroid-sparing agent. Patients presenting initially with severe ILD or rapidly progressive disease are treated with pulse or high-dose corticosteroids combined with either cyclophosphamide, rituximab, a calcineurin inhibitor, or tofacitinib (tofacitinib especially if MDA5 positive), and treatment should be tapered or intensified based on the response to therapy.

Other Connective Tissue Disease–Associated Interstitial Lung Diseases

This article briefly comments on ILDs associated with primary Sjögren syndrome (pSS), mixed CTD (MCTD), and systemic lupus erythematosus (SLE), conditions for which there are even fewer data. In these circumstances, there are 3 main guides for choosing therapy:

- Known treatments effective for the underlying systemic disease.
- Known treatments effective for the idiopathic interstitial pneumonia pattern that is present.
- Acuity/severity of the ILD presentation. The more acute/severe, the more aggressive; for example, use of pulse methylprednisolone, pulse cyclophosphamide.

Primary Sjögren syndrome–associated interstitial lung disease

Bronchiolitis and bronchiectasis are the most common pulmonary manifestations. The interstitial involvement in pSS is less common but includes NSIP, UIP, and lymphocytic interstitial pneumonia. Patients with pSS are also at an increased risk of lymphoma, amyloidosis, and pseudolymphoma.[71] Treatment recommendations for pSS-ILD are based on small case series that have tried corticosteroids, usually associated with another agent such as hydroxychloroquine, azathioprine, cyclophosphamide, or rituximab.[72–76]

Mixed connective tissue disease–associated interstitial lung disease

MCTD is defined by the combined presence of high-titer serum antiribonucleoprotein (RNP) antibodies and overlapping features of 2 or more of the CTDs: systemic sclerosis, SLE, polymyositis, and RA.[77] Treatment recommendations for MCTD-ILD are based on expert opinion and case series. The choice of drug for the ILD usually follows the recommendations for the overlapping disease feature that predominates in the lungs.[78]

Systemic lupus erythematosus–associated interstitial lung disease

ILD is a rare manifestation of SLE.[79] When present, it most often manifests as NSIP or as OP.[79] In patients with SLE with respiratory symptoms, pleuritis and the shrinking lung syndrome should be ruled out before the diagnosis of SLE-ILD is made.[79,80] There are few data to support recommendations on SLE-ILD treatment, and treatment recommendations for SLE-ILD are based on expert opinion and case series where drugs such as corticosteroids, MMF, cyclophosphamide, and rituximab have been tested.[80–83]

ANTIFIBROTICS

Nintedanib and pirfenidone, two antifibrotics approved by the US Food and Drug Administration (FDA) in 2014 for the treatment of IPF,[84] have also been investigated for CTD-ILDs.

A randomized controlled trial testing nintedanib in SSc-ILD (SENSCIS trial) showed that nintedanib use was associated with a lower rate of annual FVC decline compared with placebo (treatment difference 41 mL in 1 year), and that effect seemed additive to the effect of MMF.[27] Based on these data, nintedanib was FDA approved for SSc-ILD in 2019.[85]

Another trial investigated nintedanib in other progressive forms of non-IPF ILD, including CTD-ILDs.[86] Approximately a quarter of the trial population was composed of fibrotic CTD-ILDs (mostly RA-ILD and SSc-ILD).[86] Although the INBUILD trial was not designed or powered to provide evidence for the benefit of nintedanib in specific ILDs, a subgroup analysis suggested that nintedanib reduced the rate of ILD progression similarly in patients from all the major ILD subgroups, including CTD-ILDs.[86,87]

Pirfenidone has also been tested in the context of pulmonary fibrosis and autoimmunity.[88] In the unclassifiable ILD trial (which included fibrotic interstitial pneumonia with autoimmune features), pirfenidone slowed the rate of decline of FVC compared with placebo.[88] Further, a case series has suggested that patients with rapidly progressive CADM-associated ILD might benefit from pirfenidone 1800 mg/d added to standard-of-care treatment.[89] Another case series also suggested a possible benefit of pirfenidone for RA-ILD, but the results of an ongoing clinical trial are still pending.[90,91]

Based on these data, antifibrotics will likely be part of the treatment regimen for patients with CTD-ILD. However, these trials do not address the timing of antifibrotic therapy (eg, concurrent, sequential, or add-on therapy) and the management of concurrent immunosuppression, particularly in the context of active extrapulmonary disease. Further work is required to determine how best to include antifibrotics in the overall management of CTD-ILD.

ONGOING CLINICAL TRIALS

In **Table 1**, there is a list of recruiting and not-yet recruiting clinical trials on the pharmacologic treatment of various CTD-ILDs.

NONPHARMACOLOGIC TREATMENT

Supportive nonpharmacologic treatment is an important component in the management of CTD-ILD, especially if the disease is moderate to severe and if systemic organ involvement is present.

All patients with CTD-ILD should be vaccinated for influenza and pneumococcus and advised on tobacco cessation and on avoidance of environmental exposures theoretically capable of triggering an exacerbation (eg, fumes, dusts, chemicals, avian and fungal antigens). If patients are immunosuppressed with high-dose corticosteroids (>20 mg prednisone/d or equivalent for >4 weeks), patients should be placed on pneumocystis pneumonia prophylaxis with trimethoprim/sulfamethoxazole 1 double-strength tablet 3 times a week or 1 single-strength tablet every day, or its equivalent.[92] Strongyloides hyperinfection syndrome prophylaxis should also be considered, especially in the acute/subacute setting where higher doses of corticosteroids and/or other immunosuppressants are administered, if patients are geographically at risk for this.[93]

Oxygen Supplementation

Patients with advanced ILD frequently develop hypoxemia caused by multiple physiologic derangements, including ventilation-perfusion mismatching, loss of alveolar membrane surface area, and pulmonary vasculature abnormalities.[94–96] Hypoxemia during exercise impairs maximal workload and endurance time, attenuating the benefits gained from pulmonary rehabilitation.[97] Hypoxemia may also contribute to the development of PH, a prognostically important comorbidity.[98] Supplemental oxygen can improve many of these adverse changes; however, there is no clear consensus on the threshold below which oxygen supplementation is warranted, given the sparse and inconsistent data.[99] Despite the paucity of evidence, clinical supplemental oxygen is usually prescribed to patients with ILD.[100]

Overall, supplemental oxygen is a safe therapeutic intervention that should be considered in conjunction with patient wishes and goals. The goals of oxygen use are multifaceted, primarily aiming to improve the patient experience, targeting symptoms and/or exercise tolerance.[101–104]

Pulmonary Rehabilitation

Pulmonary rehabilitation (PR) presents a unique opportunity to implement an in-person education program tailored to patients with ILD. Besides exercise training, key educational topics of a PR program are the pathophysiology of ILD, management of symptoms, clinical tests, autonomy, oxygen use, medications, and end-of-life counseling.[105]

Table 1
List of recruiting and not-yet recruiting randomized clinical trials on the medical treatment of connective tissue disease–interstitial lung diseases

Study Title	Condition	Status	Intervention	Sponsor
APRIL (AbatacePt in Rheumatoid Arthritis-ILD) NCT03084419	RA-ILD	Recruiting	Abatacept	Cambridge University Hospitals NHS Foundation Trust, United Kingdom
Phase II Study of Pirfenidone in Patients With RAILD (TRAIL1) NCT02808871	RA-ILD	Recruiting	Pirfenidone	Brigham and Women's Hospital, United States
Effects of Tofacitinib vs Methotrexate on Rheumatoid Arthritis Interstitial Lung Disease NCT04311567	RA-ILD	Not yet recruiting	Tofacitinib	Vastra Gotaland Region (Göteborg University), Sweden
The Safety and Effects of Mesenchymal Stem Cell (MSCs) in the Treatment of Rheumatoid Arthritis NCT03798028	RA-ILD	Recruiting	Mesenchymal stem cell	Xijing Hospital, China
Efficacy and Safety of Pirfenidone in Patient With Systemic Sclerosis-associated Interstitial Lung Disease NCT03856853	SSc-ILD	Recruiting	Pirfenidone	Beijing Continent Pharmaceutical Co, Ltd, China
Scleroderma Lung Study III - Combining Pirfenidone With Mycophenolate NCT03221257	SSc-ILD	Recruiting	Pirfenidone	University of California, Los Angeles, CA
Autologous Stem Cell Transplantation in Patients With Systemic Sclerosis NCT03630211	SSc-ILD	Recruiting	Autologous stem cell transplant	University of Pittsburgh, United States
Pragmatic Clinical Trials in Scleroderma (PCTS) NCT03610217	SSc-ILD	Not yet recruiting	Rituximab or intravenous cyclophosphamide	University of West London, Ontario, Canada

(continued on next page)

Table 1
(continued)

Study Title	Condition	Status	Intervention	Sponsor
Comparing and Combining Bortezomib and Mycophenolate in SSc Pulmonary Fibrosis NCT02370693	SSc-ILD	Recruiting	Bortezomib	Northwestern University, Illinois
Efficacy and Safety of Pirfenidone in Patient With Dermatomyositis Interstitial Lung Disease (Dm-ILD) NCT03857854	DM-ILD	Recruiting	Pirfenidone	Beijing Continent Pharmaceutical Co, Ltd, China
Abatacept for the Treatment of Myositis-associated Interstitial Lung Disease NCT03215927	Antisynthetase syndrome	Recruiting	Abatacept	University of Pittsburgh, PA
Cyclophosphamide and Azathioprine vs Tacrolimus in Antisynthetase Syndrome-related Interstitial Lung Disease NCT03770663	Antisynthetase syndrome	Not yet recruiting	Cyclophosphamide and azathioprine vs tacrolimus	Assistance Publique - Hôpitaux de Paris, France
Allogeneic Bone Marrow Mesenchymal Stem Cells for Patients With Interstitial Lung Disease (ILD) & Connective Tissue Disorders (CTD) NCT03929120	CTD-ILD	Recruiting	Allogeneic Bone Marrow Derived Mesenchymal Stem Cells	Mayo Clinic, Florida
Evaluation of Efficacy and Safety of Rituximab With Mycophenolate Mofetil in Patients With Interstitial Lung Diseases NCT02990286	CTD-ILD/IPAF	Recruiting	Rituximab	University Hospital, Tours, France

| Cyclosporine A in the Treatment of Interstitial Pneumonitis Associated With Sjogren's Syndrome NCT02370550 | pSS-ILD | Recruiting | Cyclosporine | Peking University, China |

Abbreviation: IPAF, interstitial pneumonia with autoimmune features.
Data from Rosas I. Phase II Study of Pirfenidone in Patierts With RAILD (TRAIL1). Available at: https://clinicaltrials.gov/ct2/show/record/NCT02808871. Accessed Aug 3 2020.

PR seems to be safe for people with ILD. Improvements in functional exercise capacity, dyspnea, and quality of life are seen immediately following pulmonary rehabilitation.[106–109] Although little evidence is available regarding longer-term effects of PR, its safety and short-term beneficial effects suggest that PR should be considered in the care of patients with CTD-ILD.[106]

TREATMENT OF COMORBIDITIES

Comorbidities in ILDs are often underappreciated, but they are prevalent conditions with significant consequences on quality of life, morbidity, and mortality.[110,111] In CTD-ILDs, this is even more important, because extrapulmonary manifestations of CTD are common. The management of extrapulmonary manifestations of the CTD is beyond the scope of this article. However, comorbidities directly associated with the ILD or its progression, and that are not necessarily a manifestation of the underlying CTD, are briefly addressed here.

Gastroesophageal Reflux

Gastroesophageal reflux (GER) may be a consequence of the ILD[110–113] as well as a cause of ILD progression. In IPF, there are data to suggest that the identification of GER allows antireflux interventions to be taken, which may reduce the progression of ILD, although the data are conflicting.[114,115] Invasive diagnostic methods to identify the presence of GER include (1) esophageal manometry; (2) ambulatory 24-hour pH monitoring; (3) a combination of pH plus impedance monitoring in order to identify both acid and nonacid reflux events in the esophagus, as well as the height and volume of the reflux; and (4) upper endoscopy to identify erosive esophagitis and Barrett esophagus. It should be stressed that reflux episodes associated with nonesophageal symptoms (eg, cough) are not always detected by standard esophageal tests, which have low sensitivity for gaseous or aerosolized reflux.[116] The treatment of GER involves lifestyle measures (weight loss and elevation of the head end of the bed), pharmacologic treatment (proton pump inhibitors, H2-receptor antagonists, prokinetic agents), and surgical treatment.[117–119]

Cardiovascular Disease

Cardiovascular disease can represent a comorbidity but also a consequence of direct cardiac involvement in CTDs. Significant coronary artery disease has been associated with worse survival in IPF.[120] Extrapolating from IPF, patients with CTD-ILD angina or moderate to severe coronary calcifications on HRCT should be referred for cardiologic evaluation. Cardiovascular disease as a consequence of CTD is most frequent in SSc and in PM/DM, in which cardiac disease is the third most frequent cause of death after lung disease and malignancy.[121] Subclinical disease is more frequent than clinically evident cardiac disease. In PM/DM, heart failure, valvular disease, coronary artery disease, myocarditis, and bundle branch block have been reported. A low threshold for cardiac investigation is appropriate because exertional dyspnea caused by cardiac disease may be difficult to separate from dyspnea caused by ILD.

Obstructive Sleep Apnea

Sleepiness and fatigue are common symptoms in patients with ILD, indicating poorer quality of sleep.[122] In addition, nocturnal hypoxia with or without associated OSA is also common in ILD. The importance of nocturnal hypoxia has been debated, but sleep desaturation has been found to be an independent predictor of poorer prognosis.[123] To date, there is no clear evidence of worse outcomes in patients with asymptomatic OSA; hence, routine screening for OSA of all patients with ILD is not justified. Continuous positive airway pressure initiation has been shown to improve quality-of-life measures and sleep instruments in patients with IPF with comorbid moderate to severe OSA, and it may be reasonable to extrapolate this to patients with CTD-ILD.[124]

Depression

Depression is under-recognized in the ILD population.[125] There are no ILD-specific screening tools for depression, but the threshold to screen patients with ILD for depression should be low, given its impact on quality of life. Given the relationship between severity of dyspnea and depression, targeting the management of dyspnea may have beneficial effects on depressive symptoms. Short-term outpatient participation in PR has also been shown to improve depression scores.[109]

Lung Cancer and Pulmonary Lymphoma

Pulmonary fibrosis is a risk factor for carcinogenesis.[126] SSc-ILD in particular carries an additional increased risk of lung cancer (non–small cell lung cancer).[127] Distinction between malignancy and areas of confluent fibrosis may be difficult, especially when previous imaging is unavailable. Histologic diagnosis is often obtained by percutaneous CT-guided biopsy because of the peripheral location of the tumors. In some centers, annual HRCT is performed to screen for cancer, but this approach has yet to be validated. Management discussion in the appropriate multidisciplinary team setting is pivotal in order to define a suitable diagnostic algorithm, and realistic treatment decisions based on prognosis.[127,128] Pulmonary lymphoma, particularly non-Hodgkin lymphoma (NHL), has its incidence increased specially among Sjögren patients (relative risk, 13.76).[129] The pathogenetic link between Sjögren syndrome and NHL is unclear, but chronic antigenic activation of B cells is thought to play a role.[130] Overall, patients with primary Sjögren syndrome have slightly increased mortalities compared with the general population, and this is mainly accounted for by the excess lymphoproliferative disorders.[131]

LUNG TRANSPLANT

Despite concerns that patients with CTD-ILD may be at risk for worse outcomes after lung transplant because of preexisting immune dysregulation or extrapulmonary manifestations of their underlying disease, studies suggest that posttransplant outcomes in patients with CTD-ILD, both in SSc-ILD and in other CTD-ILDs, do not differ significantly from those in patients with non–CTD-ILD.[132–134] Lung transplant remains a therapy for appropriately selected candidates with treatment-refractory lung disease. Progressive disease, especially if fibrosis is present, should prompt an early referral, because these patients require a multidisciplinary evaluation before transplant consideration and optimization before listing.

SUMMARY

There is a lack of robust evidence to guide the management of patients with CTD-ILDs. Immunosuppressants are the mainstay of treatment, but there is limited evidence to support their efficacy or safety as treatments for CTD-ILDs, other than SSc-ILD. Comorbidity assessment and management and nonpharmacologic treatments are other important components in the management of CTD-ILDs. The results of ongoing clinical trials are much awaited and will provide additional valuable insights on the management of CTD-ILDs.

CLINICS CARE POINTS

- The pharmacological treatment of CTD-ILDs should be triggered by evidence of disease severity, activity and or progression.
- Methotrexate lung toxicity is unlikely to explain pulmonary fibrosis development and or progression, especially if insidious.
- Antifibrotics are a reasonable treatment option, added to immunosuppressants or in isolation, to CTD-ILDs manifested with progressive pulmonary fibrosis.

DISCLOSURE

L. Kawano-Dourado has research grants from Bristol-Myers Squibb and Boehringer Ingelheim. L. Kawano-Dourado has received personal fees from Bristol-Myers-Squibb, Roche, and Boehringer-Ingelheim. J.S. Lee has research grants from the National Institutes of Health and Boehringer Ingelheim. J.S. Lee has received personal fees from Galapagos, Boehringer-Ingelheim, Eleven P15, Bonac, Celgene, and United Therapeutics.

REFERENCES

1. Aparicio IJ, Lee JS. Connective tissue disease-associated interstitial lung diseases: unresolved issues. Semin Respir Crit Care Med 2016;37:468–76.
2. Fischer A, Chartrand S. Assessment and management of connective tissue disease-associated interstitial lung disease. Sarcoidosis Vasc Diffuse Lung Dis 2015;32(1):2–21.
3. Raimundo K, Solomon JJ, Olson AL, et al. Rheumatoid arthritis–interstitial lung disease in the United States: prevalence, incidence, and healthcare costs and mortality. J Rheumatol 2019;46:360–9.
4. Volkmann ER, Tashkin DP, Sim M, et al. Short-term progression of interstitial lung disease in systemic sclerosis predicts long-term survival in two independent clinical trial cohorts. Ann Rheum Dis 2019;78(1):122–30.
5. Solomon JJ, Ryu JH, Tazelaar HD, et al. Fibrosing interstitial lung pneumonia predicts survival in patients with rheumatoid arthritis-associated interstitial lung disease (RA-ILD). Respir Med 2013;107:1247–52.
6. Fischer A, Strek ME, Cottin V, et al. Proceedings of the American College of Rheumatology/Association of Physicians of Great Britain and Ireland

Connective Tissue Disease–associated interstitial lung disease summit: a multidisciplinary approach to address challenges and opportunities. Arthritis Rheumatol 2019;71(2):182–95.

7. Sparks JA, He X, Huang J, et al. Rheumatoid arthritis disease activity predicting incident clinically-apparent RA-associated interstitial lung disease: a prospective cohort study. Arthritis Rheumatol 2019;71(9):1472–82.

8. Khanna D, Lin CJF, Furst DE, et al. Tocilizumab in systemic sclerosis: a randomised, double-blind, placebo-controlled, phase 3 trial. Lancet Respir Med 2020. https://doi.org/10.1016/S2213-2600(20)30318-0.

9. Vij R, Strek ME. Diagnosis and treatment of connective tissue disease-associated interstitial lung disease. Chest 2013;143(3):814–24.

10. Walsh SLF, Sverzellati N, Devaraj A, et al. Connective tissue disease related fibrotic lung disease: high resolution computed tomographic and pulmonary function indices as prognostic determinants. Thorax 2014;69(3):216–22.

11. Goh N, Desai SR, Veeraraghavan S, et al. Interstitial lung disease in systemic sclerosis: a simple staging system. Am J Respir Crit Care Med 2008; 177:248–1254.

12. Khanna D, Tashkin DP, Denton CP, et al. Etiology, risk factors, and biomarkers in systemic sclerosis with interstitial lung disease. Am J Respir Crit Care Med 2020;201(6):650–60.

13. Kawano-Dourado L, Doyle TJ, Bonfiglioli K, et al. Baseline characteristics and progression of a spectrum of interstitial lung abnormalities and disease in rheumatoid arthritis. Chest 2020. https://doi.org/10.1016/j.chest.2020.04.061.

14. Putman RK, Gudmundsson G, Axelsson GT, et al. Imaging patterns are associated with interstitial lung abnormality progression and mortality. Am J Respir Crit Care Med 2019;200(2):175–83.

15. Sellarés J, Hernández-González F, Lucena CM, et al. Auscultation of Velcro crackles is associated with usual interstitial pneumonia. Medicine (Baltimore) 2016;95(5):e2573.

16. Distler O, Assassi S, Cottin V, et al. Predictors of progression in systemic sclerosis patients with interstitial lung disease. Eur Respir J 2020;55: 1902026.

17. Morisset J, Vittinghoff E, Lee BY, et al. The performance of the GAP model in patients with rheumatoid arthritis associated interstitial lung disease. Respir Med 2017;51:e56.

18. Zamora-Legoff J, Krause ML, Crowson CS, et al. Progressive decline of lung function in rheumatoid arthritis associated interstitial lung disease. Arthritis Rheumatol 2017;69(3):542–9.

19. Sambataro G, Ferro F, Orlandi M, et al. Clinical, morphological features and prognostic factors associated with interstitial lung disease in primary Sjögren's syndrome: a systematic review from the Italian Society of Rheumatology. Autoimmun Rev 2020;19:102447.

20. Jani M, Hirani N, Matteson EL, et al. The safety of biologic therapies in RA-associated interstitial lung disease. Nat Rev Rheumatol 2014;10(5):284–94.

21. Groen H, Postma DS, Kallenberg GM, et al. Interstitial lung disease and myositis in a patient with simultaneously occurring sarcoidosis and scleroderma. Chest 1993;104(4):1298–300.

22. Kawano-Dourado L, Costa AN, Carvalho CRR, et al. Environmental triggers of autoimmunity in anti-synthetase syndrome: the lungs under the spot light. Clin Exp Rheumatol 2013;31(6):950–3.

23. Meyer KC, Raghu G, Baughman RP, et al. An official American Thoracic Society Clinical Practice Guideline: the clinical utility of bronchoalveolar lavage cellular analysis in interstitial lung disease. Am J Respir Crit Care Med 2012;185(9):1004–14.

24. Roofeh D, Distler O, Allanore Y, et al. Treatment of systemic sclerosis–associated interstitial lung disease: lessons from clinical trials. J Scleroderma Relat Disord 2020;5(2S):61–71.

25. Tashkin DP, Elashoff R, Clements PJ, et al. Cyclophosphamide versus placebo in scleroderma lung disease. N Engl J Med 2006;354:2655–66.

26. Tashkin DP, Roth MD, Clements PJ, et al. Mycophenolate mofetil versus oral cyclophosphamide in scleroderma-related interstitial lung disease (SLS II): a randomised controlled, double-blind, parallel group trial. Lancet Respir Med 2016; 4(9):708–19.

27. Distler O, Highland KB, Gahlemann M, et al. Nintedanib for systemic sclerosis–associated interstitial lung disease. N Engl J Med 2019;380:2518–28.

28. Steen V, Costantino J, Shapiro A, et al. Outcome of renal crisis in systemic sclerosis: relation to availability of angiotensin-converting-enzyme (ACE) inhibitors. Ann Intern Med 1990;114(3):249–50.

29. Trang G, Steele R, Baron M, et al. Corticosteroids and the risk of scleroderma renal crisis: a systematic review. Rheumatol Int 2012;32:645–53.

30. Roofeh D, Jaafar S, Vummidi D, et al. Management of systemic sclerosis-associated interstitial lung disease. Curr Opin Rheumatol 2019;31(3):241–9.

31. Fernández-Codina A, Walker KM, Pope JE, et al. Treatment algorithms for systemic sclerosis according to experts. Arthritis Rheumatol 2018;70: 1820–8.

32. Sircar G, Goswami RP, Sircar D, et al. Intravenous cyclophosphamide vs rituximab for the treatment of early diffuse scleroderma lung disease: open label, randomized, controlled trial. Rheumatology (Oxford) 2018;57(12):2106–13.

33. Sullivan KM, Goldmuntz EA, Keyes-Elstein L, et al. Myeloablative autologous stem-cell transplantation

for severe scleroderma. N Engl J Med 2018;378(1): 35–47.

34. Burt RK, Shah SJ, Dill K, et al. Autologous non-myeloablative haemopoietic stem-cell transplantation compared with pulse cyclophosphamide once per month for systemic sclerosis (ASSIST): an open-label, randomised phase 2 trial. Lancet 2011;378(9790):498–506.

35. van Laar JM, Farge D, Sont JK, et al. Autologous hematopoietic stem cell transplantation vs intravenous pulse cyclophosphamide in diffuse cutaneous systemic sclerosis: a randomized clinical trial. JAMA 2014;311(24):2490–8.

36. Walker UA, Saketkoo LA, Distler O. Haematopoietic stem cell transplantation in systemic sclerosis. RMD Open 2018;4(1):e000533.

37. Khanna D, Denton CP, Jahreis A, et al. Safety and efficacy of subcutaneous tocilizumab in adults with systemic sclerosis (faSScinate): a phase 2, randomised, controlled trial. Ann Rheum Dis 2018;77(2): 212–20.

38. Raghu G, Depaso WJ, Cain K, et al. Azathioprine combined with prednisone in the treatment of idiopathic pulmonary fibrosis: a prospective double-blind, randomized, placebo-controlled clinical trial. Am Rev Respir Dis 1991;144(2):291–6.

39. Spagnolo P, Lee JS, Sverzellati N, et al. The lung in rheumatoid arthritis: focus on interstitial lung disease. Arthritis Rheum 2018;70(10):1544–54.

40. Raghu G, Rochwerg B, Zhang Y, et al. An official ATS/ERS/JRS/ALAT clinical practice guideline: treatment of idiopathic pulmonary fibrosis. An update of the 2011 clinical practice guideline. Am J Respir Crit Care Med 2015;192(2):e3–19.

41. The Idiopathic Pulmonary Fibrosis Clinical Research Network. Prednisone, azathioprine, and N-Acetylcysteine for pulmonary fibrosis. N Engl J Med 2012;366:1968–77.

42. Iqbal K, Kelly C. Treatment of rheumatoid arthritis-associated interstitial lung disease: a perspective review. Ther Adv Musculoskelet Dis 2015;7(6):247–67.

43. Fischer A, Brown KK, Du Bois, et al. Mycophenolate mofetil improves lung function in connective tissue disease-associated interstitial lung disease. J Rheumatol 2013;40:640–6, 87.

44. Swigris JJ, Olson AL, Fischer A, et al. Mycophenolate mofetil is safe, well tolerated, and preserves lung function in patients with connective tissue disease-related interstitial lung disease. Chest 2006;130:30–6.

45. Bendstrup E, Møller J, Kronborg-White S, et al. Interstitial lung disease in rheumatoid arthritis remains a challenge for clinicians. J Clin Med 2019;8:2038.

46. Cassone G, Manfredi A, Vacchi C, et al. Treatment of rheumatoid arthritis-associated interstitial lung disease: lights and shadows. J Clin Med 2020; 9(4):1082.

47. Mochizuki T, Ikari K, Yano K, et al. Long-term deterioration of interstitial lung disease in patients with rheumatoid arthritis treated with abatacept. Mod Rheumatol 2019;29(3):413–7.

48. Roodenrijs NMT, de Hair MJH, Wheather G, et al. The multi-biomarker disease activity score tracks response to rituximab treatment in rheumatoid arthritis patients: a post hoc analysis of three cohort studies. Arthritis Res Ther 2018;20(1): 256.

49. Vadillo C, Asuncion-Nieto M, Romero-Bueno F. Efficacy of rituximab in slowing down progression of rheumatoid arthritis–related interstitial lung disease: data from the NEREA Registry. Rheumatology (Oxford) 2020;59(8):2099–108.

50. Holroyd C, Seth R, Marwan B, et al. The British Society for Rheumatology biologic DMARD safety guidelines in inflammatory arthritis-Executive summary. Rheumatology (Oxford) 2019;58(2):220–6.

51. Salliot C, van der Heijde D. Long-term safety of methotrexate monotherapy in patients with rheumatoid arthritis: a systematic literature research. Ann Rheum Dis 2009;68:1100–4.

52. Smolen JS, Aletaha D, McInnes IB. Rheumatoid arthritis. Lancet 2016;388:2023–38.

53. Fragoulis G, Conway R, Nikiphorou E. Methotrexate and interstitial lung disease: controversies and questions. A narrative review of the literature. Rheumatology 2019;58:1900–6.

54. Conway R, Low C, Coughlan RJ, et al. Methotrexate and lung disease in rheumatoid arthritis: a meta-analysis of randomized controlled trials. Arthritis Rheumatol 2014;66:803–12.

55. Juge PA, Lee JS, Lau J, et al. Methotrexate and rheumatoid arthritis associated interstitial lung disease. Eur Respir J 2020. https://doi.org/10.1183/13993003.00337-2020.

56. Long K, Danoff SK. Interstitial lung disease in polymyositis and dermatomyositis. Clin Chest Med 2019;40(3):561–72.

57. Betteridge Z, Mchugh N. Myositis-specific autoantibodies: an important tool to support diagnosis of myositis. J Intern Med 2016;280(1):8–23.

58. Hoshino K, Muro Y, Sugiura K, et al. Anti-MDA5 and anti-TIF1-g antibodies have clinical significance for patients with dermatomyositis. Rheumatology 2010;49(9):1726–33.

59. Morisset J, Johnson C, Rich E, et al. Management of myositis-related interstitial lung disease. Chest 2016;150(5):1118–28.

60. Takada T, Suzuki E, Nakano M, et al. Clinical features of polymyositis/dermatomyositis with steroid-resistant interstitial lung disease. Intern Med 1998;37(8):669–73.

61. Shimojima Y, Ishii W, Matsuda M, et al. Effective use of calcineurin inhibitor in combination therapy for interstitial lung disease in patients with

dermatomyositis and polymyositis. J Clin Rheumatol 2017;23(2):87–93.

62. Mira-Avendano IC, Parambil JG, Yadav R, et al. A retrospective review of clinical features and treatment outcomes in steroid-resistant interstitial lung disease from polymyositis/dermatomyositis. Respir Med 2013;107(6):890–6.

63. Takada K, Kishi J, Miyasaka N. Step-up versus primary intensive approach to the treatment of interstitial pneumonia associated with dermatomyositis/polymyositis: a retrospective study. Mod Rheumatol 2007;17(2):123–30.

64. Go DJ, Park JK, Kang EH, et al. Survival benefit associated with early cyclosporine treatment for dermatomyositis-associated interstitial lung disease. Rheumatol Int 2015;36(1): 125–31.

65. Ge Y, Peng Q, Zhang S, et al. Cyclophosphamide treatment for idiopathic inflammatory myopathies and related interstitial lung disease: a systematic review. Clin Rheumatol 2014;34(1):99–105.

66. Ge Y, Zhou H, Shi J, et al. The efficacy of tacrolimus in patients with refractory dermatomyositis/polymyositis: a systematic review. Clin Rheumatol 2015;34(12):2097–103.

67. Bauhammer J, Blank N, Max R, et al. Rituximab in the treatment of Jo1 antibody–associated antisynthetase syndrome: anti-Ro52 positivity as a marker for severity and treatment response. J Rheumatol 2016;43(8):1566–74.

68. Andersson H, Sem M, Lund MB, et al. Long-term experience with rituximab in anti-synthetase syndrome-related interstitial lung disease. Rheumatology 2015;54(8):1420–8.

69. Hallowell RW, Amariei D, Danoff SK. Intravenous immunoglobulin as potential adjunct therapy for interstitial lung disease. Ann Am Thorac Soc 2016;13(10):1682–8.

70. Chen Z, Wang X, Ye S. Tofacitinib in amyopathic dermatomyositis–associated interstitial lung disease. N Engl J Med 2019;381(3):291–3.

71. Highland K, Kreider M. Pulmonary involvement in Sjögren syndrome. Semin Respir Crit Care Med 2014;35(02):255–64.

72. Roca F, Dominique S, Schmidt J, et al. Interstitial lung disease in primary Sjögren's syndrome. Autoimmun Rev 2017;16(1):48–54.

73. Parambil JG, Myers JL, Lindell RM, et al. Interstitial lung disease in primary Sjögren syndrome. Chest 2006;130(5):1489–95.

74. Isaksen K, Jonsson R, Omdal R. Anti-CD20 treatment in primary Sjögren's syndrome. Scand J Immunol 2008;68(6):554–64.

75. Swartz MA, Vivino FB. Dramatic reversal of lymphocytic interstitial pneumonitis in Sjögren's syndrome with rituximab. J Clin Rheumatol 2011; 17(8):454.

76. Lee AS, Scofield RH, Hammitt KM, et al. Consensus guidelines for evaluation and management of pulmonary disease in Sjögren's. Chest 2020. S0012-3692(20)34902-34903. Epub ahead of print. PMID: 33075377.

77. Tani C, Carli L, Vagnani S, et al. The diagnosis and classification of mixed connective tissue disease. J Autoimmun 2014;48–49:46–9.

78. Reiseter S, Gunnarsson R, Corander J, et al. Disease evolution in mixed connective tissue disease: results from a long-term nationwide prospective cohort study. Arthritis Res Ther 2017;19:284.

79. Mittoo S, Fischer A, Strand V, et al. Systemic lupus erythematosus-related interstitial lung disease. Curr Rheumatol Rev 2010;6:99–107.

80. D'Cruz DP, Hannah JR. Pulmonary complications of systemic lupus erythematosus. Semin Respir Crit Care Med 2019;40(02):227–34.

81. Enomoto N, Egashira R, Tabata K, et al. Analysis of systemic lupus erythematosus-related interstitial pneumonia: a retrospective multicentre study. Sci Rep 2019;9:7355.

82. Hanata N, Shoda H, Fujio K. Successful treatment by mycophenolate mofetil of subacute progressive interstitial lung disease associated with systemic lupus erythematosus. Curr Rheumatol Rev 2010; 6:99–107.

83. Reynolds JA, Toescu V, Yee CS, et al. Effects of rituximab on resistant SLE disease including lung involvement. Lupus 2009;18(1):67–73.

84. Karimi-Shah BA, Chowdhury BA. Forced vital capacity in idiopathic pulmonary fibrosis — FDA review of Pirfenidone and Nintedanib. N Engl J Med 2015;372:1189–91.

85. FDA press announcements. Available at: https://nam03.safelinks.protection.outlook.com/?url= https:%2F%2Fwww.fda.gov%2Fnews-events% 2Fpress-announcements%2Ffda-approves-first-treatment-group-progressive-interstitial-lung-diseases%23: ~ :text%3DThe%2520U.S.%2520 Food%2520and%2520Drug%2Cdiseases%2520 that%2520worsen%2520over%2520time& data=04%7C01%7Cr.mayakrishnan%40elsevier. com%7C17b667c39f4046e436c508d8fa9fe62e% 7C9274ee3f94254109a27f9fb15c10675d%7C0% 7C0%7C637534912445257626%7CUnknown% 7CTWFpbGZsb3d8eyJWIjoiMC4wLjAwMDAi LCJQIjoiV2luMzIiLCJBTil6Ik1haWwiLCJXVC I6Mn0%3D%7C3000&sdata=su%2F% 2BIB7RBNGTkD%2B51xBTghMEf2ULHmDnsE rP66mKFmg%3D&reserved=0. Accessed April 8, 2021.

86. Flaherty KR, Wells AU, Cottin V, et al. Nintedanib in progressive fibrosing interstitial lung diseases. N Engl J Med 2019;381:1718–27.

87. Wells AU, Flaherty KR, Brown KK, et al. Nintedanib in patients with progressive fibrosing interstitial

lung diseases—subgroup analyses by interstitial lung disease diagnosis in the INBUILD trial: a randomised, double-blind, placebo-controlled, parallel-group trial. Lancet Respir Med 2020;8(5):453–60.

88. Maher TM, Corte TJ, Fischer A, et al. Pirfenidone in patients with unclassifiable progressive fibrosing interstitial lung disease: a double-blind, randomised, placebo-controlled, phase 2 trial. Lancet Respir Med 2020;8(2):147–57.

89. Li T, Guo L, Chen Z, et al. Pirfenidone in patients with rapidly progressive interstitial lung disease associated with clinically amyopathic dermatomyositis. Sci Rep 2016;6:33226.

90. Cassone G, Sebastiani M, Vacchi C, et al. Pirfenidone for the treatment of interstitial lung disease associated to rheumatoid arthritis: a new scenario is coming? Respir Med Case Rep 2020;30:101051.

91. Phase II Study of Pirfenidone in Patients with RAILD (TRAIL1). Clinicaltrials.gov: NCT02808871. Available at: https://nam03.safelinks.protection.outlook.com/?url=https%3A%2F%2Fclinicaltrials.gov%2Fct2%2Fshow%2FNCT02808871&data=04%7C01%7Cr.mayakrishnan%40elsevier.com%7C17b667c39f4046e436c508d8fa9fe62e%7C9274ee3f94254109a27f9fb15c10675d%7C0%7C0%7C637534912445257626%7CUnknown%7CTWFpbGZsb3d8eyJWIjoiMC4wLjAwMDAiLCJQIjoiV2luMzIiLCJBTiI6Ik1haWwiLCJXVCI6Mn0%3D%7C3000&sdata=S%2FgaOarJ%2BkxeLA8dsVU7PYVO9gFeLSwXzp9aFX0L75Q%3D&reserved=0. Accessed April 8, 2021.

92. Park JW, Curtis JR, Moon J, et al. Prophylactic effect of trimethoprim-sulfamethoxazole for pneumocystis pneumonia in patients with rheumatic diseases exposed to prolonged high-dose glucocorticoids. Ann Rheum Dis 2018;77(5):644–9.

93. Marcos LA, Terashima A, Dupont HL, et al. Strongyloides hyperinfection syndrome: an emerging global infectious disease. Trans R Soc Trop Med Hyg 2008;102(4):314–8.

94. Johannson KA, Pendharkar SR, Mathison K, et al. Supplemental oxygen in interstitial lung disease: an art in need of science. Ann Am Thorac Soc 2017;14(9):1373–7.

95. Agustí AG, Roca J, Gea J, et al. Mechanisms of gas-exchange impairment in idiopathic pulmonary fibrosis. Am Rev Respir Dis 1991;143:219–25.

96. Risk C, Epler GR, Gaensler EA. Exercise alveolar-arterial oxygen pressure difference in interstitial lung disease. Chest 1984;85:69–74.

97. Dowman LM, McDonald CF, Hill CJ, et al. The evidence of benefits of exercise training in interstitial lung disease: a randomised controlled trial. Thorax 2017;72:610–9.

98. Nathan SD, Barbera JA, Gaine SP, et al. Pulmonary hypertension in chronic lung disease and hypoxia. Eur Respir J 2019;53(1):1801914.

99. Sharp C, Adamali H, Millar AB. Ambulatory and short-burst oxygen for interstitial lung disease. Cochrane Database Syst Rev 2016;(7):CD011716.

100. Khor YH, Renzoni EA, Visca D, et al. Oxygen therapy in COPD and interstitial lung disease: navigating the knowns and unknowns. ERJ Open Res 2019;5(3):00118–2019.

101. Lim RK, Humphreys C, Morisset J, et al, O2 Delphi Collaborators. Oxygen in patients with fibrotic interstitial lung disease: an international Delphi survey. Eur Respir J 2019;54(2):1900421.

102. Magnet FS, Schwarz SB, Callegari J, et al. Long-term oxygen therapy: comparison of the German and British Guidelines. Respiration 2017;93(4):253–63.

103. Bradley B, Branley HM, Egan JJ, et al. Interstitial lung disease guideline: the British Thoracic Society in collaboration with the Thoracic Society of Australia and New Zealand and the Irish Thoracic Society. Thorax 2008;63(Suppl 5):v1–58 [published correction appears in Thorax 2008;63(11):1029. multiple author names added].

104. Raghu G, Collard HR, Egan JJ, et al. An official ATS/ERS/JRS/ALAT statement: idiopathic pulmonary fibrosis: evidence-based guidelines for diagnosis and management. Am J Respir Crit Care Med 2011;183(6):788–824.

105. Morisset J, Dubé BP, Garvey C, et al. The unmet educational needs of patients with interstitial lung disease. setting the stage for tailored pulmonary rehabilitation. Ann Am Thorac Soc 2016;13(7):1026–33.

106. Dowman L, Hill CJ, Holland AE. Pulmonary rehabilitation for interstitial lung disease. Cochrane Database Syst Rev 2014;(10):CD006322.

107. Deniz S, Şahin H, Yalnız E. Does the severity of interstitial lung disease affect the gains from pulmonary rehabilitation? Clin Respir J 2018;12(6):2141–50.

108. Sciriha A, Lungaro-Mifsud S, Fsadni P, et al. Pulmonary rehabilitation in patients with interstitial lung disease: the effects of a 12-week programme. Respir Med 2019;146:49–56.

109. Ferreira A, Garvey C, Connors GL, et al. Pulmonary rehabilitation in interstitial lung disease: benefits and predictors of response. Chest 2009;135(2):442–7.

110. Margaritopoulos GA, Kokosi MA, Wells AU. Diagnosing complications and co-morbidities of fibrotic interstitial lung disease. Expert Rev Respir Med 2019;13(7):645–58.

111. Schwarzkopf L, Witt S, Waelscher J, et al. Associations between comorbidities, their treatment and

survival in patients with interstitial lung diseases - a claims data analysis. Respir Res 2018;19(1):73.

112. Cantu E III, Appel JZ III, Hartwig MG, et al. Early fundoplication prevents chronic allograft dysfunction in patients with gastroesophageal reflux disease. Ann Thorac Surg 2004;78:1142–51.

113. Lee JS, Song JW, Wolters PJ, et al. Bronchoalveolar lavage pepsin in acute exacerbation of idiopathic pulmonary fibrosis. Eur Respir J 2012;39: 352–8.

114. Tcherakian C, Cottin V, Brillet PY, et al. Progression of idiopathic pulmonary fibrosis: lessons from asymmetrical disease. Thorax 2011;66:226–31.

115. Raghu G, Pellegrini CA, Yow E, et al. Laparoscopic anti-reflux surgery for the treatment of idiopathic pulmonary fibrosis (WRAP-IPF): a multicentre, randomised, controlled phase 2 trial. Lancet Respir Med 2018;6:707–14.

116. Faruqi S, Sedman P, Jackson W, et al. Fundoplication in chronic intractable cough. Cough 2012;8:3.

117. Lee JS, Ryu JH, Elicker BM, et al. Gastroesophageal reflux therapy is associated with longer survival in patients with idiopathic pulmonary fibrosis. Am J Respir Crit Care Med 2011;184: 1390–4.

118. Linden PA, Gilbert RJ, Yeap BY, et al. Laparoscopic fundoplication in patients with end-stage lung disease awaiting transplantation. J Thorac Cardiovasc Surg 2006;131:438–46.

119. Macaluso C, Furcada JM, Alzaher O, et al. The potential impact of azithromycin in idiopathic pulmonary fibrosis. Eur Respir J 2019;53(2):1800628.

120. Nathan SD, Basavaraj A, Reichner C, et al. Prevalence and impact of coronary artery disease in idiopathic pulmonary fibrosis. Respir Med 2010;104: 1035–41.

121. Van Gelder H, Charles-Schoeman C. The heart in inflammatory myopathies. Rheum Dis Clin North Am 2014;40:1–10.

122. Krishnan V, McCormack MC, Mathai SC, et al. Sleep quality and health-related quality of life in idiopathic pulmonary fibrosis. Chest 2008;134: 693–8, 160.

123. Corte TJ, Wort SJ, Talbot S, et al. Elevated nocturnal desaturation index predicts mortality in interstitial lung disease. Sarcoidosis Vasc Diffuse Lung Dis 2012;29:41–50.

124. Mermigkis C, Bouloukaki I, Antoniou K, et al. Obstructive sleep apnea should be treated in patients with idiopathic pulmonary fibrosis. Sleep Breath 2015;19:385–91.

125. Ryerson CJ, Donesky D, Pantilat SZ, et al. Dyspnea in idiopathic pulmonary fibrosis: a systematic review. J Pain Symptom Manage 2012;43:771–82.

126. Tzouvelekis A, Gomatou G, Bouros E, et al. Common pathogenic mechanisms between idiopathic pulmonary fibrosis and lung cancer. Chest 2019; 156(2):383–91.

127. Bonifazi M, Tramacere I, Pomponio G, et al. Systemic sclerosis (scleroderma) and cancer risk: systematic review and meta-analysis of observational studies. Rheumatology (Oxford) 2013;52(1):143–54.

128. Tomassetti S, Gurioli C, Ryu JH, et al. The impact of lung cancer on survival of idiopathic pulmonary fibrosis. Chest 2015;147:157–64.

129. Liang Y, Yang Z, Qin B, et al. Primary Sjogren's syndrome and malignancy risk: a systematic review and meta-analysis. Ann Rheum Dis 2014;73: 1151–6.

130. Bernatsky S, Ramsey-Goldman R, Clarke A. Malignancy and autoimmunity. Curr Opin Rheumatol 2006;18:129–34.

131. Voulgarelis M, Tzioufas AG, Moutsopoulos HM. Mortality in Sjögren's syndrome. Clin Exp Rheumatol 2008;26(Suppl. 51):S66–71.

132. Saggar R, Khanna D, Furst DE, et al. Systemic sclerosis and bilateral lung transplantation: a single centre experience. Eur Respir J 2010;36:893–900.

133. Bernstein EJ, Peterson ER, Sell JL, et al. Survival of adults with systemic sclerosis following lung transplantation: a nationwide cohort study. Arthritis Rheumatol 2015;67:1314–22.

134. Courtwright AM, El-Chemaly S, Dellaripa PF, et al. Survival and outcomes after lung transplantation for non-scleroderma connective tissue-related interstitial lung disease. J Heart Lung Transplant 2017;36(7):763–9.

Management of Fibrotic Hypersensitivity Pneumonitis

Hayley Barnes, MBBS, MPH[a,b,]*, Kerri A. Johannson, MD, MPH[c,d]

KEYWORDS

- Pulmonary fibrosis • Extrinsic allergic alveolitis • Environmental medicine
- Occupational lung disease

KEY POINTS

- Fibrotic hypersensitivity pneumonitis is a chronic, often progressive form of interstitial lung disease, arising in susceptible individuals from exposure to inhaled inciting antigens.
- Antigen identification is a critical component of diagnosis and management.
- Immunosuppression with mycophenolate or azathioprine is suggested for active or severe disease; cautious use of steroids is advised; antifibrotics may be considered in progressive fibrosis.
- Nonpharmacologic treatments, including pulmonary rehabilitation, oxygen therapy for hypoxemia, and early referral for lung transplant, should be considered where indicated.
- Future research should focus on the genetic and immunologic risk factors for disease, and develop biomarkers to guide therapeutic decision making.

INTRODUCTION

Hypersensitivity pneumonitis (HP) is an immune-mediated interstitial lung disease (ILD) that arises because of repeated inhalational exposure to 1 or more environmental antigens. Although likely under-reported, HP is thought to affect approximately 2 to 3 per 100,000 people per year, or 11.5 per 100,000 people more than 65 years of age per year.[1] It is one of the most commonly diagnosed forms of ILD at specialty ILD clinics[2,3] and its associated mortality is increasing over time.[4] In particular at-risk populations, the prevalence of HP is higher than in the general population, with estimates of 3.7% to 10.4%[5,6] in bird breeders and 1.3% to 12.9%[7,8] in farmers.

HP has a heterogeneous clinical presentation and has previously been described using multiple subcategories. These subcategories have included time-based definitions (ie, acute, subacute, chronic) and those founded in disease behavior (ie, stable vs progressive).[9,10] However, a robust body of evidence indicates that the most important prognostic factor that determines clinical outcomes and responses to specific management approaches is the presence or absence of fibrosis on chest imaging. The presence and extent of fibrosis on chest computed tomography (CT) is associated with symptoms, disease progression, and mortality in patients with HP, with greater fibrosis extent associated with worse outcomes.[11,12] Recently, international consensus guidelines on HP diagnosis were published, proposing the conceptualization of HP into 2 distinct phenotypes: nonfibrotic and fibrotic.[10] Nonfibrotic HP can be considered a typically acute and predominantly inflammatory, potentially reversible form of disease, whereas fibrotic HP (fHP) is typically a chronic and more often progressive form.[9,10] It has been presumed that nonfibrotic HP

a Department of Respiratory Medicine, Alfred Hospital, Melbourne, Australia; b Central Clinical School, Monash University, Melbourne, Australia; c Department of Medicine, University of Calgary, Calgary, Alberta, Canada; d Department of Community Health Sciences, University of Calgary, Calgary, Alberta, Canada
* Corresponding author. Department of Respiratory Medicine, Alfred Hospital, 34 Commercial Rd, Melbourne 3004, Australia.
E-mail address: hayleynbarnes@gmail.com

Clin Chest Med 42 (2021) 311–319
https://doi.org/10.1016/j.ccm.2021.03.007

develops into fHP given a sufficient duration of exposure; however, patients with fHP may also present without a clear acute episode of exposure or illness, and it may be that distinct genetic and/or immunologic pathways contribute to fHP development. Its insidious onset and frequent lack of obvious exposure leads to challenges in establishing an accurate diagnosis of fHP. fHP is frequently misdiagnosed as other forms of fibrotic ILD, with the diagnosis recognized only after case reevaluation[13] or after pathologic examination of explanted lung tissue.[14] Delays in diagnosis may lead to missed opportunities for antigen remediation or inappropriate treatment or prognostication. It is essential to accurately differentiate fHP from other forms of ILD to ensure appropriate disease management and optimal patient outcomes. This article focuses on the approach to diagnosis and management of patients with fHP.

ESTABLISHING AN ACCURATE DIAGNOSIS

The current gold standard for diagnosis of fHP includes review of all available information in the context of a formal multidisciplinary discussion (MDD), where such resources are available. The main diagnostic domains include exposure identification, radiologic chest imaging, and data from bronchoscopy with cellular analysis and/or histopathologic findings from lung biopsy.[10,15]

Exposure identification begins with screening for known exposures linked to fHP using clinical history or formal questionnaires. Use of established HP-specific exposure questionnaires[16] and databases (eg, www.hplung.com) may be useful, but, to date, none have been clinically validated. Despite a thorough exposure history, an inciting exposure may go unidentified in up to 50% of cases seen at ILD referral centers.[17] Additional testing may be considered to support the identification of an inciting antigen, including serum specific antibody tests or specific inhalational challenge testing.[18] However, these tests have important limitations: a positive result does not equal causation (poor specificity), and a negative result does not exclude a potentially causative exposure (poor sensitivity).[19] Because of this, the authors do not routinely recommend serum specific antibody testing in the evaluation of fHP. When a causal exposure cannot be readily identified, or has occurred in a workplace setting, consultation with an industrial hygienist and/or occupational medicine specialist may be informative to guide environmental assessment and exposure abatement.

Although exposure identification is typically dichotomized as present or absent, it may be helpful to consider exposures along a gradient of probability.[20] Not all exposures are equally relevant for causation of HP. For example, breeding pigeons is likely to confer a higher pretest probability of HP compared with a small amount of mold in the home, or a remote history of farming. Although most approaches to exposure identification in HP conceptualize single agents as causal, remote exposures may contribute to the sensitization necessary to trigger the HP-related immune response. In addition, reports of multiple exposures may complicate the otherwise simplistic view of exposure assessment. Multidisciplinary approaches to exposure assessment should be considered, particularly when exposures may occur in the occupational setting.

High-resolution CT (HRCT) imaging informs both the diagnosis of fHP and also the identification of prognostic factors.[10] Typical HP findings on HRCT include parenchymal infiltration with ground-glass opacities, and mosaic attenuation on inspiratory films or air trapping on expiratory films. Lung fibrosis with coarse reticulation, septal thickening, traction bronchiectasis, and honeycombing is present in patients with fHP, and portends worse survival.[11] HRCT is useful in differentiating fHP from other ILDs; idiopathic pulmonary fibrosis (IPF) typically shows a basal predominance, honeycombing, and an absence of relative subpleural sparing and centrilobular nodules; nonspecific interstitial pneumonia (NSIP) shows relative subpleural sparing, absence of lobular areas with increased attenuation, and lack of honeycombing.[21]

Bronchoalveolar lavage (BAL) with a predominant lymphocytosis on differential cell count (>30% lymphocytes; healthy controls 8%–15%) favors a diagnosis of HP, with the degree of lymphocytosis thought to reflect the degree of alveolitis.[22] Lymphocytosis is less marked in fHP, and the extent of radiologic fibrosis negatively correlates with BAL lymphocytosis.[23] Therefore, its test accuracy in distinguishing fHP from other ILDs is reduced (68% sensitivity and 65% specificity when using a >20% threshold).[24] The finding of BAL lymphocytosis may add to the overall clinical picture and should be incorporated into the diagnostic algorithm, but alone does not rule in or rule out a diagnosis of fHP. Where diagnostic uncertainty remains, a lung biopsy showing poorly formed noncaseating granulomas with peribronchiolar interstitial inflammation or dense collagen fibrosis and presence of fibroblastic foci supports the diagnosis of fHP.[25] The recent consensus guideline on HP diagnosis outlines radiologic and histopathologic findings that are characteristic of fHP.[10] Histologic sampling of the lung may be obtained via transbronchial lung cryobiopsy or surgical lung biopsy via a video-assisted thoracoscopic surgical approach. The diagnostic yield of surgical biopsy is high in fibrotic ILD, with the associated perioperative risks minimized when performed in select patient populations and at experienced centers.[10,26] Cryobiopsy is increasingly used for diagnosis of ILD, with recent data supporting high accuracy and lower complications compared with surgical biopsy.[27] Whether to use transbronchial or surgical lung biopsy should be determined based on the local ILD center's technical experience and the resources available. Most importantly, the decision to pursue lung biopsy should be considered after review of all available clinical information in an MDD, and weighing the procedural risks against the anticipated benefit of diagnostic accuracy. The patient's values and preferences are of critical importance in such decision making.

ASSOCIATED RISK FACTORS

Certain risk factors for the development of HP have been identified, with specific features associated with the fibrotic form of disease. Previous lower respiratory tract infections (Epstein-Barr virus, human herpes virus 7 and 8, cytomegalovirus, and parvovirus B19) may increase risk of HP,[28] whereas a paradoxic relationship with smoking has been described.[29] Genetic variants identified in patients with HP include HP-specific pathways and pathways shared with other ILDs. Susceptibility to the development of HP has been associated with genes encoding the major histocompatibility complex, including human leukocyte antigen (HLA)–DR3 alleles (bird-related HP); HLA-DQ3 (summer-type HP); and HLA-A, HLA-B, and HLA-C loci antigens (farmer's lung).[30] Genes encoding for chemokine-mediated signaling pathways and cytokine-to-cytokine receptors are specifically upregulated in fHP.[31]

Certain genetic variants have been associated with fHP. Similar to IPF, MUC5B gain-of-function variants (rs35705950) have been shown to occur at greater frequency in patients with fHP compared with healthy controls.[32] Overexpression of MUC5B in the distal airways, respiratory bronchioles, and bronchiolar epithelium may lead to mucociliary dysfunction, retention of viral or chemical particles, endoplasmic reticulum stress, and disruption of normal repair mechanisms in the lung. Protein-altering telomere-related gene variants, including telomerase reverse transcriptase (TERT), regulator of telomere elongation helicase 1 (RTEL1), and poly[A]-specific RNase (PARN), have been identified in genetic studies of patients

with fHP, and these variants were associated with a significantly shorter peripheral blood leukocyte telomere length.[33] Telomere dysfunction likely leads to DNA-damage pathways, premature cellular senescence, inappropriate apoptosis, and stimulation of lung remodeling and lung fibrosis. Patients with telomere-related gene variants showed significantly worse transplant-free survival than their counterparts, identifying a subpopulation of patients at highest risk of clinical deterioration.[33] Familial forms of HP have been described, occurring in kinship cohorts but also occurring sporadically in families whose affected members manifest other forms of fibrotic ILD.[33,34] There seems to be an important familial component to some patients' fHP diagnoses, but how the genetic predisposition combines with antigen exposure and other risk factors has yet to be determined. Specific genetic testing has yet to be incorporated into routine clinical care in the diagnostic and prognostic evaluation of patients with suspected fHP, but this is anticipated to become increasingly available and relevant in the upcoming years.

MANAGEMENT

The approach to the management of fHP is shown in **Fig. 1**.

Exposure Remediation

The initial management step for all patients diagnosed with fHP centers on identification and remediation of the implicated exposure. Although some patients with fHP continue to develop lung function decline following removal of the inciting antigen, the rate of decline is faster in those who have ongoing exposure compared with those who do not.[35–37]

There is a paucity of evidence to guide exposure remediation in fHP, with most data derived from the asthma literature.[22] Removal without additional environmental cleaning may be insufficient, because antigenic dust may persist in the environment without proper remediation.[38,39] Changes in workplace practices may reduce occupation-related exposures. Addition of biocides at contaminated swimming pools and increased exhaust ventilation to reduce the aerosolization of contaminated metalworking fluids has halted outbreaks of HP.[40,41] Industrial fans to accelerate hay drying and wrapping hay bales in plastic may reduce mold contamination.[42] Respiratory-protective equipment such as helmet respirators used in farming also limits exposure, although at potential cost of discomfort and low compliance.[43]

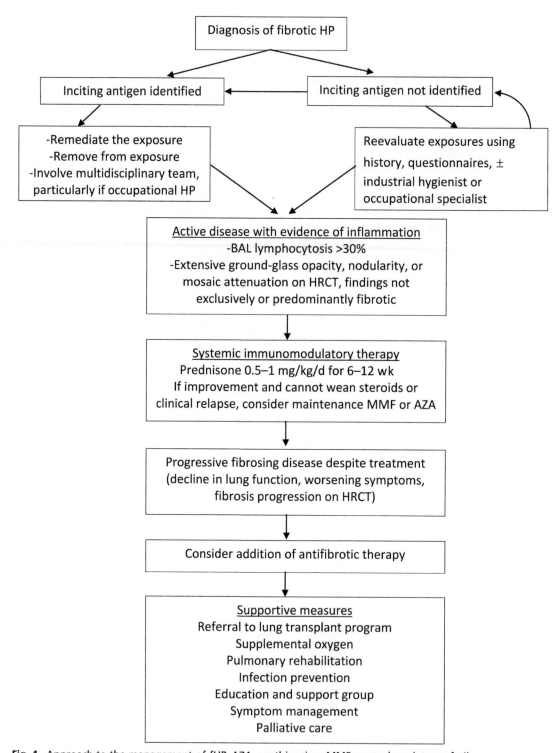

Fig. 1. Approach to the management of fHP. AZA, azathioprine; MMF, mycophenolate mofetil.

In cases of progressive fHP, patients may be advised to relocate or change jobs, particularly if the antigen is unidentified or there is concern about ongoing exposure that cannot be remediated. These interventions are prohibitively expensive or not feasible for some patients and may not necessarily improve clinical outcomes. Such recommendations should be made in conjunction with patient values and preferences, considering the overall impact of relocation or job change. Job changes and workplace modifications should be established in collaboration with occupational medicine experts and/or industrial hygienists in order to minimize exposure to the affected individual and reduce the risk of occupational outbreaks in other exposed workers.

Pharmacologic Management

Immunomodulatory therapies

For patients with persistent symptoms despite cessation of exposure, impaired lung function, or hypoxemia, the initiation of pharmacologic therapy should be considered. In acute, symptomatic, or inflammatory-predominant cases, a short tapering course of 0.5 to 1 mg/kg daily of oral prednisone over 4 to 6 weeks has been recommended. This approach is based primarily on observational data and 1 randomized controlled study in acute farmer's lung that found the use of prednisolone compared with placebo improved forced vital capacity (FVC) and diffusing capacity of the lungs for carbon monoxide (DLCO) in the short term, but with no sustained benefits.[44] To date, there are no randomized or prospective studies of corticosteroid therapy in patients with fHP. Few retrospective studies have addressed the role of steroids in fHP. The presence of BAL lymphocytosis (>20%) has been associated with improvements in FVC with corticosteroid treatment, but, in patients with low BAL lymphocyte levels or radiographic honeycombing, no clear benefit was found,[45] so the role of corticosteroids in fHP remains unclear. Corticosteroids carry potential risk of side effects and complications and should be used judiciously in patients with fHP, after careful consideration of the risks and benefits. Fibrotic forms of lung disease are not classically steroid responsive and steroids may have deleterious effects on patients. The authors encourage clinicians to establish a priori metrics that will inform responses to therapy, in order to guide subsequent clinical decision making. Stability of lung function after a steroid trial may or may not indicate treatment success, because the outcome may be influenced by other factors, such as exposure status. Similarly, worsening lung function may not herald treatment failure, because outcomes may have been worse without steroid treatment.

In patients who have had a clinical response to steroids, or in whom long-term immunomodulation is anticipated to be of benefit, the cell cycle inhibitors mycophenolate mofetil (MMF) and azathioprine (AZA) have been used. Although the data for their primary efficacy in fHP are scarce, they are often used as steroid-sparing agents to treat certain forms of ILD. Two retrospective studies showed the efficacy and tolerability of MMF and AZA in patients with fHP. In a multicenter study of 70 patients, the use of MMF or AZA was associated with no change in FVC%, but improved DLCO % in the year after drug initiation in patients with fHP.[46] Six months after drug initiation, patients on MMF or AZA were on lower mean daily prednisone doses (12.3 ± 14 vs 3.8 ± 5.3 mg), with few treatment-related adverse events, although more patients were switched from AZA to MMF during the follow-up period. In another large study of 131 patients with fHP, the use of MMF or AZA was associated with a marginally slowed FVC% decline compared with patients on prednisone alone.[47] MMF or AZA was associated with fewer treatment emergent adverse events compared with prednisone alone in this cohort. However, these data are limited by their retrospective nature and cannot inform treatment decisions on a more granular scale when considering disease severity, bronchoscopic findings, or antigen status (eg, identified vs unidentified, remediated vs ongoing exposure). Taken together, the data support a role for MMF or AZA as steroid-sparing agents in select patients with fHP, but prospective randomized studies are needed to fully address this question.

Other immunosuppressive agents have been used to treat patients with fHP. In small retrospective studies, intravenous cyclophosphamide has been shown to slow lung function decline in selected patients.[48,49] In 1 case series of 64 patients, the mean decline in FVC% and DLCO% in the preceding 12 months was −8% ± 18% and −18.3% ± 18% respectively, whereas, following cyclophosphamide treatment, it decreased to −1.2% ± 15% and −3.8% ± 17% (P = .02).[49] However, the effectiveness on lung function stabilization was not as marked as their connective tissue disease–ILD counterparts, and cyclophosphamide carries risk of serious infection, side effects, and toxicity.[49] Rituximab use has been reported in patients with progressive fHP in small retrospective studies. In 3 of 6 patients with fHP treated with rituximab, lung function stabilized, whereas the other 3 patients developed progressive respiratory failure and died.[50] A larger retrospective study reported its use in patients with fHP, but limitations of the data preclude robust conclusions about its efficacy, safety, or role.[51]

The management of fHP is largely extrapolated from the treatment approach of nonfibrotic HP and other acute inflammatory lung conditions; however, the efficacy and safety of these approaches is unclear. Combined immunosuppression with prednisone, n-acetylcysteine, and AZA was at one time considered routine care for patients with IPF, until it was discovered to be potentially harmful and associated with higher mortality risk.[52] Further analyses of the data found that patients with a genetic variant resulting in a shorter peripheral blood leukocyte telomere length (TERT, TERC, RTEL1, and PARN) were more likely to die, require lung transplant, experience an FVC decline, or become hospitalized when treated with combined immunosuppression compared with placebo-treated controls.[53] Given that a proportion of patients with fHP are known to have these genetic variants,[33] this raises important questions about the current approach to management. Further research into the relationships between genetic variants and treatments responses in these patients is urgently needed. Notably, there are no data to inform the safety or appropriateness of reducing or discontinuing immunomodulatory therapy in patients with fHP, representing another important area for future research.

Antifibrotic therapy

Immunomodulatory treatments may target the proinflammatory pathways in some forms of fHP, but do not address profibrotic mechanisms, and, despite immunomodulatory treatment and even apparent antigen remediation, many patients with fHP experience progressive disease.

The antifibrotic agents pirfenidone and nintedanib are recommended for the treatment of patients with IPF and have now been studied in other progressive fibrosing ILDs, including fHP. In a small retrospective cohort study, pirfenidone slowed lung function decline in patients with chronic HP, when FVC% decline was compared before and after treatment initiation.[54] However, these findings have important limitations, and the role of pirfenidone will be clarified with data from an ongoing randomized controlled trial in patients with fHP.[55] The INBUILD study recruited patients with non-IPF progressive fibrosing ILDs, finding that nintedanib slowed disease progression compared with placebo as measured by FVC decline at 52 weeks. In the subgroup analysis of patients with HP (84 received nintedanib, 89 received placebo), nintedanib reduced the rate of FVC decline by 73.1 mL/y (95% confidence interval, 8.6–154.8) compared with placebo. This effect was consistent across the other diagnostic subgroups.[56] Notably, INBUILD patients were not permitted to be on baseline immunomodulatory therapy at time of trial enrollment.

To further inform the role of antifibrotics as treatment of fHP, future studies should carefully endotype and phenotype patients to provide clinically applicable treatment algorithms to this subgroup of patients with PF-ILD. More data are needed to guide the use of combination MMF and nintedanib therapy in this patient population, and to better inform their efficacy and when treatment regimens should be changed. It is hoped that patients with fHP will be included in upcoming trials of novel therapeutics for pulmonary fibrosis.

Other medical therapies

There are no clear data supporting a role for antifungal or antimycobacterial therapy in patients with fHP, although case reports have described the use of antimycobacterial therapy in MAC-associated hot tub lung or humidifier lung.[57] The use of macrolide therapy is being studied in IPF[58] but has not been assessed in human trials of fHP. Pulmonary hypertension as a result of fHP is an indication of advanced disease, but, similar to other forms of fibrotic ILD, PH-specific treatments are not currently recommended for these patients.

Nonpharmacologic management

Pulmonary rehabilitation is an important component to general ILD management, and improves dyspnea, functional capacity, and quality of life in the short term,[59] but with less robust evidence for longer-term benefit.[60] Oxygen supplementation should be considered in patients with resting or exertional hypoxemia; limited evidence suggests it improves dyspnea and exercise tolerance, and theoretically reduces the development of secondary pulmonary hypertension and right heart failure.[61] All other forms of supportive care should be considered in patients with fHP, given the frequency of advanced and progressive disease. Patients with fHP have worse health-related quality of life compared with patients with IPF.[54] A recent mixed-methods study explored reasons for this, finding that complex psychosocial problems associated with antigen avoidance and identification contributed to patients' unique experience with this disease.[62,63] These considerations are important in comprehensive patient management.

Lung transplant

Lung transplant should be considered for appropriate patients with fHP with advanced disease or a progressive phenotype despite optimal treatment. Survival after lung transplant in patients with fHP seems better than in their IPF counterparts; 1 case series analyzing 31 HP and 91 IPF cases found survival was significantly better in the HP group compared with the IPF group at 1, 3, and

5 years with transplant-related HP survival 96%, 89%, and 89% and transplant-related IPF survival 85%, 67%, and 49% respectively.[14] HP can reoccur in the transplanted lung, reported in 2 out of 31 cases after reexposure to the inciting antigen.[14,64]

SUMMARY

FHP represents an important phenotype of ILD and is important to accurately diagnose. Patients with fHP experience disease progression, early mortality, and impaired disease-related quality of life. The mainstay of disease management remains antigen remediation and cessation of exposure where possible. Systemic immunomodulatory therapies should be considered in symptomatic or progressive disease, with antifibrotics showing efficacy in slowing the rate of disease progression in patients with a progressive phenotype. Early referral for lung transplant should be considered in select patients given the high rates of progressive disease, with supportive and nonpharmacologic care offered similarly to other forms of pulmonary fibrosis. Future work should focus on understanding the genetic and immunologic risk factors for disease, the relationship with antigen exposure, and developing biomarkers to guide therapeutic decision making.

CLINICS CARE POINTS

- Review of clinical, HRCT and pathological information at a multi-disciplinary meeting is recommended.
- Identification of potential exposures through clinical history and questionnaires is recommended for both diagnosis and exposure remediation.
- Steroids may benefit those with BAL lymphocytosis; but should be used judiciously in those with fHP, after consideration of risks and benefits.
- MMF and AZA may be used as steroid-sparing agents or in those who long-term immunosuppression may be of benefit.
- Limited data suggests anti-fibrotic therapy may be of benefit in fHP.
- Non-pharmacological treatment including pulmonary rehabilitation, and oxygen therapy and lung transplantation should be considered where appropriate.

DISCLOSURE

The authors have nothing to disclose.

REFERENCES

1. Fernandez Perez ER, Kong AM, Raimundo K, et al. Epidemiology of hypersensitivity pneumonitis among an insured population in the United States: a claims-based cohort analysis. Ann Am Thorac Soc 2018;15(4):460–9.
2. Cottin V, Hirani NA, Hotchkin DL, et al. Presentation, diagnosis and clinical course of the spectrum of progressive-fibrosing interstitial lung diseases. Eur Respir Rev 2018;27(150). https://doi.org/10.1183/16000617.0076-2018.
3. Barber CM, Wiggans RE, Carder M, et al. Epidemiology of occupational hypersensitivity pneumonitis; reports from the SWORD scheme in the UK from 1996 to 2015. Occup Environ Med 2017;74:528–30.
4. Bang KM, Weissman DN, Pinheiro GA, et al. Twenty-three years of hypersensitivity pneumonitis mortality surveillance in the United States. Am J Ind Med 2006;49(12):997–1004.
5. Charitopoulos K, Gioulekas D, Sichletidis L, et al. Hypoxemia: an early indication of pigeon breeders' disease. Clinical and laboratory findings among pigeon breeders in the Salonica area. J Investig Allergol Clin Immunol 2005;15(3):211–5.
6. Banham SW, McSharry C, Lynch PP, et al. Relationships between avian exposure, humoral immune response, and pigeon breeders' disease among Scottish pigeon fanciers. Thorax 1986;41(4):274–8.
7. Hoppin JA, Umbach DM, Kullman GJ, et al. Pesticides and other agricultural factors associated with self-reported farmer's lung among farm residents in the Agricultural Health Study. Occup Environ Med 2007;64(5):334–41.
8. Stanford CF, Hall G, Chivers A, et al. Farmer's lung in Northern Ireland. Br J Ind Med 1990;47(5):314–6.
9. Vasakova M, Morell F, Walsh S, et al. Hypersensitivity pneumonitis: perspectives in diagnosis and management. Am J Respir Crit Care Med 2017;196(6):680–9.
10. Raghu G, Document S, Remy-Jardin M, et al. Diagnosis of hypersensitivity pneumonitis in adults: an official ATS/JRS/ALAT clinical practice guideline. Am J Respir Crit Care Med 2020. https://doi.org/10.1164/rccm.202005-2032ST.
11. Salisbury ML, Gu T, Murray S, et al. Hypersensitivity pneumonitis: radiologic phenotypes are associated with distinct survival time and pulmonary function trajectory. Chest 2019;155(4):699–711.
12. Mooney JJ, Elicker BM, Urbania TH, et al. Radiographic fibrosis score predicts survival in hypersensitivity pneumonitis. Chest 2013;144(2):586–92.

13. Morell F, Villar A, Montero M, et al. Chronic hypersensitivity pneumonitis in patients diagnosed with idiopathic pulmonary fibrosis: a prospective case-cohort study. Lancet Respir Med 2013; 1(9):685–94.

14. Kern RM, Singer JP, Koth L, et al. Lung transplantation for hypersensitivity pneumonitis. Chest 2015; 147(6):1558–65.

15. Jo HE, Prasad JD, Troy LK, et al. Diagnosis and management of idiopathic pulmonary fibrosis: Thoracic Society of Australia and New Zealand and Lung Foundation Australia position statements summary. Med J Aust 2018;208(2):82–8.

16. Barnes H, Morisset J, Molyneaux P, et al. A systematically derived exposure assessment instrument for chronic hypersensitivity pneumonitis. Chest 2020;157(6):1506–12.

17. Fernandez Perez ER, Swigris JJ, Forssen AV, et al. Identifying an inciting antigen is associated with improved survival in patients with chronic hypersensitivity pneumonitis. Chest 2013;144(5):1644–51.

18. Jenkins AR, Chua A, Chami HA, et al. Questionnaires or Serum IgG testing in the diagnosis of hypersensitivity pneumonitis among patients with interstitial lung disease. Ann Am Thorac Soc 2020. https://doi.org/10.1513/AnnalsATS.202005-419OC.

19. Suhara K, Miyazaki Y, Okamoto T, et al. Utility of immunological tests for bird-related hypersensitivity pneumonitis. Respir Invest 2015;53(1):13–21.

20. Johannson KA, Barnes H, Bellanger A-P, et al. Exposure assessment tools for hypersensitivity pneumonitis. an official American Thoracic Society Workshop Report. Ann Am Thorac Soc 2020;17(12):1501–9.

21. Lynch DA, Sverzellati N, Travis WD, et al. Diagnostic criteria for idiopathic pulmonary fibrosis: a Fleischner Society white paper. Lancet Respir Med 2018; 6(2):138–53.

22. Ohtani Y, Hisauchi K, Sumi Y, et al. Sequential changes in bronchoalveolar lavage cells and cytokines in a patient progressing from acute to chronic bird Fancier's lung disease. Intern Med 1999;38(11): 896–9.

23. Ohtani Y, Saiki S, Kitaichi M, et al. Chronic bird fancier's lung: histopathological and clinical correlation. An application of the 2002 ATS/ERS consensus classification of the idiopathic interstitial pneumonias. Thorax 2005;60(8):665–71.

24. Adderley N, Humphreys CJ, Barnes H, et al. Bronchoalveolar lavage fluid lymphocytosis in chronic hypersensitivity pneumonitis: a systematic review and meta-analysis. Eur Respir J 2020;2000206. https://doi.org/10.1183/13993003.00206-2020.

25. Churg A, Bilawich A, Wright JL. Pathology of chronic hypersensitivity pneumonitis what is it? what are the diagnostic criteria? why do we care? Arch Pathol Lab Med 2018;142(1):109–19.

26. Fisher JH, Shapera S, To T, et al. Procedure volume and mortality after surgical lung biopsy in interstitial lung disease. Eur Respir J 2019;53(2). https://doi.org/10.1183/13993003.01164-2018.

27. Troy LK, Grainge C, Corte TJ, et al. Diagnostic accuracy of transbronchial lung cryobiopsy for interstitial lung disease diagnosis (COLDICE): a prospective, comparative study. Lancet Respir Med 2019. https://doi.org/10.1016/s2213-2600(19)30342-x.

28. Wuyts WA, Agostini C, Antoniou KM, et al. The pathogenesis of pulmonary fibrosis: a moving target. Eur Respir J 2013;41(5):1207–18.

29. Blanchet MR, Israel-Assayag E, Cormier Y. Inhibitory effect of nicotine on experimental hypersensitivity pneumonitis in vivo and in vitro. Am J Respir Crit Care Med 2004;169(8):903–9.

30. Falfan-Valencia R, Camarena A, Pineda CL, et al. Genetic susceptibility to multicase hypersensitivity pneumonitis is associated with the TNF-238 GG genotype of the promoter region and HLA-DRB1*04 bearing HLA haplotypes. Respir Med 2014;108(1): 211–7.

31. Furusawa H, Cardwell JH, Okamoto T, et al. Chronic hypersensitivity pneumonitis, an interstitial lung disease with distinct molecular signatures. Am J Respir Crit Care Med 2020. https://doi.org/10.1164/rccm. 202001-0134OC.

32. Ley B, Newton CA, Arnould I, et al. The MUC5B promoter polymorphism and telomere length in patients with chronic hypersensitivity pneumonitis: an observational cohort-control study. Lancet Respir Med 2017;5(8):639–47.

33. Ley B, Torgerson DG, Oldham JM, et al. Rare protein-altering telomere-related gene variants in patients with chronic hypersensitivity pneumonitis. Am J Respir Crit Care Med 2019;200(9): 1154–63.

34. Okamoto T, Miyazaki Y, Tomita M, et al. A familial history of pulmonary fibrosis in patients with chronic hypersensitivity pneumonitis. Respiration 2013;85(5): 384–90.

35. Inase N, Ohtani Y, Usui Y, et al. Chronic summer-type hypersensitivity pneumonitis: clinical similarities to idiopathic pulmonary fibrosis. Sarcoidosis Vasc Diffuse Lung Dis 2007;24(2):141–7.

36. Sema M, Miyazaki Y, Tsutsui T, et al. Environmental levels of avian antigen are relevant to the progression of chronic hypersensitivity pneumonitis during antigen avoidance. Immun Inflamm Dis 2018;6(1): 154–62.

37. Gimenez A, Storrer K, Kuranishi L, et al. Change in FVC and survival in chronic fibrotic hypersensitivity pneumonitis. Thorax 2018;73(4):391–2.

38. Baverstock AM, White RJ. A hazard of christmas: bird fancier's lung and the christmas tree. Respir Med 2000;94(2):176.

39. Greinert U, Lepp U, Becker W. Bird Keeper's lung without bird keepinge. Eur J Med Res 2000;5(3):124.

40. Rose CS, Martyny JW, Newman LS, et al. Lifeguard lung": Endemic granulomatous pneumonitis in an indoor swimming pool. Am J Public Health 1998;88(12):1795–800.

41. Ross AS, Teschke K, Brauer M, et al. Determinants of exposure to metalworking fluid aerosol in small machine shops. Ann Occup Hyg 2004;48(5):383–91.

42. Cormier Y. Hypersensitivity pneumonitis (extrinsic allergic alveolitis): a Canadian historical perspective. Can Respir J 2014;21(5):277–8.

43. Muller-Wening D, Schmitt M. Comparison of the effectiveness of two respirators in farmers suffering from farmer's lung. [German]. Pneumologie 1990;44(5):781–6.

44. Kokkarinen JI, Tukiainen HO, Terho EO. Effect of corticosteroid treatment on the recovery of pulmonary function in farmer's lung. Am Rev Respir Dis 1992;145(1):3–5.

45. De Sadeleer LJ, Hermans F, De Dycker E, et al. Effects of corticosteroid treatment and antigen avoidance in a large hypersensitivity pneumonitis cohort: a single-centre cohort study. J Clin Med 2018;8(1):14.

46. Morisset J, Johannson KA, Vittinghoff E, et al. Use of mycophenolate mofetil or azathioprine for the management of chronic hypersensitivity pneumonitis. Chest 2017;151(3):619–25.

47. Adegunsoye A, Oldham JM, Fernandez Perez ER, et al. Outcomes of immunosuppressive therapy in chronic hypersensitivity pneumonitis. ERJ Open Res 2017;3(3). https://doi.org/10.1183/23120541.00016-2017.

48. Wiertz IA, van Moorsel CHM, Van Moorsel CHM, et al. Cyclophosphamide in steroid-refractory hypersensitivity pneumonitis and non-classifiable interstitial lung disease. Eur Respir J 2017;50(suppl 61):PA3828.

49. Hastings RA, Saunders P, Hogben C, et al. P164 Cyclophosphamide for the treatment of refractory chronic hypersensitivity pneumonitis. Thorax 2018;73(Suppl 4):A191.

50. Lota HK, Keir GJ, Hansell DM, et al. Novel use of rituximab in hypersensitivity pneumonitis refractory to conventional treatment. Thorax 2013;68(8):780.

51. Ferreira M, Borie R, Crestani B, et al. Efficacy and safety of rituximab in patients with chronic hypersensitivity pneumonitis (cHP): a retrospective, multicentric, observational study. Respir Med 2020;106146. https://doi.org/10.1016/j.rmed.2020.106146.

52. The Idiopathic Pulmonary Fibrosis Clinical Research Network. Prednisone, azathioprine, and N-acetylcysteine for pulmonary fibrosis. N Engl J Med 2012;366(21):1968–77.

53. Newton CA, Zhang D, Oldham JM, et al. Telomere length and use of immunosuppressive medications in idiopathic pulmonary fibrosis. Am J Respir Crit Care Med 2019;200(3):336–47.

54. Shibata SFH, Inase N. Pirfenidone in chronic hypersensitivity pneumonitis: a real-life experience. Sarcoidosis Vasc Diffuse Lung Dis 2018;35:139–42.

55. ClinicalTrials.gov [Internet]. Bethesda (MD): National Library of Medicine (US) Identifier: NCT02958917. Study of Efficacy and Safety of Pirfenidone in Patients With Fibrotic Hypersensitivity Pneumonitis 2016. Available at: https://www.clinicaltrials.gov/ct2/show/NCT02958917.

56. Wells AU, Flaherty KR, Brown KK, et al. Nintedanib in patients with progressive fibrosing interstitial lung diseases-subgroup analyses by interstitial lung disease diagnosis in the INBUILD trial: a randomised, double-blind, placebo-controlled, parallel-group trial. Lancet Respir Med 2020;8(5):453–60.

57. Hanak V, Kalra S, Aksamit TR, et al. Hot tub lung: presenting features and clinical course of 21 patients. Respir Med 2006;100(4):610–5.

58. Anstrom KJ, Noth I, Flaherty KR, et al. Design and rationale of a multi-center, pragmatic, open-label randomized trial of antimicrobial therapy - the study of clinical efficacy of antimicrobial therapy strategy using pragmatic design in Idiopathic Pulmonary Fibrosis (CleanUP-IPF) clinical trial. Respir Res 2020;21(1):68.

59. Dowman L, Hill CJ, Holland AE. Pulmonary rehabilitation for interstitial lung disease. Cochrane Database Syst Rev 2014;10. https://doi.org/10.1002/14651858.CD006322.pub3.

60. Perez-Bogerd S, Wuyts W, Barbier V, et al. Short and long-term effects of pulmonary rehabilitation in interstitial lung diseases: a randomised controlled trial. Respir Res 2018;19(1):182.

61. Bell EC, Cox NS, Goh N, et al. Oxygen therapy for interstitial lung disease: a systematic review. Eur Respir Rev 2017;26(143):160080.

62. Lubin M, Chen H, Elicker B, et al. A comparison of health-related quality of life in idiopathic pulmonary fibrosis and chronic hypersensitivity pneumonitis. Chest 2014;145(6):1333–8.

63. Aronson KI, Hayward BJ, Robbins L, et al. 'It's difficult, it's life changing what happens to you' patient perspective on life with chronic hypersensitivity pneumonitis: a qualitative study. BMJ Open Respir Res 2019;6(1):e000522.

64. Winstone T, Hague CJ, Churg A, et al. Biopsy-proven recurrent, acute, familial hypersensitivity pneumonitis: a case report and literature review. Respir Med Case Rep 2018;24:173–5.

Diagnosis and Management of Fibrotic Interstitial Lung Diseases

Bridget F. Collins, MD[a,*], Fabrizio Luppi, MD, PhD[b,c]

KEYWORDS

- Idiopathic pulmonary fibrosis • Progressive fibrotic interstitial lung disease • Antifibrotic treatment
- Pirfenidone • Nintedanib • Fibrotic hypersensitivity pneumonitis
- Connective tissue disease-interstitial lung disease • Unclassifiable interstitial lung disease

KEY POINTS

- Nonidiopathic pulmonary fibrosis (non-IPF) fibrotic interstitial lung diseases (ILDs) may progress and have clinical behavior similar to that of IPF. It is not yet known how to best predict which non-IPF ILDs will evolve to fibrosis and progress.
- The definition of progression in non-IPF fibrotic lung disease requires further study.
- Although antifibrotic drugs may slow the rate of lung function decline in patients with a variety of fibrotic lung diseases, accurate diagnosis remains critical when considering other facets of treatment and prognosis.
- Nonpharmacologic treatment options for progressive fibrotic lung diseases are essential and should be broadly considered.

INTRODUCTION

Although idiopathic pulmonary fibrosis (IPF) is the most well studied among the fibrotic interstitial lung diseases (ILDs), non-IPF fibrotic lung diseases may also have a progressive phenotype, hereafter referred to as non-IPF PF-ILD (progressive fibrotic interstitial lung disease).[1–3] In addition to IPF, the usual interstitial pneumonia (UIP) pattern on high-resolution computed tomography (HRCT) chest occurs in other ILDs such as connective tissue disease–associated ILD (CTD-ILD), fibrotic hypersensitivity pneumonitis (FHP), asbestosis, and others with substantial morbidity and mortality.[4,5] In fact, as is the case with UIP, among patients with fibrotic lung disease the underlying pattern and extent of fibrosis often influence outcomes and prognosis more strongly than the specific clinical diagnosis.[6–9]

There has been increasing interest in non-IPF PF-ILD, specifically characterizing fibrotic lung disease with a focus on clinical and pathophysiologic behavior rather than separating diagnoses based on specific cause.[10–12] Although accurate diagnosis is important, invasive procedures such as surgical lung biopsy are not without risk (mortality 1.7% for elective surgical lung biopsy) and some patients are too ill to tolerate or do not wish to undergo surgical lung biopsy or other invasive procedures.[13–15] Making a clear diagnosis can remain challenging and it is important to note that even when performed, surgical lung biopsy does not always yield a specific diagnosis, particularly in centers without access to expert multidisciplinary discussion (MDD).[14,15] ILD may remain unclassifiable in 10% to 15% of patients in spite of evaluation at an ILD center.[16,17] Some patients may therefore be left without a clear specific ILD diagnosis. Even among those who do

[a] Department of Medicine, Center for Interstitial Lung Diseases, University of Washington Medical Center, 1959 NE Pacific Street, Box 356166, Seattle, WA 98195-6166, USA; [b] Department of Medicine and Surgery, University of Milan Bicocca; [c] Pneumology Unit, Ospedale "S. Gerardo", ASST Monza, Monza, Italy
* Corresponding author.
E-mail addresses: bfc3@uw.edu; bfc3@medicine.washington.edu

Clin Chest Med 42 (2021) 321–335
https://doi.org/10.1016/j.ccm.2021.03.008
0272-5231/21/© 2021 Elsevier Inc. All rights reserved.

chestmed.theclinics.com

have a specific ILD diagnosis, little is known regarding the frequency with which nonfibrotic ILD may evolve to fibrotic disease or the frequency and rate at which such fibrotic lung disease will progress. The INBUILD study, a phase 3 clinical trial, demonstrated a decreased rate of decline in forced vital capacity (FVC) over 52 weeks among patients with non-IPF progressive fibrotic lung disease (PFLD) treated with nintedanib.[18] However, much remains unknown regarding optimal diagnosis and treatment of non-IPF-PFLD, particularly surrounding the role for immunosuppressive versus antifibrotic treatment. Debate continues regarding risks and benefits of "lumping" and "splitting" fibrotic ILDs and whether IPF itself is in fact a distinct clinical entity.[10,11,19] Given that non-IPF PF-ILD is not well defined, management is often challenging. In this review, we discuss facets of diagnosis and management of non-IPF fibrotic lung disease with a focus on patients with a progressive phenotype.

DEFINITION OF NON–IDIOPATHIC PULMONARY FIBROSIS PROGRESSIVE FIBROTIC LUNG DISEASE

Non-IPF PF-ILD can be defined in a variety of ways. The most basic description is of lung diseases with fibrosis on HRCT chest with accompanying worsening of symptoms, lung function, and radiographic evidence of fibrosis over time in spite of treatment directed at the underlying disease. Various definitions of the term "progressive" have been proposed in the context of fibrotic lung disease. In the INBUILD study, among patients with fibrosing lung disease affecting greater than 10% lung volume on HRCT, progression was defined as meeting at least 1 of the following within 24 months: (1) relative decline of FVC of 10% predicted, (2) relative decline in FVC of 5% to <10% and worsening respiratory symptoms or increased fibrosis on HRCT, (3) worsening respiratory symptoms and increased fibrosis on HRCT.[18] Cottin and colleagues[1] defined "progressive" as characterizing patients with fibrotic lung disease meeting 1 the following criteria within 24 months: (1) relative decline of ≥10% FVC, (2) relative decline of ≥15% diffusing capacity of carbon monoxide (DLCO), or (3) worsening symptoms or worsening radiographic appearance *with* ≥5% to 10% relative decline in FVC. A recent position statement from the Erice ILD working group defined progressive fibrosis in clinical practice as demonstration of 1 or more of the following over 24 months in spite of treatment: (1) relative decline of ≥10% FVC, (2) relative decline of ≥5% FVC with decline in DLCO of ≥15%, (3) relative decline of FVC of

≥5% with increased fibrosis on HRCT, (4) relative decline of FVC ≥5% with progressive symptoms, (5) progressive symptoms with increased fibrosis on HRCT.[20] A primary challenge of such criteria surrounds how to measure and quantify worsening of respiratory symptoms as well as other factors that may signify progression, such as reductions in exercise capacity and worsening quality of life. There is not one universally accepted definition of PFLD at this time.

SUBSETS OF PROGRESSIVE FIBROTIC INTERSTITIAL LUNG DISEASE

Epidemiology of non-IPF PF-LD is challenging to characterize due to innate heterogeneity in how diagnoses are and in disease behavior.[21] Unlike IPF, in which fibrotic lung disease is uniformly progressive, albeit at varying rates, some ILDs have both nonfibrotic, fibrotic, and progressive fibrotic phenotypes, as shown in **Fig. 1**.[2,5,10,21–26] FHP, CTD-ILD such as rheumatoid arthritis (RA)-ILD or scleroderma ILD, interstitial pneumonia with autoimmune features (IPAF), idiopathic nonspecific interstitial pneumonia (iNSIP), occupational ILD and other

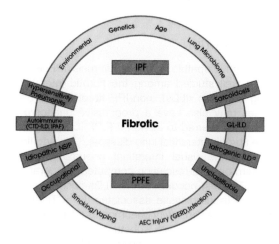

Nonfibrotic

Fig. 1. Types of ILD with both nonfibrotic and fibrotic phenotypes and only fibrotic phenotypes. Factors influencing disease development and clinical course with associated examples include environmental (air pollution, individual level domestic and occupational exposures), genetic (presence of MUC5B promotor polymorphism, mutations in telomere maintenance genes, sex by birth), age, lung microbiome, alveolar epithelial cell injury (via gastroesophageal reflux, infection), cigarette smoking and vaping. [a]Iatrogenic: refers to medication-induced and radiation-associated interstitial lung diseases. AEC, alveolar epithelial cell; NSIP, nonspecific interstitial pneumonia; PPFE, pleuroparenchymal fibroelastosis. (*Courtesy of* Sean McLaughlin.)

fibrotic ILDs may stabilize or may progress despite treatment.[2,10,27] The frequency and timing with which such diseases progress is not well understood or described.[21,28] Environmental factors (occupational, domestic, air pollution), recurrent alveolar epithelial injury (via gastroesophageal reflux), and host factors (genetics, lung microbiome) likely interact to influence which patients develop PFLD (see **Fig. 1**).[29–33] Regardless of cause, some patients with non-IPF PF-ILD will have clinical behavior similar to those with IPF; among patients with progressive fibrotic ILD in the placebo group of the INBUILD study, 1-year rates in decline in FVC were similar to those seen among IPF patients in the placebo group of the INPULSIS trial (**Fig. 2**).[18,34] Mortality was also similar between non-IPF PF-ILD and IPF groups, particularly for patients with a UIP like pattern of fibrosis.[34] These data lend support to the concept that clinical behavior, underlying pattern, and extent of fibrosis may have greater influence on outcomes such as survival than does underlying cause of disease.[11,28,35] However, a limitation of INBUILD and subsequent analyses is that the population of patients studied was quite heterogeneous and factors other than UIP that may identify patients and disease groups at greatest risk of progression were not studied.

Little is known regarding which patients with nonfibrotic ILD may evolve to a fibrotic phenotype.[9,20] A recent study of 245 patients with fibrosing ILD followed at 2 Italian ILD referral centers found that 31% had progressive disease with iNSIP, CTD-ILD, chronic HP, and sarcoidosis most likely be progressive.[36] Progression was defined based on the INBUILD trial criteria; most

of the patients met criteria for progression based on FVC decline of $\geq 10\%$.[36] A study of physicians who routinely manage patients with ILD reported physician estimates that 18% to 32% of patients with non-IPF ILD will have progressive fibrosis.[37] Physicians identified unclassifiable ILD, RA-ILD, iNSIP, and systemic sclerosis (SSc)-ILD as non-IPF ILDs most often evolving to a progressive fibrotic phenotype.[37] Although chronic HP was not one of the non-IPF ILDs predicted to most frequently evolve to a progressive fibrotic phenotype in the aforementioned study, chronic HP may progress relatively rapidly, particularly if an offending antigen is not identified and avoided.[26,38,39] A study of patients with chronic HP recently demonstrated that monthly decline in FVC % predicted over 1 year was similar to decline among patients with IPF.[40] Morell and colleagues[41] found that 20 of 46 patients diagnosed with IPF based on 2011 guideline criteria actually had HP after detailed exposure history and further evaluation, raising the possibility that there is a larger group of patients diagnosed with IPF who actually have progressive fibrotic chronic HP.

Other ILDs, such as sarcoidosis or occupational associated lung disease, may have a progressive fibrotic phenotype.[22,42] Approximately 20% of patients with sarcoidosis will develop fibrotic lung disease, some of whom will progress.[22] Among patients with stage IV sarcoidosis, survival is reduced, with 75% of deaths attributable to respiratory causes.[43] Patients with sarcoidosis and UIP have been described with median survival similar to that of patients with IPF, although further study is needed to determine whether this represents a coincidence, a distinct phenotype or a final

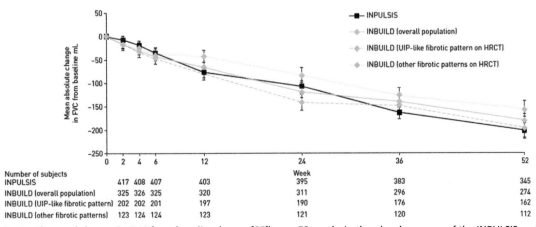

Fig. 2. Observed change in FVC from baseline (mean [SE]) over 52 weeks in the placebo group of the INPULSIS and INBUILD trials. (*From*: KK Brown et al. The natural history of progressive fibrosing interstitial lung diseases. Eur Respir J. 2020; 55(6). Reproduced with permission of the © ERS 2020: European Respiratory Journal 2020 55: 2000085; https://doi.org/10.1183/13993003.00085-2020.)

common pathway in fibrotic lung disease.[44,45] Occupational exposures may also be associated with progressive pulmonary fibrosis. In addition to classic progressive massive fibrosis, interstitial fibrosis was seen on histopathology, including some areas of UIP like fibrosis among coal miners with rapidly progressive pneumoconiosis in the setting of silica exposure.[42]

Although unclassifiable pulmonary fibrosis (PF) may fall under the umbrella of non-IPF PF-ILD, unclassifiable PF is a distinct entity encompassing 10% of patients with ILD despite MDD and evaluation at an ILD center.[16] Iatrogenic causes of ILD include medication-related nonfibrotic and fibrotic ILD and radiation pneumonitis and fibrosis.[46,47] Granulomatous ILD (GL-ILD), occurring in some patients with common variable immunodeficiency (CVID), may manifest with progressive fibrosis.[48] IPAF has been shown behave similarly to IPF in some studies, particularly among patients with IPAF with UIP, although IPAF is not universally fibrotic.[49,50] Cystic lung disease such as pulmonary Langerhans cell histiocytosis may progress to a fibrotic phenotype.[51] Smoking-related ILDs include respiratory bronchiolitis–associated ILD (RB-ILD) and desquamative interstitial pneumonia (DIP); patients with DIP may manifest progressive pulmonary fibrosis.[52] Smoking-related interstitial fibrosis has also been described as a distinct entity.[52–54] E-cigarette or vaping-related acute lung injury (EVALI) is a recently described form of lung injury related to vaping; various patterns of ILD such as organizing pneumonia, peribronchiolar granulomatous pneumonitis, diffuse alveolar damage, and eosinophilic pneumonia have been described in patients with EVALI, which could have long-term consequences resulting in fibrotic lung disease.[55–57]

DIAGNOSIS

Making a precise ILD diagnosis can be challenging and multiple diagnostic tests are often obtained, placing a burden on patients as well as health care systems.[58] Tools in making an accurate diagnosis of ILD include clinical history, physical examination, HCRT chest, serologic/laboratory evaluation, lung function testing, bronchoscopy for bronchoalveolar lavage, and in some cases histopathology. MDD, particularly in cases in which diagnosis is not clear, is essential to ILD diagnosis and is recommended by the IPF and HP diagnostic guidelines as well as statements on classification of idiopathic interstitial pneumonias and progressive fibrotic ILDs.[2,20,59,60] Although patients with some non-IPF PF-ILD may have clinical behavior similar to patients with IPF, accurate diagnosis

remains critical in most cases, especially surrounding treatment decisions and prognosis. For instance, fibrotic HP is often underrecognized, yet in some cases antigen identification and avoidance may lead to improvement and stabilization in clinical course.[23,26,41] Likewise, immunosuppressive medications have been shown to be associated with increased risk of death and hospitalization in most patients with IPF, whereas immunosuppression may lead to stabilization or even improvement in lung function in other fibrotic lung diseases such as scleroderma ILD.[61–63]

Clinical history is the key element to an accurate diagnosis of ILD and is emphasized in the American Thoracic Society/European Respiratory Society/Japanese Respiratory Society/Latin American Thoracic Association (ATS/ERS/JRS/ALAT) clinical practice guidelines for diagnosis of IPF as well as the recently published ATS/JRS/ALAT clinical practice guideline for diagnosis of hypersensitivity pneumonitis.[5,23,59] The importance of a detailed exposure history was illustrated in a study by Morell and colleagues,[41] in which nearly half of patients diagnosed with IPF based on 2011 guideline criteria were reclassified as having HP after a detailed exposure history and additional testing was obtained. There is not yet a standardized and validated questionnaire to aid in taking a detailed exposure history, although this was emphasized as an important area of future study in recently published guideline for diagnosis of hypersensitivity pneumonitis.[23] Providers should perform a thorough inquiry regarding both domestic and occupational exposures with particular attention to geographic and cultural factors that may influence exposures by region.[23,64] Physical examination focused on identifying signs of connective tissue disease, lung function testing, and serologic studies for CTD as well as immunoglobulin G antibodies to antigens known to be associated with HP further aid in making an accurate ILD diagnosis.[23,59] When histopathology is needed, transbronchial lung cryobiopsy has been shown to have relatively high levels of histopathologic agreement in comparison to surgical lung biopsy among patients with ILD and increase diagnostic confidence, although use is not yet universal.[65,66]

Development of biomarkers and genetic tests to aide in ILD diagnosis is ongoing. The envisia genomic classifier is one such tool that takes small amounts of lung tissue via transbronchial biopsy and classifies patients as having UIP or non-UIP with 88% specificity and 70% sensitivity.[67] A recent study in a second validation cohort demonstrated similar sensitivity and specificity of the envisia molecular classifier to detect UIP with diagnostic yield further increased when results were interpreted in conjunction with HRCT findings.[68] Quantitative HRCT chest as well as other advanced imaging tools and machine learning may facilitate ILD diagnosis in the future and inform prognosis.[69–71] Shaish and colleagues[72] recently described a machine learning algorithm using a convolutional neural network to predict histopathologic UIP through a virtual surgical lung biopsy wedge resection in a proof of concept study. Future studies of machine learning techniques in ILD diagnosis are eagerly awaited. An international working group recently proposed an ontological framework for classifying fibrotic ILDs.[73] A confident diagnosis was one for which the diagnosis met guideline criteria or in which the provider had ≥90% confidence based on clinical judgment, a provisional diagnosis may be high confidence (70%–89% confidence) or low confidence (51%–69% confidence), and if confidence was ≤50% the fibrotic ILD was considered unclassifiable.[73] It is important to note that the acceptable level of diagnostic confidence will vary based on patient preferences and characteristics; in the setting of advanced disease or significant comorbidities, some patients are not able to safely undergo diagnostic procedures or may not be willing. Although achieving as accurate a diagnosis as safely as possible is the goal, a critical question to consider is how management will or will not change with additional data. For some patients, more specific characterization of PFLD through additional diagnostic testing may be helpful in terms of qualifying for various treatments or clinical trials. Informed shared decision making and MDD between providers and patients is often helpful when making complex decisions regarding next steps in diagnosis and treatment of non-IPF PF-ILD.[74]

TREATMENT

Treatment of fibrotic lung disease is both pharmacologic and nonpharmacologic as outlined in **Table 1**. There are few randomized controlled clinical trials of immunosuppressive medications to treat fibrotic ILD outside of scleroderma ILD, in which immunosuppression has been helpful in some cases, and IPF, in which immunosuppression has been harmful.[61–63] A recent study of patients with fibrotic lung disease seen at 2 Italian referral centers demonstrated that most patients (93%) with progressive disease were prescribed pharmacologic treatment after diagnosis (most common diagnoses: iNSIP, CTD-ILD, sarcoidosis and hypersensitivity pneumonitis).[36] Corticosteroids were frequently utilized, with 40% of patients treated with steroids alone and 52% treated with

both steroids and a steroid-sparing immunosuppressive agent; 2 patients received an antifibrotic drug as part of a clinical trial.[36]

Pharmacologic Treatment

Targeting the fibrotic cascade has been a cornerstone of treatment for IPF. Two antifibrotic drugs, pirfenidone and nintedanib, were approved by the US Food and Drug Administration for treatment of IPF in 2014 and previously by the European EMA, after both drugs were shown to reduce the rate of decline in lung function over 52 weeks among patients with IPF who have a moderately reduced FVC.[75,76] These drugs are conditionally recommended for treatment of IPF in the most recent IPF evidence-based guidelines.[59] Pirfenidone and nintedanib effects on rate of decline in FVC have been similar among patients with IPF who have mild or severe disease in subsequent studies.[77–80] Pirfenidone exerts antifibrotic, anti-inflammatory, and antioxidative effects through a mechanism that while not well understood, leads to suppression of transforming growth factor beta (TGFB) and reduction in collagen synthesis and deposition.[81–83] Nintedanib is an intracellular tyrosine kinase inhibitor that inhibits the platelet derived growth factor receptor, vascular endothelial growth factor receptor and fibroblast growth factor receptor resulting in inhibition of downstream signaling pathways that stimulate proliferation, migration and maturation of lung fibroblasts.[84] Given overlap in predisposing genetic factors, molecular mechanisms of fibrosis and clinical course between IPF and non-IPF PF, nintedanib and pirfenidone have recently been studied in non-IPF PFLD.[18,28]

Among non-IPF fibrotic lung diseases, scleroderma ILD is the best studied. Scleroderma ILD has been shown to share similar pathophysiologic mechanisms with IPF, particularly surrounding the role of TGFB upregulation and deposition of excess extracellular matrix.[85–87] The SENSCIS trial randomized patients with scleroderma and ILD affecting at least 10% of the lungs on HRCT to nintedanib versus placebo.[87,88] This trial demonstrated reduced rate of decline in FVC over 52 weeks in the nintedanib group compared with the placebo group (adjusted annual rate of change in FVC −52.4 mL in the nintedanib group, −93.3 mL in the placebo group) although there were not significant effects on skin sclerosis.[87] The study did include some patients on stable doses of ≤10 mg prednisone, mycophenolate, or methotrexate in the 6 months leading up to enrollment. The SLS III study, randomizing patients to pirfenidone and mycophenolate versus

Table 1
Pharmacologic and nonpharmacologic treatment of progressive pulmonary fibrosis

Pharmacologic	Nonpharmacologic
Disease modifying	Pulmonary rehab
Antifibrotics (pirfenidone, nintedanib)	Supplemental oxygen (O2)
Immunomodulatory medications	Avoidance of potential environmental contributors
Diagnosis and treatment of comorbid conditions (ie, GERD, PH, CAD)	Lifestyle modification (smoking cessation, conservative measures to reduce GERD, weight loss)
Symptom modifying-identify and treat:	Appropriate vaccinations
Contributors to cough (asthma, postnasal drip, GERD)	Education and support
Contributors to fatigue (OSA, hypothyroidism)	Lung transplant referral when appropriate
Anxiety and depression	Advance care planning
Dyspnea (low-dose opiates)	Dyspnea (hand-held fans, modification of O2 carrying devices, breathing techniques)
Participation in clinical trials and registries	

Abbreviations: CAD, coronary artery disease; GERD, gastroesophageal reflux disease; OSA, obstructive sleep apnea; PH, pulmonary hypertension.

mycophenolate alone is currently ongoing.[89] A previous study, the LOTUSS study, showed that pirfenidone had acceptable safety and tolerability among patients with SSc-ILD although the study was not designed to assess potential effects on lung function.[90]

The INBUILD study randomized patients with PF-ILD with greater than 10% lung volume occupied by fibrosis on HRCT chest who met criteria for progression as described above to nintedanib or placebo. This study demonstrated reduced annual rate of decline in FVC among patients in the nintedanib group (−80 mL/y) compared with the placebo group (−187.8 mL/y).[18] This effect persisted among subsets of patients with UIP-like and non-UIP fibrotic patterns although was slightly more pronounced among patients with a UIP-like pattern.[18] The INBUILD study was not powered to assess potential benefit of nintedanib by specific diagnostic subgroup, although effects on reduced annual rate of FVC decline were maintained across prespecified groups of ILD diagnoses (chronic hypersensitivity pneumonitis, autoimmune-ILD, iNSIP, unclassifiable idiopathic interstitial pneumonias, and other ILDs) on subgroup analysis.[91]

A recent phase 2 study of pirfenidone versus placebo among patients with unclassifiable PFLD did not meet the primary endpoint (change in FVC measured by home spirometry) due to intraindividual variability in home spirometry measurements.[92] However, there was a reduced rate of decline in FVC measured by site spirometry in the pirfenidone group compared with the placebo group over 24 weeks (−17.8 mL/24 weeks in pirfenidone vs −113 mL/24 weeks in placebo) suggesting a beneficial effect of pirfenidone in the study population.[92] Additional clinical trials assessing efficacy of antifibrotic medications in other specific non-IPF pulmonary fibrotic diseases are ongoing and well described elsewhere.[93]

Although antifibrotic drugs may reduce the rate of decline in lung function among patients with PFLD, there are some cases in which immunosuppressive medications may be beneficial. Further study is needed in this area, as the combination of prednisone/azathioprine/N-acetylcysteine has been associated with increased risk of mortality and hospitalization compared with placebo among patients with IPF.[61] Effects of immunosuppressive medications on non-IPF progressive PF are largely unknown outside of SSc-ILD and likely vary by disease subtype. Diseases with more inflammatory features such as organizing pneumonia or subsets of CTD-ILD will likely be more responsive than others to steroids and other immunosuppressive medications such as cyclophosphamide, although further study is needed.[62,94,95] In some cases, treatment with both immunomodulatory medications and antifibrotics may be appropriate. Given the lack of clinical trials and studies addressing this question at present, MDD as well as shared decision making with patients and close clinical follow-up for changes in physiology as well as potential medication adverse effects will be essential.

Identification and treatment of comorbid conditions among patients with PF is necessary, with treatment of comorbidities conferring a survival benefit in some cases.[96,97] Common comorbid conditions include gastroesophageal reflux disease (GERD), ischemic heart disease (IHD), pulmonary hypertension (PH), obstructive sleep apnea (OSA), and lung cancer.[98,99] Treatment of these conditions may also provide some mitigation of symptoms such as cough, fatigue, and dyspnea.

Precision medicine may be useful in the future to guide pharmacologic treatment in PFLD. This is particularly appealing given heterogeneity within frequency of development and progression of fibrotic lung disease as well as potential differences in treatment response. This is illustrated by N-acetylcysteine (NAC), an antioxidant and glutathione precursor studied in IPF without effects on FVC in a randomized controlled trial.[100] A subsequent study demonstrated that among patients with IPF with a particular toll interacting protein (TOLLIP) genotype (TT), NAC was associated with improvement in composite endpoint-free survival (time from enrollment to death, transplant, hospitalization, decreased FVC $\geq$10%), whereas among patients with a CC genotype, NAC was associated with a trend toward harm.[101] TOLLIP genotype is not routinely checked in clinical practice at present. In the anticipated PRECISIONS study, a multicenter clinical trial, patients with IPF who have a TOLLIP TT genotype will be randomized to NAC or placebo and time to a composite endpoint (relative decline in FVC, first respiratory hospitalization, lung transplant, or all-cause mortality) will be assessed.[102] Future studies such as this, that leverage genetics or other biomarkers to identify patients most likely to respond to a medication, are particularly appealing for patients who fall into the broad and heterogeneous category of non-IPF PF-ILD.

Nonpharmacologic Treatment

Pulmonary rehabilitation has been shown to reduce dyspnea and improve quality of life and 6-minute walk distance among patients with various ILDs.[103–105] Patients who have more severe disease and exercise impairment have been shown to benefit the most from pulmonary rehabilitation, suggesting that significant limitations to exercise capacity should not be a deterrent when referring patients.[103,104,106] The IPF guidelines strongly recommend long-term supplemental oxygen use for patients with resting hypoxemia.[5] Some studies have shown improved quality of life and decreased shortness of breath associated with supplemental oxygen use among patients with IPF, whereas others have shown reduced quality of life, largely related to physical challenges

associated with using supplemental oxygen.[107–110] Further study of optimizing supplemental oxygen use to maximize potential benefits while minimizing associated challenges (such as the rapidity at which tanks require replacement) are needed. Additional important nonpharmacologic measures include education and communication surrounding diagnosis, treatment options, prognosis, and advanced care planning.[111–113] Low-dose opioids may be used for dyspnea among patients with progressive fibrotic ILD with careful monitoring. Cough is often difficult to treat and other causes of cough such as asthma, postnasal drip, and GERD should be considered and treated if present. Thalidomide has been the only medication thus far shown to reduce cough among patients with IPF, although these data are from a small single-center study.[114] Thalidomide has substantial potential adverse effects and should not routinely be used for treatment of cough among patients with progressive PF until further studies are conducted.[114] Inhaled sodium cromoglicate (PA101) was shown to reduce cough in comparison with placebo among patients with IPF in a recent small pilot study; results of a phase 2B study are anticipated.[115,116]

The IPF guidelines recommend considering lung transplant as a treatment for IPF, although there is a paucity of data to guide timing of lung transplant referral and listing.[5,117] Among patients with non-IPF PFLD, even less is known regarding optimal timing of lung transplant referral as well as lung transplant outcomes; further study is needed. The International Society for Heart and Lung Transplantation has published guidelines for lung transplant referral and listing timing for patients with ILD, although in practicality, this may vary by center or geographic location depending on lung transplant wait times and overall organ availability. In general, among patients without contraindication to lung transplant, referral is recommended for patients with ILD with the following: (1) histopathologic or radiographic evidence of UIP or fibrosing NSIP regardless of lung function; (2) FVC <80% predicted or DLCO <40% predicted; (3) any oxygen requirement, (4) any dyspnea or functional limitation related to lung disease; or (5) failure to improve dyspnea, O2 requirement, and/or lung function after a trial of appropriate medical therapy among patients with inflammatory ILD.[117] Listing is recommended at the time of the following: (1) decrease in FVC $\geq$10% over 6 months, (2) decrease in DLCO$\geq$15% over 6 months, (3) desaturation to <88% or distance <250 m on 6-minute walk test or >50 m decline in 6-minute walk distance over 6 months, (4) PH on RHC or TTE, or

(5) hospitalization because of respiratory decline, pneumothorax, or acute exacerbation.[117]

CLINICAL COURSE/PROGNOSIS

Discussion of clinical course and prognosis with patients and caretakers are important aspects of managing fibrotic lung disease. IPF, the most well studied ILD, has a poor prognosis, with median survival 3 to 5 years from time of diagnosis.[5] Although other fibrotic ILDs are often thought to have a better prognosis than IPF, more data are emerging that this is not universally the case. Particularly when a UIP pattern is present, survival rates among patients with non-IPF PF-ILD can be similar to those seen in IPF.[34] For instance, a study of patients with RA-ILD found a median time of 3.2 years from initial clinic visit to death among patients with a UIP pattern, similar to that seen in a comparison cohort of patients with IPF, whereas median survival among all included patients with RA-ILD was 5 years.[118] Prognosis can similarly be poor in fibrotic HP, with worse survival seen among patients with UIP and among those for whom an inciting antigen cannot be identified.[6,26]

Despite the preceding studies, overall clinical course among patients with non-IPF PF-ILD is not well described and is likely more heterogeneous than among patients with IPF. Certain features such as the presence of a UIP pattern, honeycombing on HRCT, older age, lower baseline FVC, and history of acute exacerbation have been associated with increased mortality among patients with various non-IPF PF-ILDs.[119–124] A UIP pattern on CT chest or histopathology is not only associated with worse prognosis but also more rapid disease progression compared with other patterns such as NSIP.[27,125,126] Extent of fibrosis on HRCT chest has similarly been associated with higher mortality risk in scleroderma ILD and there has been increasing interest in quantitative CT techniques to aid in estimating prognosis.[16,121,127,128] Among a variety of fibrotic lung diseases as well as IPF, lower baseline FVC and DLCO, as well as declines in FVC and DLCO, have been associated with increased mortality.[5,27,129,130] The IPF guidelines note that a decrease in FVC by $\geq$10% or DLCO by $\geq$15% are associated with increased mortality risk.[5] These thresholds are often extrapolated to other fibrotic lung diseases, although are not broadly studied. Among patients with fibrotic progressive ILD included in the INBUILD study, FVC decline of greater than 10% predicted was associated with increased mortality.[18] A $\geq$10% decline in FVC over 6 to 12 months has been associated with decreased survival among patients with chronic fibrotic HP.[131] Similarly, a decline in FVC by $\geq$10% from baseline has been associated with increased mortality among patients with RA-ILD.[27] Some studies including among patients with IPF have suggested that smaller changes in FVC are also associated with survival.[129] Although lower baseline FVC and decline in FVC have been associated with mortality risk among patients with various fibrotic lung diseases including IPF, current or recent rate of decline does not consistently predict future rate of decline.[25,129,132]

Genetic changes and biomarkers may be useful in predicting prognosis in the future. Genetic changes leading to shortened telomeres have been associated with progression and reduced transplant-free survival among patients with PF-ILD as well as IPF.[133,134] Alternatively, a single nucleotide polymorphism in the MUC5B minor allele has been associated with lower mortality risk among patients with IPF, higher mortality among patients with IPAF, and shown no association with mortality risk in chronic HP or CTD-ILD.[33,135,136] Further study is needed to delineate whether the MUC5B polymorphism truly has differential associations with mortality among various fibrotic ILDs. Serum biomarkers have been evaluated as a means to determine both diagnosis and prognosis among patients with fibrotic lung diseases. There has been ongoing research in to how levels of and changes in serum biomarkers such as matrix metalloproteinase 7 (MMP-7), surfactant protein D (SPD), CC chemokine ligand 18 (CCL-18), and Krebs von den Lungen-6 protein (KL-6) may correlate with disease course and prognosis among patients with ILD.[137–140] Data have not been robust enough yet for use in general and routine clinical practice, nor is testing for such serum biomarkers routinely available or recommended.[59]

Scoring systems such as the Gender, Age and Physiology (GAP) index and the Composite Physiology Index (CPI) have been created to predict mortality among patients with IPF.[141,142] The ILD-GAP score was modified to provide prognostic information for patients with non-IPF ILD.[143] Although these scoring systems may predict overall mortality, they do not predict which patients with a particular ILD will develop PFLD nor do they predict rate of progression. There is increasing interest in quantitative CT and radiologic scoring systems in predicting prognosis, although this is not yet used in routine clinical practice.[128,144]

Acute exacerbations (AE) may occur in non-IPF PF-ILD but are best described among patients with IPF. An international working group described AE-IPF as acute respiratory deterioration less than

1 month in duration with new bilateral ground glass opacities or consolidation on CT chest that are not completely explained by heart failure.[145] After exclusion of extraparenchymal causes (eg, pulmonary embolism, pleural effusion) of worsening, AE-IPF were described as triggered (infection, aspiration) or untriggered (idiopathic).[145] AE-IPF occur in approximately 5% to 10% of patients, more frequently among patients with advanced disease.[5,145–147] Mortality from AE-IPF is high; 46% of IPF deaths follow AE-IPF and median survival after AE-IPF is 3 to 4 months.[145,147–149] Acute exacerbations have been described in non-IPF PF-ILD including FHP, CTD-ILD, and others.[150–152] There has not been a clearly proposed definition for AE among patients with non-IPF PF-ILD, although a similar definition to that used for AE-IPF is reasonable and was used to define AE as an endpoint in the INBUILD study.[18,151] Among patients with non-IPF progressive fibrotic lung disease, those with a UIP pattern of disease have higher rates of acute exacerbation. Mortality is high, similar to that seen among patients with AE-IPF.[150,151,153]

The presence of comorbid conditions has been shown to influence prognosis in fibrotic lung disease.[98,99] The frequency and impact of comorbid conditions has primarily been studied among patients with IPF. Particular comorbidities of note that occur at increased rates in patients with IPF and fibrotic lung disease with adverse effects on survival include lung cancer, IHD and PH.[96,154,155] More study is needed regarding the frequency and effects of comorbid conditions in non-IPF fibrotic lung disease.

FUTURE DIRECTIONS

There is more to learn about non-IPF PF-ILD. An important step will be development and validation of an accepted definition of progression. Research is needed to identify distinguishing early features including biomarkers or gene expression profiles that may predict which patients are more likely to develop progressive fibrosis and which patients may respond to particular treatments. The INBUILD study set the stage for studies of non-IPF PF-ILD, which potentially opens up clinical trials and treatments to a wider range of patients. That said, accurate and timely diagnosis is critical. Ongoing development of tools such as the envisia molecular classifier and machine learning algorithms may allow distinction of fibrotic ILDs by less invasive means. It remains unknown whether and when to choose an immunosuppressive agent or an antifibrotic for non-IPF PF-ILD. Further trials are needed to identify which patients are most

likely to potentially benefit from immunosuppression and whether to use such medications with an antifibrotic drug. Identification and treatment of comorbid conditions and nonpharmacologic treatments are important considerations in treatment of patients with fibrotic lung disease. Discussion of potential clinical course and prognosis with patients and caretakers is also an essential aspect of management.

CLINICS CARE POINTS

- NonIPF PF ILD may have clinical behavior similar to that of IPF; it is not yet known how to best distinguish which non-IPF ILDs will evolve to fibrosis and progress.

- Accurate diagnosis of non-IPF PF ILD has implications for treatment and prognosis.

- Pharmacologic and non-pharmacologic treatments have a role in treatment of non-IPF PF ILD. However, the best pharmacologic strategy is not always clear. Further study is needed in this area.

DISCLOSURE

B.F. Collins declares personal fees from Boehringer-Ingelheim outside of the submitted work. F. Luppi declares grants and personal fees from Roche and personal fees from Boehringer-Ingelheim outside of the submitted work.

REFERENCES

1. Cottin V, Hirani NA, Hotchkin DL, et al. Presentation, diagnosis and clinical course of the spectrum of progressive-fibrosing interstitial lung diseases. Eur Respir Rev 2018;27:11.

2. Travis WD, Costabel U, Hansell DM, et al. An official American Thoracic Society/European Respiratory Society statment: update of the international multidisciplinary classification of the idiopathic interstitial pneumonias. Am J Respir Crit Care Med 2013;188:10.

3. Richeldi L, Collard HR, Jones MG. Idiopathic pulmonary fibrosis. Lancet 2017;389:1941–52.

4. Wuyts WA, Cavazza A, Rossi G, et al. Differential diagnosis of usual interstitial pneumonia: when is it truly idiopathic? Eur Respir Rev 2014;23:12.

5. Raghu G, Collard HR, Egan JJ. An official ATS/ERS/JRS/ALAT statement: idiopathic pulmonary fibrosis: evidence-based guidelines for diagnosis

and management. Am J Respir Crit Care Med 2011;183:37.

6. Churg A, Sin DD, Everett D, et al. Pathologic patterns and survival in chronic hypersensitivity pneumonitis. Am J Surg Pathol 2009;33:1765–70.

7. Yunt ZX, Chung JH, Hobbs S, et al. High resolution computed tomography pattern of usual interstitial pneumonia in rheumatoid arthritis-associated interstitial lung disease: relationship to survival. Respir Med 2017;126:100–4.

8. Hoffmann-Vold AM, Fretheim H, Halse AK, et al. Tracking impact of interstitial lung disease in systemic sclerosis in a complete nationwide cohort. Am J Respir Crit Care Med 2019;200: 1258–66.

9. Cottin V, Wollin L, Fischer A, et al. Fibrosing interstitial lung diseases: knowns and unknowns. Eur Respir Rev 2019;28:180100.

10. Wells AU, Brown KK, Flaherty KR, et al. What's in a name? That which we call IPF, by any other name would act the same. Eur Respir J 2018;51: 1800692.

11. Wolters PJ, Blackwell TS, Eickelberg O, et al. Time for a change: is idiopathic pulmonary fibrosis still idiopathic and only fibrotic? Lancet Respir Med 2018;6:154–60.

12. Wijsenbeek M, Cottin V. Spectrum of fibrotic lung diseases. N Engl J Med 2020;383:958–68.

13. Hutchinson JP, Fogarty AW, McKeever TM, et al. In-hospital mortality after surgical lung biopsy for interstitial lung disease in the United States. 2000 to 2011. Am J Respir Crit Care Med 2016;193: 1161–7.

14. Hutchinson J, Hubbard R, Raghu G. Surgical lung biopsy for interstitial lung disease: when considered necessary, should these be done in larger and experienced centres only? Eur Respir J 2019;53:1900023.

15. Cottin V. Lung biopsy in interstitial lung disease: balancing the risk of surgery and diagnostic uncertainty. Eur Respir J 2016;48:1274–7.

16. Ryerson CJ, Urbania TH, Richeldi L, et al. Prevalence and prognosis of unclassifiable interstitial lung disease. Eur Respir J 2013;42:750–7.

17. Guler SA, Ellison K, Algamdi M, et al. Heterogeneity in unclassifiable interstitial lung disease. A systematic review and meta-analysis. Ann Am Thorac Soc 2018;15:854–63.

18. Flaherty KR, Wells AU, Cottin V, et al. Nintedanib in progressive fibrosing interstitial lung diseases. N Engl J Med 2019;381:1718–27.

19. Raghu G. Idiopathic pulmonary fibrosis: shifting the concept to irreversible pulmonary fibrosis of many entities. Lancet Respir Med 2019;7:926–9.

20. George PM, Spagnolo P, Kreuter M, et al. Progressive fibrosing interstitial lung disease: clinical uncertainties, consensus recommendations, and research priorities. Lancet Respir Med 2020;8: 925–34.

21. Olson AL, Gifford AH, Inase N, et al. The epidemiology of idiopathic pulmonary fibrosis and interstitial lung diseases at risk of a progressive-fibrosing phenotype. Eur Respir Rev 2018;27:180077.

22. Patterson KC, Strek ME. Pulmonary fibrosis in sarcoidosis. Clinical features and outcomes. Ann Am Thorac Soc 2013;10:362–70.

23. Raghu G, Remy-Jardin M, Ryerson CJ, et al. Diagnosis of hypersensitivity pneumonitis in adults. An official ATS/JRS/ALAT clinical practice guideline. Am J Respir Crit Care Med 2020;202:e36–69.

24. Reiseter S, Gunnarsson R, Mogens Aaløkken T, et al. Progression and mortality of interstitial lung disease in mixed connective tissue disease: a long-term observational nationwide cohort study. Rheumatology (Oxford) 2018;57:255–62.

25. Guler SA, Winstone TA, Murphy D, et al. Does systemic sclerosis-associated interstitial lung disease burn out? Specific phenotypes of disease progression. Ann Am Thorac Soc 2018;15:1427–33.

26. Fernández Pérez ER, Swigris JJ, Forssén AV, et al. Identifying an inciting antigen is associated with improved survival in patients with chronic hypersensitivity pneumonitis. Chest 2013;144: 1644–51.

27. Solomon JJ, Chung JH, Cosgrove GP, et al. Predictors of mortality in rheumatoid arthritis-associated interstitial lung disease. Eur Respir J 2016;47: 588–96.

28. Flaherty KR, Brown KK, Wells AU, et al. Design of the PF-ILD trial: a double-blind, randomised, placebo-controlled phase III trial of nintedanib in patients with progressive fibrosing interstitial lung disease. BMJ Open Respir Res 2017;4:e000212.

29. Wuyts WA, Agostini C, Antoniou KM, et al. The pathogenesis of pulmonary fibrosis: a moving target. Eur Respir J 2013;41:1207–18.

30. Harari S, Raghu G, Caminati A, et al. Fibrotic interstitial lung diseases and air pollution: a systematic literature review. Eur Respir Rev 2020;29:200093.

31. Sack C, Raghu G. Idiopathic pulmonary fibrosis: unmasking cryptogenic environmental factors. Eur Respir J 2019;53:1801699.

32. Paolocci G, Folletti I, Torén K, et al. Occupational risk factors for idiopathic pulmonary fibrosis in Southern Europe: a case-control study. BMC Pulm Med 2018;18:75.

33. Newton CA, Oldham JM, Ley B, et al. Telomere length and genetic variant associations with interstitial lung disease progression and survival. Eur Respir J 2019;53:1801641.

34. Brown KK, Martinez FJ, Walsh SLF, et al. The natural history of progressive fibrosing interstitial lung diseases. Eur Respir J 2020;55:2000085.

35. Wijsenbeek M. Progress in the treatment of pulmonary fibrosis. Lancet Respir Med 2020;8:424–5.

36. Faverio P, Piluso M, De Giacomi F, et al. Progressive fibrosing interstitial lung diseases: prevalence and characterization in two Italian referral centers. Respiration 2020;99(10):838–45.

37. Wijsenbeek M, Kreuter M, Fischer A, et al. Non-IPF progressive fibrosing interstitial lung disease (PF-ILD): The patient journey. 2018;197:A167.

38. Salisbury M, Myers JL, Belloi EA, et al. Diagnosis and treatment of fibrotic hypersensitivity pneumonitis. Am J Respir Crit Care Med 2018;196:10.

39. Vasakova M, Morell F, Walsh S, et al. Hypersensitivity pneumonitis: perspectives in diagnosis and management. Am J Respir Crit Care Med 2018;196:10.

40. Adegunsoye A, Oldham JM, Chung JH, et al. Phenotypic clusters predict outcomes in a longitudinal interstitial lung disease cohort. Chest 2018; 153:349–60.

41. Morell F, Villar A, Montero MA, et al. Chronic hypersensitivity pneumonitis in patients diagnosed with idiopathic pulmonary fibrosis: a prospective case-cohort study. Lancet Respir Med 2013;1:10.

42. Cohen RA, Petsonk EL, Rose C, et al. Lung pathology in U.S. coal workers with rapidly progressive pneumoconiosis implicates silica and silicates. Am J Respir Crit Care Med 2016;193:673–80.

43. Nardi A, Brillet PY, Letoumelin P, et al. Stage IV sarcoidosis: comparison of survival with the general population and causes of death. Eur Respir J 2011;38:1368–73.

44. Collins BF, McClelland RL, Ho LA, et al. Sarcoidosis and IPF in the same patient-a coincidence, an association or a phenotype? Respir Med 2018;144s: S20–7.

45. Shigemitsu H, Oblad JM, Sharma OP, et al. Chronic interstitial pneumonitis in end-stage sarcoidosis. Eur Respir J 2010;35:695–7.

46. Skeoch S, Weatherley N, Swift AJ, et al. Drug-induced interstitial lung disease: a systematic review. J Clin Med 2018;7:30.

47. Hanania AN, Mainwaring W, Ghebre YT, et al. Radiation-induced lung injury: assessment and management. Chest 2019;156:150–62.

48. Bates CA, Ellison MC, Lynch DA, et al. Granulomatous-lymphocytic lung disease shortens survival in common variable immunodeficiency. J Allergy Clin Immunol 2004;114:415–21.

49. Fischer A, Antoniou KM, Brown KK, et al. An official European Respiratory Society/American Thoracic Society research statement: interstitial pneumonia with autoimmune features. Eur Respir J 2015;46: 976–87.

50. Oldham JM, Adegunsoye A, Valenzi E, et al. Characterisation of patients with interstitial pneumonia with autoimmune features. Eur Respir J 2016;47: 1767–75.

51. Tazi A. Adult pulmonary Langerhans's cell histiocytosis. Eur Respir J 2006;27:14.

52. Konopka KE, Myers JL. A review of smoking-related interstitial fibrosis, respiratory bronchiolitis, and desquamative interstitial pneumonia: overlapping histology and confusing terminology. Arch Pathol Lab Med 2018;142:1177–81.

53. Chae KJ, Jin GY, Jung HN, et al. Differentiating smoking-related interstitial fibrosis (SRIF) from usual interstitial pneumonia (UIP) with emphysema using CT features based on pathologically proven cases. PLoS One 2016;11:15.

54. Katzenstein AL, Mukhopadhyay S, Zanardi C, et al. Clinically occult interstitial fibrosis in smokers: classification and significance of a surprisingly common finding in lobectomy specimens. Hum Pathol 2010;41:316–25.

55. Layden JE, Ghinai I, Pray I, et al. Pulmonary illness related to E-cigarette use in Illinois and Wisconsin - Final Report. N Engl J Med 2020;382:903–16.

56. Blagev DP, Harris D, Dunn AC, et al. Clinical presentation, treatment, and short-term outcomes of lung injury associated with e-cigarettes or vaping: a prospective observational cohort study. Lancet 2019;394:2073–83.

57. Arter ZL, Wiggins A, Hudspath C, et al. Acute eosinophilic pneumonia following electronic cigarette use. Respir Med Case Rep 2019;27:100825.

58. Cosgrove GP, Bianchi P, Danese S, et al. Barriers to timely diagnosis of interstitial lung disease in the real world: the INTENSITY survey. BMC Pulm Med 2018;18:9.

59. Raghu G, Remy-Jardin M, Myers JL, et al. Diagnosis of idiopathic pulmonary fibrosis: an official ATS/ERS/JRS/ALAT clinical practice guideline. Am J Respir Crit Care Med 2018;198:25.

60. Flaherty KR, King TE Jr, Raghu G, et al. Idiopathic interstitial pneumonia: what is the effect of a multidisciplinary approach to diagnosis? Am J Respir Crit Care Med 2004;170:7.

61. Raghu G, Anstrom KJ, King TE Jr, et al. Prednisone, azathioprine, and N-Acetylcysteine for pulmonary fibrosis. N Engl J Med 2012;366:10.

62. Tashkin DP, Elashoff R, Clements PJ, et al. Cyclophosphamide versus placebo in scleroderma lung disease. N Engl J Med 2006;354:2655–66.

63. Tashkin DP, Roth MD, Clements PJ, et al. Mycophenolate mofetil versus oral cyclophosphamide in scleroderma-related interstitial lung disease (SLS II): a randomised controlled, double-blind, parallel group trial. Lancet Respir Med 2016;4: 708–19.

64. Johannson KA, Barnes H, Bellanger AP, et al. Exposure assessment tools for hypersensitivity pneumonitis. An official American Thoracic Society workshop report. Ann Am Thorac Soc 2020;17: 1501–9.

65. Troy LK, Grainge C, Corte TJ, et al. Diagnostic accuracy of transbronchial lung cryobiopsy for interstitial lung disease diagnosis (COLDICE): a prospective, comparative study. Lancet Respir Med 2020;8:171–81.

66. Hetzel J, Wells AU, Costabel U, et al. Transbronchial cryobiopsy increases diagnostic confidence in interstitial lung disease: a prospective multicenter trial. Eur Respir J 2020;56(6):1901520.

67. Raghu G, Flaherty KR, Lederer DJ, et al. Use of a molecular classifier to identify usual interstitial pneumonia in conventional transbronchial lung biopsy samples: a prospective validation study. Lancet Respir Med 2019;7:487–96.

68. Richeldi L, Scholand MB, Lynch DA, et al. Utility of a molecular classifier as a complement to HRCT to identify usual interstitial pneumonia. Am J Respir Crit Care Med 2021;203(2):211–20.

69. Weatherley ND, Eaden JA, Stewart NJ, et al. Experimental and quantitative imaging techniques in interstitial lung disease. Thorax 2019;74:611–9.

70. Walsh SLF, Devaraj A, Enghelmayer JI, et al. Role of imaging in progressive-fibrosing interstitial lung diseases. Eur Respir Rev 2018;27(150):180073.

71. Walsh SLF, Calandriello L, Silva M, et al. Deep learning for classifying fibrotic lung disease on high-resolution computed tomography: a case-cohort study. Lancet Respir Med 2018;6:837–45.

72. Shaish H, Ahmed FS, Lederer D, et al. Deep learning of CT Virtual wedge resection for prediction of histologic usual interstitial pneumonitis. Ann Am Thorac Soc 2021;18(1):51–9.

73. Ryerson CJ, Corte TJ, Lee JS, et al. A standardized diagnostic ontology for fibrotic interstitial lung disease. An International Working Group Perspective. Am J Respir Crit Care Med 2017;196:1249–54.

74. Wijsenbeek MS, Holland AE, Swigris JJ, et al. Comprehensive supportive care for patients with fibrosing interstitial lung disease. Am J Respir Crit Care Med 2019;200:152–9.

75. King TE Jr, Bradford WZ, Castro-Bernardini S, et al. A phase 3 trial of pirfenidone in patients with idiopathic pulmonary fibrosis. N Engl J Med 2014; 370:10.

76. Richeldi L, du Bois RM, Raghu G, et al. Efficacy and safety of nintedanib in idiopathic pulmonary fibrosis. N Engl J Med 2014;370:12.

77. Sakamoto K, Itoh T, Muramatsu Y, et al. Efficacy of pirfenidone in patients with advanced-stage idiopathic pulmonary fibrosis. Intern Med 2013;52:7.

78. Noble PW, Albera C, Bradford WZ, et al. Pirfenidone for idiopathic pulmonary fibrosis: analysis of pooled data from three multinational phase 3 trials. Eur Respir J 2016;47:243–53.

79. Kolb M, Richeldi L, Behr J, et al. Nintedanib in patients with idiopathic pulmonary fibrosis and preserved lung volume. Thorax 2017;72:7.

80. Harari S, Caminati A, Poletti V, et al. A real-life multicenter national study on nintedanib in severe idiopathic pulmonary fibrosis. Respiration 2018; 95:8.

81. Macias-Barragan J, Sandoval-Rodriguez A, Navarro-Partida J, et al. The multifaceted role of pirfenidone and its novel targets. Fibrogenesis Tissue Repair 2010;3:11.

82. Iyer SN, Gurujeyalakshmi G, Giri SN. Effects of pirfenidone on transforming growth factor-beta gene expression at the transcriptional level in bleomycin hamster model of lung fibrosis. J Pharmacol Exp Ther 1999;291:9.

83. Nakayama S, Mukae H, Sakamoto N, et al. Pirfenidone inhibits the expression of HSP47 in TGF-beta 1-stimulated human lung fibroblasts. Life Sci 2008; 82:8.

84. Wollin L, Wex E, Pautsch A, et al. Mode of action of nintedanib in the treatment of idiopathic pulmonary fibrosis. Eur Respir J 2015;45:12.

85. Herzog EL, Mathur A, Tager AM, et al. Interstitial lung disease associated with systemic sclerosis and idiopathic pulmonary fibrosis. How similar and how distinct? Arthritis Rheumatol 2014;66:12.

86. Lafyatis R. Transforming growth factor beta–at the centre of systemic sclerosis. Nat Rev Rheumatol 2014;10:706–19.

87. Distler O, Highland KB, Gahlemann M, et al. Nintedanib for systemic sclerosis-associated interstitial lung disease. N Engl J Med 2019;380:2518–28.

88. Distler O, Brown KK, Distler JHW, et al. Design of a randomised, placebo-controlled clinical trial of nintedanib in patients with systemic sclerosis-associated interstitial lung disease (SENSCIS). Clin Exp Rheumatol 2017;35(Suppl 106):75–81.

89. National Institutes of Health Clinical Center. Scleroderma lung study III - Combining pirfenidone with mycophenolate (SLSIII). 2018. Available at: https://clinicaltrials.gov/ct2/show/NCT03221257. Accessed February 9, 2019.

90. Khanna D, Albera C, Fischer A, et al. An open-label, phase II study of the safety and tolerability of pirfenidone in patients with scleroderma-associated interstitial lung disease: the LOTUSS trial. J Rheumatol 2016;43:1672–9.

91. Wells AU, Flaherty KR, Brown KK, et al. Nintedanib in patients with progressive fibrosing interstitial lung diseases-subgroup analyses by interstitial lung disease diagnosis in the INBUILD trial: a randomised, double-blind, placebo-controlled, parallel-group trial. Lancet Respir Med 2020;8:453–60.

92. Maher TM, Corte TJ, Fischer A, et al. Pirfenidone in patients with unclassifiable progressive fibrosing interstitial lung disease: a double-blind, randomised, placebo-controlled, phase 2 trial. Lancet Respir Med 2020;8:147–57.

93. Collins BF, Raghu G. Antifibrotic therapy for fibrotic lung disease beyond idiopathic pulmonary fibrosis. Eur Respir Rev 2019;28:190022.

94. Wiertz IA, van Moorsel CHM, Vorselaars ADM, et al. Cyclophosphamide in steroid refractory unclassifiable idiopathic interstitial pneumonia and interstitial pneumonia with autoimmune features (IPAF). Eur Respir J 2018;51:1702519.

95. Wong AW, Ryerson CJ, Guler SA. Progression of fibrosing interstitial lung disease. Respir Res 2020; 21:32.

96. Kreuter M, Ehlers-Tenenbaum S, Palmowski K, et al. Impact of comorbidities on mortality in patients with idiopathic pulmonary fibrosis. PLoS One 2016;11:18.

97. Schwarzkopf L, Witt S, Waelscher J, et al. Associations between comorbidities, their treatment and survival in patients with interstitial lung diseases-a claims data analysis. Respir Res 2018;19:15.

98. Raghu G, Amatto VC, Behr J, et al. Comorbidities in idiopathic pulmonary fibrosis patients: a systematic literature review. Eur Respir J 2015;46:18.

99. Wälscher J, Gross B, Morisset J, et al. Comorbidities and survival in patients with chronic hypersensitivity pneumonitis. Respir Res 2020;21:12.

100. Martinez FJ, de Andrade JA, Anstrom KJ, et al. Randomized trial of acetylcysteine in idiopathic pulmonary fibrosis. N Engl J Med 2014;370:9.

101. Oldham JM, Ma SF, Martinez FJ, et al. TOLLIP, MUC5B, and the response to N-Acetylcysteine among individuals with idiopathic pulmonary fibrosis. Am J Respir Crit Care Med 2015;192:8.

102. National Institutes of Health Clinical Center. Prospective treatment efficacy in IPF using genotype for Nac Selection (PRECISIONS) Trial (PRECISIONS). 2020. Available at: https://clinicaltrials.gov/ct2/show/NCT04300920. Accessed September 1, 2020.

103. Ferreira A, Garvey C, Connors GL, et al. Pulmonary rehabilitation in interstitial lung disease: benefits and predictors of response. Chest 2009;135: 442–7.

104. Tonelli R, Cocconcelli E, Lanini B, et al. Effectiveness of pulmonary rehabilitation in patients with interstitial lung disease of different etiology: a multicenter prospective study. BMC Pulm Med 2017;17:130.

105. Perez-Bogerd S, Wuyts W, Barbier V, et al. Short and long-term effects of pulmonary rehabilitation in interstitial lung diseases: a randomised controlled trial. Respir Res 2018;19:182.

106. Ryerson CJ, Cayou C, Topp F, et al. Pulmonary rehabilitation improves long-term outcomes in interstitial lung disease: a prospective cohort study. Respir Med 2014;108:203–10.

107. Dowman LM, McDonald CF, Bozinovski S, et al. Greater endurance capacity and improved dyspnoea with acute oxygen supplementation in idiopathic pulmonary fibrosis patients without resting hypoxaemia. Respirology 2017;22:957–64.

108. Visca D, Mori L, Tsipouri V, et al. Effect of ambulatory oxygen on quality of life for patients with fibrotic lung disease (AmbOx): a prospective, open-label, mixed-method, crossover randomised controlled trial. Lancet Respir Med 2018;6:759–70.

109. Graney BA, Wamboldt FS, Baird S, et al. Informal caregivers experience of supplemental oxygen in pulmonary fibrosis. Health Qual Life Outcomes 2017;15:133.

110. Swigris JJ, Stewart AL, Gould MK, et al. Patients' perspectives on how idiopathic pulmonary fibrosis affects the quality of their lives. Health Qual Life Outcomes 2005;3:61.

111. van Manen MJ, Kreuter M, van den Blink B, et al. What patients with pulmonary fibrosis and their partners think: a live, educative survey in The Netherlands and Germany. ERJ Open Res 2017;3(1):00065–2016.

112. Senanayake S, Harrison K, Lewis M, et al. Patients' experiences of coping with Idiopathic Pulmonary Fibrosis and their recommendations for its clinical management. PLoS One 2018;13:e0197660.

113. Zou RH, Kass DJ, Gibson KF, et al. The role of palliative care in reducing symptoms and improving quality of life for patients with idiopathic pulmonary fibrosis: a review. Pulm Ther 2020;6:35–46.

114. Horton MR, Santopietro V, Mathew L, et al. Thalidomide for the treatment of cough in idiopathic pulmonary fibrosis: a randomized trial. Ann Intern Med 2012;157:398–406.

115. Birring SS, Wijsenbeek MS, Agrawal S, et al. A novel formulation of inhaled sodium cromoglicate (PA101) in idiopathic pulmonary fibrosis and chronic cough: a randomised, double-blind, proof-of-concept, phase 2 trial. Lancet Respir Med 2017;5:806–15.

116. National Institutes of Health Clinical Center. A phase 2b study of inhaled RVT-1601 for the treatment of persistent cough in IPF (SCENIC). 2019. Available at: https://clinicaltrials.gov/ct2/show/NCT03864328. Accessed March 18, 2019.

117. Weill D, Benden C, Corris PA, et al. A consensus document for the selection of lung transplant candidates: 2014–an update from the pulmonary transplantation council of the International Society for Heart and Lung Transplantation. J Heart Lung Transplant 2015;34:1–15.

118. Kim EJ, Elicker BM, Maldonado F, et al. Usual interstitial pneumonia in rheumatoid arthritis-associated interstitial lung disease. Eur Respir J 2010;35: 1322–8.

119. Yamakawa H, Sato S, Tsumiyama E, et al. Predictive factors of mortality in rheumatoid arthritis-associated interstitial lung disease analysed by modified HRCT classification of idiopathic

pulmonary fibrosis according to the 2018 ATS/ERS/JRS/ALAT criteria. J Thorac Dis 2019;11:5247–57.

120. Adegunsoye A, Oldham JM, Bellam SK, et al. Computed tomography honeycombing identifies a progressive fibrotic phenotype with increased mortality across diverse interstitial lung diseases. Ann Am Thorac Soc 2019;16:580–8.

121. Winstone TA, Assayag D, Wilcox PG, et al. Predictors of mortality and progression in scleroderma-associated interstitial lung disease: a systematic review. Chest 2014;146:422–36.

122. Ojanguren I, Morell F, Ramón MA, et al. Long-term outcomes in chronic hypersensitivity pneumonitis. Allergy 2019;74:944–52.

123. Walsh SL, Sverzellati N, Devaraj A, et al. Chronic hypersensitivity pneumonitis: high resolution computed tomography patterns and pulmonary function indices as prognostic determinants. Eur Radiol 2012;22:1672–9.

124. Salisbury ML, Gu T, Murray S, et al. Hypersensitivity pneumonitis: radiologic phenotypes are associated with distinct survival time and pulmonary function trajectory. Chest 2019;155:699–711.

125. Chan C, Ryerson CJ, Dunne JV, et al. Demographic and clinical predictors of progression and mortality in connective tissue disease-associated interstitial lung disease: a retrospective cohort study. BMC Pulm Med 2019;19:192.

126. Wang P, Jones KD, Urisman A, et al. Pathologic findings and prognosis in a large prospective cohort of chronic hypersensitivity pneumonitis. Chest 2017;152:502–9.

127. Jacob J, Bartholmai BJ, Rajagopalan S, et al. Automated computer-based CT stratification as a predictor of outcome in hypersensitivity pneumonitis. Eur Radiol 2017;27:3635–46.

128. Jacob J, Bartholmai BJ, Rajagopalan S, et al. Predicting outcomes in idiopathic pulmonary fibrosis using automated computed tomographic analysis. Am J Respir Crit Care Med 2018;198:767–76.

129. Zappala CJ, Latsi PI, Nicholson AG, et al. Marginal decline in forced vital capacity is associated with a poor outcome in idiopathic pulmonary fibrosis. Eur Respir J 2010;35:830–6.

130. Volkmann ER, Tashkin DP, Sim M, et al. Short-term progression of interstitial lung disease in systemic sclerosis predicts long-term survival in two independent clinical trial cohorts. Ann Rheum Dis 2019;78:122–30.

131. Gimenez A, Storrer K, Kuranishi L, et al. Change in FVC and survival in chronic fibrotic hypersensitivity pneumonitis. Thorax 2018;73:391–2.

132. Schmidt SL, Tayob N, Han MK, et al. Predicting pulmonary fibrosis disease course from past trends in pulmonary function. Chest 2014;145:579–85.

133. Newton CA, Batra K, Torrelba J, et al. Telomere-related lung fibrosis is diagnostically heterogeneous but uniformly progressive. Eur Respir J 2016;48:11.

134. Ley B, Torgerson DG, Oldham JM, et al. Rare protein-altering telomere-related gene variants in patients with chronic hypersensitivity pneumonitis. Am J Respir Crit Care Med 2019;200:1154–63.

135. Peljto AL, Zhang W, Fingerlin TE, et al. Association between the MUC5B promoter polymorphism and survival in patients with idiopathic pulmonary fibrosis. JAMA 2013;309:8.

136. Ley B, Newton CA, Arnould I, et al. The MUC5B promoter polymorphism and telomere length in patients with chronic hypersensitivity pneumonitis: an observational cohort-control study. Lancet Respir Med 2017;5:9.

137. Zhang H, Chen L, Wu L, et al. Diagnostic and prognostic predictive values of circulating KL-6 for interstitial lung disease: a PRISMA-compliant systematic review and meta-analysis. Medicine 2020;99:e19493.

138. Kennedy B, Branagan P, Moloney F, et al. Biomarkers to identify ILD and predict lung function decline in scleroderma lung disease or idiopathic pulmonary fibrosis. Sarcoidosis Vasc Diffuse Lung Dis 2015;32:228–36.

139. Tiev KP, Hua-Huy T, Kettaneh A, et al. Serum CC chemokine ligand-18 predicts lung disease worsening in systemic sclerosis. Eur Respir J 2011;38:1355–60.

140. Hoffmann-Vold AM, Tennøe AH, Garen T, et al. High level of chemokine CCL18 is associated with pulmonary function deterioration, lung fibrosis progression, and reduced survival in systemic sclerosis. Chest 2016;150:299–306.

141. Wells AU, Desai SR, Rubens MB, et al. Idiopathic pulmonary fibrosis: a composite physiologic index derived from disease extent observed by computed tomography. Am J Respir Crit Care Med 2003;167:962–9.

142. Ley B, Ryerson CJ, Vittinghoff E, et al. A multidimensional index and staging system for idiopathic pulmonary fibrosis. Ann Intern Med 2012;156:8.

143. Ryerson CJ, Vittinghoff E, Ley B, et al. Predicting survival across chronic interstitial lung disease: the ILD-GAP model. Chest 2014;145:723–8.

144. Walsh SLF. Imaging biomarkers and staging in IPF. Curr Opin Pulm Med 2018;24:445–52.

145. Collard HR, Ryerson CJ, Corte TJ, et al. Acute exacerbation of idiopathic pulmonary fibrosis. An international working group report. Am J Respir Crit Care Med 2016;194:11.

146. Collard HR, Richeldi L, Kim DS, et al. Acute exacerbations in the INPULSIS trials of nintedanib in idiopathic pulmonary fibrosis. Eur Respir J 2017;49:7.

147. Song JW, Hong SB, Lim CM, et al. Acute exacerbation of idiopathic pulmonary fibrosis: incidence, risk factors and outcome. Eur Respir J 2011;37:356–63.

148. Natsuizaka M, Chiba H, Kuronuma K, et al. Epidemiologic survey of Japanese patients with idiopathic pulmonary fibrosis and investigation of ethnic differences. Am J Respir Crit Care Med 2014;190:773–9.

149. Collard HR, Yow E, Richeldi L, et al. Suspected acute exacerbation of idiopathic pulmonary fibrosis as an outcome measure in clinical trials. Respir Res 2013;14:73.

150. Olson AL, Huie TJ, Groshong SD, et al. Acute exacerbations of fibrotic hypersensitivity pneumonitis: a case series. Chest 2008;134:844–50.

151. Kolb M, Bondue B, Pesci A, et al. Acute exacerbations of progressive-fibrosing interstitial lung diseases. Eur Respir Rev 2018;27:180071.

152. Tachikawa R, Tomii K, Ueda H, et al. Clinical features and outcome of acute exacerbation of interstitial pneumonia: collagen vascular diseases-related versus idiopathic. Respiration 2012;83:20–7.

153. Park IN, Kim DS, Shim TS, et al. Acute exacerbation of interstitial pneumonia other than idiopathic pulmonary fibrosis. Chest 2007;132:214–20.

154. Tomassetti S, Gurioli C, Ryu JH, et al. The impact of lung cancer on survival of idiopathic pulmonary fibrosis. Chest 2015;147:157–64.

155. Choi WI, Park SH, Park BJ, et al. Interstitial lung disease and lung cancer development: a 5-year nationwide population-based study. Cancer Res Treat 2018;50:8.

Providing Patient-Centered Care in Interstitial Lung Disease

Alyson W. Wong, MD, MHSc[a,b], Sonye K. Danoff, MD, PhD[c],*

KEYWORDS

- Patient-centered care • Patient-reported outcome measures • Interstitial lung disease

KEY POINTS

- Patient-centered care (PCC) is foundational to quality health care and should be applied in both the clinical and research settings.
- PCC frameworks help facilitate the application of a patient-centered approach in clinical care.
- Patient-reported outcome measures identify important health outcomes from the patient perspective and are important PCC tools in research.

INTRODUCTION

The culture of health care has shifted over time toward the concept of patient-centered care (PCC), which focuses on providing not only medically appropriate care but also care that is respectful and responsive to patient preferences, needs, and values. With PCC, an individual's specific health needs and desired health outcomes are the drivers of health care decisions and outcome measurements. PCC improves the patient experience, encourages people to lead healthier lifestyles, empowers patients to be more involved in decisions, has impact on health outcomes, reduces the use of health care services, and improves the confidence and satisfaction of health professionals with the care that they provide.[1,2]

Health care systems and organizations around the world are attempting to improve health quality through PCC.[3] There often is a gap, however, between its conceptual framework and actual implementation in the real world. Many different PCC frameworks exist and the decision on how and which one to implement should be customized to the specific setting, with consideration of the disease, health care setting, and available resources. This article discusses the PCC principles and how they can be integrated into clinical care as well as research within the field of interstitial lung disease (ILD).

PATIENT-CENTERED APPROACH IN CLINICAL CARE

PCC previously has been organized into 8 attributes, including (1) respect for a patient's values, preferences, and expressed needs; (2) information and education; (3) access to care; (4) emotional support to relieve fear and anxiety; (5) involvement of family and friends (caregivers); (6) continuity and secure transition between health care settings; (7) physical comfort; and (8) coordination of care.[4] Many PCC frameworks exist that include these principles to varying degrees. A scoping review was performed to determine common themes that could be integrated into a single framework.[3]

a Department of Medicine, University of British Columbia, Vancouver, British Columbia, Canada; b Centre for Heart Lung Innovation, St. Paul's Hospital, Ward 8B – 1081 Burrard Street, Vancouver, British Columbia V6Z 1Y6, Canada; c Division of Pulmonary and Critical Care Medicine, Johns Hopkins Medicine, 1830 East Monument Street, Suite 500, Baltimore, MD 21287, USA
* Corresponding author.
E-mail address: sdanoff@jhmi.edu

Clin Chest Med 42 (2021) 337–346
https://doi.org/10.1016/j.ccm.2021.03.003
0272-5231/21/© 2021 Published by Elsevier Inc.

These themes then were categorized into 1 of the following domains: structure, process, and outcome (**Fig. 1**). This article summarizes the PCC domains and discusses how they can be applied in an ILD health care setting (**Table 1**).

Patient-Centered Care Structure

The structural domains refer to the necessary materials, health care resources, and organizational characteristics required to support PCC process and outcomes. These domains include supporting patient and caregiver education, establishing a PCC-focused culture and environment, and integrating health technology.[3]

In a survey of 1488 patients with idiopathic pulmonary fibrosis (IPF), two-thirds of respondents reported a lack of information and resources on pulmonary fibrosis at the time of diagnosis. In addition, fewer than half the respondents felt well-informed about treatment options, the role of supplemental oxygen, pulmonary rehabilitation, and transplantation.[5] Patient education is a cornerstone of treating chronic illnesses, such as ILD, and the opportunities to provide patient education extend beyond health care provider–patient interactions. Peer support groups, patient-focused and caregiver-focused conferences, and written and online resources specifically designed for patients and caregivers are different modalities that can help inform patients. Information ideally is evidence-based and reviewed by specialists because frequently there is inaccurate information.[6,7] **Table 2** provides a list of some currently available educational resources for common fibrotic ILDs that have been reviewed by ILD specialists and could be provided to patients and caregivers.

Another major structural component is a supportive clinical environment and culture with adequate resources for staff to practice PCC. An example of PCC structure in ILD is the use of multidisciplinary teams with allied health professionals, such as a clinical nurse specialist, pharmacist, and respiratory therapist. Lack of resources and budget to establish such a care model, however,

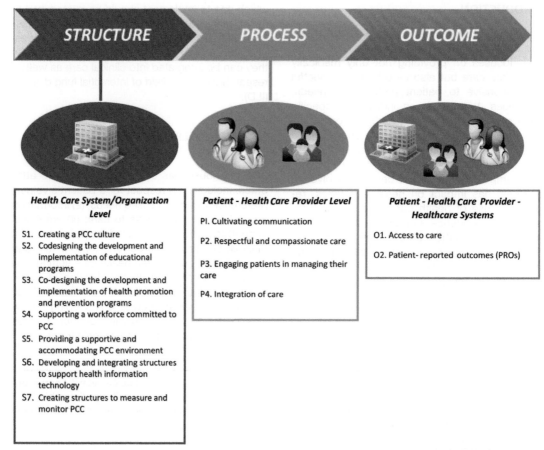

Fig. 1. PCC conceptual framework. (*From* "How to practice person-centred care: A conceptual framework.," by Santana MJ, Manalili K, Jolley RJ, Zelinsky S, Quan H, and Lu M, 2018, *Health Expect.* 21(2):429-440. CC by 4.0.)

Table 1
Integrating patient-centered care domains into interstitial lung disease care

Domain	Examples of Integrating Patient-Centered Care Domains into Interstitial Lung Disease Care
Structure	• Core values and philosophy of ILD programs reflect PCC • Include patient representatives when planning and implementing clinical and research programs. • Create partnerships with ILD community organizations. • Patient education and self-management through patient support groups and conferences • Financial models that support the time needed for health care teams to review complex patients
Process	• Ensure opportunity for patients to ask questions. • Provide credible resources. • Address questions that are important to patients (eg, treatment options, the role of supplemental oxygen, pulmonary rehabilitation, and transplantation) • Address advanced care planning with continual reassessment
Outcomes	• Ensure timely, accurate diagnosis. • Access to ILD interdisciplinary teams, including ILD clinician, other specialists (palliative care, rheumatology, etc.), clinical nurse specialist, respiratory therapist, physiotherapist, dietician, and pharmacist • Integration of PROs in clinical care and research

is a frequent barrier. In addition, current payment systems for clinicians typically encourage seeing more patients with less time spent with each individual. This payment model is not conducive to providing the time needed to foster relationships and address the many health needs of patients with complex chronic diseases. In order for PCC to be at the center of a health system, policy makers need to endorse the infrastructure and payment methods that encourage and support such practice.

Health information technology is another important structural component for providing PCC as it increases access to patient information, facilitates communication, and increases efficiency (eg, minimizes duplication of investigations if providers can see what previously has been ordered). Telehealth is a form of health information and communication technology that employs videoconferencing to provide patient care remotely. An advantage of telehealth is increased access to ILD specialty care and multidisciplinary conferences, with earlier access shown to improve survival in patients with IPF.[8] There is limited evidence on the use of telehealth in ILD; however, its use has been shown to decrease exacerbations and emergency department visits in chronic obstructive pulmonary disease (COPD).[9] In addition, there was no significant difference in survival among patients who received post–lung transplant follow-up via telehealth versus in-person.[10] A pilot study also demonstrated feasibility of a home monitoring program that included real-time wireless home spirometry in IPF.[11]

Patient-Centered Care Process

Process refers to the interaction between patients and health care providers and includes several features that promote PCC. The first feature is cultivating communication. Provider communication skills are associated with increased patient satisfaction, recall, understanding, and adherence to therapy.[12,13] The second feature is respectful and compassionate care. This entails acknowledging a patient's personal, cultural, religious, and spiritual values with empathy, which then promotes relationship building and better outcomes.[2,12] Additionally, acknowledging and engaging caregivers in communication provide added support to patients. Lastly, empowering patients in their care has been shown to improve health outcomes, quality of care, and patient safety.[14,15]

Effective communication is an integral part of a collaborative patient-caregiver-provider relationship and facilitates respectful and compassionate care. When a patient's values, needs, and preferences are incorporated into their care, communication has been shown to enhance patient engagement.[16] Communication around shared decisions is relevant particularly when discussing ILD diagnosis and treatment. The 3-talk model of shared decision making is based on team talk, option talk, and decision talk.[17] Shared decision making begins with team talk, where support is provided to patients when they are made aware of choices, and patient goals are identified in order to guide the decision-making process. Option talk

Table 2
List of interstitial lung disease resources that can be provided to patients

Organization	Overview	Online Resource
Canadian Lung Association	Causes, symptoms, and treatment of IPF	https://www.lung.ca/lung-health/lung-disease/idiopathic-pulmonary-fibrosis
American Thoracic Society	Fact sheet on IPF	https://www.thoracic.org/patients/patient-resources/resources/idiopathic-pulmonary-fibrosis.pdf
European Lung Foundation	Factsheets on IPF and sarcoidosis	https://www.europeanlung.org/en/lung-disease-and-information/factsheets/english/
UCSF	Information on various ILDs, comorbidities, and symptom management	https://www.ucsfhealth.org/education/ild-patient-resources
Pulmonary Fibrosis Foundation	General information including clinical trials, support groups, presentations by ILD specialists	https://www.pulmonaryfibrosis.org/

The information from these resources have been reviewed by ILD specialists.

then discusses alternatives, including the risks and benefits of each option. The final stage is decision talk, when a decision is made based on the informed preferences of patients, which has been guided by the experience and expertise of health professionals.

Patient and caregiver engagement is an integral part of the PCC process in which patients become invested in their own health and actively participate in codesigning their care plans. Caregivers provide integral support to patients in this process. Diagnosis and treatment of ILD are complex, with frequent misdiagnoses,[18] and can be an overwhelming process for patients and their caregivers who may not know what to ask providers, how to keep track of investigations, or follow-up with access to medications. One way to improve processes is to use patient pathways, which could include written or online information designed for patients (written at an appropriate level and with necessary explanations) about the main components of ILD diagnosis and treatment, instructions on how to prepare for appointments or tests, and contact information for team members who can help with patient navigation (eg, ILD nurse coordinator). Integrating caregivers in this process adds to the levels of support for the patient. Patient engagement also requires that medical information be readily accessible, including test results, clinic notes, and hospital records. These results may require additional interpretation to facilitate

patient understanding. Using an e-health platform is 1 way to link health care components that often are disjointed and also could support communication between health care team members, including the patient and caregiver.

Patient-Centered Care Outcomes

Indicators that can measure the quality of PCC structure and process are important to ensure that the implemented model is effective and valuable. An example of a PCC outcome is access to care, which refers to a health system's capacity to provide care efficiently after a need is recognized. Another example of a PCC outcome is the use of patient-reported outcomes (PROs), which enable patients to communicate their perceived health status including quality of life, symptoms, functionality, physical, mental, and social health.[19]

Access to care includes features that improve timely access to care and care availability and minimize financial barriers for patients. Some of these features have been evaluated in ILD. In a prospective study of 129 patients with IPF, the median time from onset of dyspnea to initial evaluation at a tertiary care center was 2.2 years (interquartile range [IQR] 1.0–3.8). This delay in access to care was associated with worse survival.[8] Furthermore, there have been studies evaluating the economic burden in ILD and highlighting the financial barriers faced by patients.[20,21]

Patient-reported outcomes (PROs), which include PRO measures (PROMs) and patient-reported experience measures, are an important clinical and research tool. PROs have been used to better understand the ILD diagnostic experience, which can include frequent misdiagnosis, exposure to costly and invasive diagnostic procedures, and use of substantial health care resources.[18] Understanding the patient perspective is critical to ensuring that health care priorities are based on importance to and impact on patients.[22]

PATIENT-CENTERED CARE IN RESEARCH

The use of PROMs increases patient engagement and maximizes the relevance and value of research to patients. PROMs are standardized, validated questionnaires that are completed by patients to measure their perception of their health status.[23] There are a multitude of PROMs, which include instruments looking at health-related quality of life (HRQOL), symptoms, health-related behaviors such as anxiety or depression, and functional status. An overview of PROMs that communicate common health status impairments experienced by patients with ILD is presented (**Table 3**). The PROMs discussed have not all been validated in ILD; however, as these PROMs are more fully understood and validated in ILD, they increasingly will offer additional insight into the success of PCC programs in clinical practice. Thus, understanding of the strengths and weaknesses of the PROMs indirectly may advance PCC care in ILD.

DYSPNEA
University of California San Diego Shortness of Breath Questionnaire

The University of California San Diego (UCSD) Shortness of Breath Questionnaire (SOBQ) is a 24-item questionnaire that assesses self-reported shortness of breath while performing various activities of daily living. Patients indicate the severity of shortness of breath for each question on a 6-point scale, which then are summed to generate a total SOBQ score. The score ranges from 0 to 120, with a higher score indicating greater severity of dyspnea. The SOBQ was validated in a cohort of 54 patients with different pulmonary disorders (cystic fibrosis, COPD, and post–lung transplant) who were participating in the UCSD pulmonary rehabilitation program.[24] The cohort included 1 patient with IPF who was post–lung transplant.

The SOBQ has been used to study dyspnea in various ILD subtypes. In a randomized controlled trial investigating pirfenidone in unclassifiable ILD, there was no difference in dyspnea using the SOBQ in patients with unclassifiable ILD who received pirfenidone versus placebo over 24 weeks.[25] Dyspnea also has been shown to predict physical function, psychological well-being, and fatigue in patients with connective tissue disease–associated ILD.[26]

Others

Other PROMs that have been used to assess dyspnea in ILD include the Dyspnea-12 (D-12) questionnaire and Medical Research Council (MRC) dyspnea scale. The D-12 consists of 12 physical and affective statements related to dyspnea, where patients grade their severity from 0 to 3, with a total score ranging between 0 and 36, and has been validated in patients with various ILDs.[27] The MRC dyspnea scale quantifies the disability associated with breathlessness when it should not occur (grades 1 and 2) or when there is associated exercise limitation (grades 3–5).[28] The MRC dyspnea scale has been associated with lung function, walk distance, and survival in patients with respiratory diseases.[29–31]

COUGH
Visual Analog Scale

The 100-mm visual analog scale (VAS) allows patients to report their cough severity by placing an X on a line measuring 100 mm. The point where the 2 lines of the X intersect is the VAS value, with higher values representing greater cough severity.[32] The VAS has been used to compare cough intensity between ILD subtypes. Patients with idiopathic interstitial pneumonias had higher cough severity compared with patients with connective tissue disease–associated ILD and fibrotic hypersensitivity pneumonitis.[33] Cough severity similarly was found greatest in patients with IPF, with a median VAS score of 39 (IQR 17–65) compared with 29 (IQR 11–48) in fibrotic hypersensitivity pneumonitis and of 18 (IQR 0–33) in systemic sclerosis–associated (SSc)-ILD ($P<.0001$).[34]

Leicester Cough Questionnaire

The Leicester Cough Questionnaire (LCQ) was developed based on patients who were seen in an adult respiratory outpatient clinic for chronic cough.[35] It contains 19 items that assess how cough affects quality of life in physical, psychological, and social domains. Items are summed to create a domain score that ranges between 1

Table 3
Overview of select patient-reported outcome measures that have been used in interstitial lung disease studies[27,38,48,49,57–63]

PROM	Validated in Interstitial Lung Disease	Number of Items	Score Range	Minimal Clinically Important Difference	Minimal Clinically Important Difference Study Population
Dyspnea					
UCSD SOBQ	Yes	24	0–120	8	IPF
MRC	Yes	1	1–5	—	—
D-12	Yes	12	0–36	—	—
Cough					
VAS	No	1	0–100	17	Acute cough
LCQ	No	19	0–21	1.3	Chronic cough
Health-related quality of life					
EQ-5D-5L	Yes	5	N/A	0.1	Fibrotic ILD
EQ VAS	Yes	1	0–100	10	Fibrotic ILD
SF-36	Yes	36	0–100	2–4	IPF
K-BILD	Yes	15	0–100	4	ILD
SGRQ	Yes	50	0–100	4–8	IPF
ATAQ-IPF-cA	Yes	43	43–172	—	—
Fatigue and sleep					
FAS	Yes	10	10–50	4	Sarcoidosis
PSQI	No	19	0–21	—	—
Anxiety and depression					
HADS	No	42	0–21	Anxiety 1.3–1.8[a] Depression 1.5–1.7[a]	COPD

Abbreviations: N/A, not applicable; OLD, obstructive lung disease; URTI, upper respiratory tract infection.

The minimal clinically important difference is the smallest change in a questionnaire score that indicates a meaningful change perceived by patients. A validated questionnaire means it has been psychometrically tested for reliability, validity, and sensitivity. The highest reported minimal clinically important differences for EQ-5D-5L and EQ VAS in fibrotic ILD are shown.

[a] HADS anxiety and depression subscales.

and 7. The 3 domain scores then are added together to generate a total score (range 3–21), with a higher score indicating lower cough severity. There is a strong correlation between objective cough frequency and LCQ (r = −0.80) in patients with IPF.[36]

HEALTH-RELATED QUALITY OF LIFE
EQ-5D

The 5-level Euroquol EQ-5D (EQ-5D-5L) is a generic tool that assesses HRQOL.[37] The EQ-5D-5L comprises a descriptive system, the EQ-5D, with 5 dimensions (mobility, self-care, usual activity, pain/discomfort, and anxiety/depression), and the EQ-VAS (ranging from 0 to 100, reflecting a patient's overall perceived health). Each dimension has 5

levels that the patient selects from: no problems, slight problems, moderate problems, severe problems, and extreme problems. The final score is a 5-digit number representing the levels selected for each dimension. Using country-specific value sets, the EQ-5D-5L score then can be converted to health utilities, which are preference values that patients attach to their overall health status (higher values represent better health status).[37]

A benefit of using a generic tool, such as the EQ-5D-5L, is that it allows comparison of HRQOL between different diseases and patient populations as well as enabling cost utility analyses to be conducted. The EQ-5D-5L and EQ-VAS have been validated in fibrotic ILD.[38] A range of values for the minimum important difference was determined using different statistical techniques, with the largest minimum important differences 0.1 and 10 for the EQ-5D-5L and EQ VAS, respectively. The EQ-5D has been used to evaluate the cost-effectiveness of antifibrotics in IPF,[39] in addition to assessing quality of life in ILD. A higher forced vital capacity (FVC)–percent predicted, older age, higher education, and working full time have been shown associated with higher HRQOL across all EQ-5D dimensions in ILD.[40] The FVC–percent predicted is associated with higher utility scores and EQ VAS, whereas only a higher diffusing capacity of the lung for carbon monoxide (DLCO)–percent predicted is associated with higher utility scores in SSc-ILD.[41]

King's Brief Interstitial Lung Disease

The King's Brief Interstitial Lung Disease (K-BILD) is a disease-specific, validated HRQOL questionnaire that comprises 3 domains: breathlessness and activities, chest symptoms, and psychological.[42] There are 15 items using a 7-point response scale, with the total score ranging between 0 and 100 (higher score represents better health status). It currently is the only ILD-specific HRQOL questionnaire that has been validated using patients with various ILD subtypes. The K-BILD has moderate correlation with lung function (r = 0.30 for FVC–percent predicted, and r = 0.45 for DLCO–percent predicted) and high correlation with health utilities derived from the generic EQ-5D (r = 0.71).[40,43]

The K-BILD has been applied in ILD clinical trials. In the AmbOx study, a randomized controlled trial evaluating supplemental oxygen in ILD, patients who received 2 weeks of supplemental oxygen had significantly higher HRQOL compared with those who did not receive oxygen, with a mean difference in total K-BILD score of 3.7 (95% CI, 1.8–5.6; P<.0001).[44] It also has been used to compare HRQOL between different ILD subtypes.[45] Patients with SSc-ILD had significantly better scores for the psychological domain of the K-BILD compared with IPF. There were no significant differences in the breathlessness and chest symptoms domains after adjusting for age, sex, FVC, and DLCO.[45]

Others

The Medical Outcomes Study 36-Item Short Form Health Survey (SF-36) is a commonly used generic HRQOL questionnaire that measures 8 key health concepts: physical functioning, role limitations due to physical health problems, bodily pain, general health, vitality, social functioning, role limitations due to emotional problems, and mental health.[46] Scores for each domain range from 0 to 100,

with a higher score reflecting a more favorable health state. There also is a specific version of the St George's Respiratory Questionnaire (SGRQ) for IPF, which retains 34 items from the original SGRQ and covers 3 domains: impacts, activities, and symptoms.[47] The A Tool to Assess Quality of Life in Idiopathic Pulmonary Fibrosis Cross-Atlantic (ATAQ-IPF-cA) is another IPF-specific HRQOL questionnaire that has been validated using study cohorts from the United States and United Kingdom. It comprises 43 items and 10 domains.[48]

SLEEP AND FATIGUE
Fatigue Assessment Scale

The Fatigue Assessment Scale (FAS) contains 10 items that allow patients to report their physical and mental fatigue using a 5-point scale.[49] These items then are added together to generate a total FAS score between 10 and 50, with a higher score indicating more fatigue. Fatigue is indicated by a score greater than or equal to 22 points, with greater than or equal to 34 points indicating severe fatigue. In patients with sarcoidosis, fatigue was associated with various domains of quality of life (physical, psychological, social, and environmental).[50]

Pittsburgh Sleep Quality Index

The Pittsburgh Sleep Quality Index (PSQI) assesses sleep quality and disturbances over a 1-month period.[51] There are 19 items that are used to generate 7 component scores, which then are added together to determine a global score that ranges between 0 and 21, where higher scores reflect worse sleep quality. In a cross-sectional analysis of 101 patients with ILD participating in a pulmonary rehabilitation program, poor sleep quality was common (67% of cohort reported poor sleep quality, with a median PSQI of 8 units [IQR 4–11]). Poor sleep quality also was independently associated with increasing symptoms of depression and sleepiness.[52]

ANXIETY AND DEPRESSION
Hospital Anxiety and Depression Scale

The Hospital Anxiety and Depression Scale (HADS) was created in 1983 and commonly is used in research studies.[53] It comprises 14 items (7 items each for anxiety and depression), with a score ranging between 0 and 21 for the anxiety and depression subscales. Scores between 8 and 10 indicate a moderate presence of symptoms, whereas a score greater than 11 indicates a significant number of symptoms that likely correspond with a clinical diagnosis.[54]

Using the HADS, the prevalence rates of clinically significant anxiety and depression are 12% and 7%, respectively, in patients with ILD.[55] A higher dyspnea score has been shown an independent predictor of anxiety (odds ratio [OR 2.60]; 95% CI, 1.37–4.92) and depression (OR 3.84; 95% CI, 1.25–11.78) among patients with ILD.[55] A greater number of comorbidities also is an independent predictor of depression (OR 2.02; 95% CI, 0.97–4.21).[55] Furthermore, depression also may have an impact on exercise capacity, with higher depression scores associated with fewer step counts in patients with fibrotic ILD.[56]

FUTURE DIRECTIONS

The priority of implementing PCC has increased over time and, as a result, various frameworks have been created. The multitude of different PCC approaches, however, makes it challenging to know which to follow and if one is preferable over others. The PCC framework described in this article seeks to incorporate common features shared by many models identified from a scoping review; however, it requires further validation and integration of patient perspectives. Further research also is needed to determine how best to evaluate PCC practices in order to guide quality improvement. Within research, studies incorporating PROMs will add to the outcome measures available to assess PCC clinical practices. Lastly, engaging patients throughout the process of implementing PCC in clinical care and research, including the design of PROMs, is critical to the success of any PCC program.

SUMMARY

PCC is essential to improving health care quality in the clinical and research setting. From a clinical perspective, features of PCC can be categorized into structural, process, or outcome domains and are interdependent on one another. For research, the use of PROMs is one method of integrating PCC.

An important consideration is how PCC frameworks and tools can be integrated into ILD care. Many questions remain unanswered. Should PROMs be used routinely in clinical care? Should only PROMs that have been validated in ILD be used? How can respondent fatigue from completing surveys and participating in research be minimized? In addition, the delivery of PCC requires more time between providers and patients, but it leads to increased quality of care and satisfaction with health care delivery. The appropriate infrastructure and reimbursement to support PCC are critical components to the success of this care model. There are examples of well-established PCC processes in ILD care, such as the use of multidisciplinary discussion and working in interdisciplinary teams with other specialists and allied health professionals. There are many areas, however, to improve PCC further, requiring stakeholders, including patients, caregivers, hospital administrators, and policy makers, to come together and work toward this important common goal.

CLINICS CARE POINTS

- PCC is part of the foundation of improving health care quality.
- PCC features can be categorized into 3 domains: structure, process, and outcomes.
- PCC structure refers to the necessary materials, health care resources, and organizational characteristics required to support PCC processes and outcomes.
- PCC process refers to the interaction between patients and health care providers.
- PCC outcomes are indicators that can measure the quality of PCC structure and process to ensure that the implemented model is effective and valuable.
- PROMs provide patient perspectives on their health status and should be integrated into clinical care and research.

DISCLOSURE

A.W. Wong and S.K. Danoff report no conflicts of interest.

REFERENCES

1. McMillan SS, Kendall E, Sav A, et al. Patient-centered approaches to health care: a systematic review of randomized controlled trials. Med Care Res Rev 2013;70(6):567–96.
2. Mead N, Bower P. Patient-centred consultations and outcomes in primary care: a review of the literature. Patient Educ Couns 2002;48(1):51–61.
3. Santana MJ, Manalili K, Jolley RJ, et al. How to practice person-centred care: a conceptual framework. Health Expect 2018;21(2):429–40.
4. National center for Interprofessional practice and education. Picker Institute's eight principles of

patient-centered care. Available at: https://nexusipe. org/informing/resource-center/picker-institute%E2% 80%99s-eight-principles-patient-centered-care. Accessed September 24, 2020.

5. Collard HR, Tino G, Noble PW, et al. Patient experiences with pulmonary fibrosis. Respir Med 2007; 101(6):1350–4.

6. Goobie GC, Guler SA, Johannson KA, et al. YouTube videos as a source of misinformation on idiopathic pulmonary fibrosis. Ann Am Thorac Soc 2019; 16(5):572–9.

7. Fisher JH, O'Connor D, Flexman AM, et al. Accuracy and reliability of internet resources for information on idiopathic pulmonary fibrosis. Am J Respir Crit Care Med 2016;194(2):218–25.

8. Lamas DJ, Kawut SM, Bagiella E, et al. Delayed access and survival in idiopathic pulmonary fibrosis: a cohort study. Am J Respir Crit Care Med 2011; 184(7):842–7.

9. Vasilopoulou M, Papaioannou AI, Kaltsakas G, et al. Home-based maintenance tele-rehabilitation reduces the risk for acute exacerbations of COPD, hospitalisations and emergency department visits. Eur Respir J 2017;49(5):1602129.

10. Sidhu A, Chaparro C, Chow CW, et al. Outcomes of telehealth care for lung transplant recipients. Clin Transplant 2019;33(6):e13580.

11. Moor CC, Wapenaar M, Miedema JR, et al. A home monitoring program including real-time wireless home spirometry in idiopathic pulmonary fibrosis: a pilot study on experiences and barriers. Respir Res 2018;19(1):105.

12. King A, Hoppe RB. Best practice" for patient-centered communication: a narrative review. J Grad Med Educ 2013;5(3):385–93.

13. Roter DL, Hall JA, Katz NR. Relations between physicians' behaviors and analogue patients' satisfaction, recall, and impressions. Med Care 1987;25(5):437–51.

14. Coulter A. Patient engagement–what works? J Ambul Care Manage 2012;35(2):80–9.

15. Coulter A, Ellins J. Effectiveness of strategies for informing, educating, and involving patients. BMJ 2007;335(7609):24–7.

16. Beck RS, Daughtridge R, Sloane PD. Physician-patient communication in the primary care office: a systematic review. J Am Board Fam Pract 2002;15(1):25–38.

17. Elwyn G, Durand MA, Song J, et al. A three-talk model for shared decision making: multistage consultation process. BMJ 2017;359:j4891.

18. Cosgrove GP, Bianchi P, Danese S, et al. Barriers to timely diagnosis of interstitial lung disease in the real world: the INTENSITY survey. BMC Pulm Med 2018; 18(1):9.

19. Santana MJ, Feeny D. Framework to assess the effects of using patient-reported outcome measures in chronic care management. Qual Life Res 2014; 23(5):1505–13.

20. Frank AL, Kreuter M, Schwarzkopf L. Economic burden of incident interstitial lung disease (ILD) and the impact of comorbidity on costs of care. Respir Med 2019;152:25–31.

21. Zhou Z, Fan Y, Thomason D, et al. Economic burden of illness among commercially insured patients with systemic sclerosis with interstitial lung disease in the USA: a claims data analysis. Adv Ther 2019;36(5): 1100–13.

22. Swigris JJ, Brown KK, Abdulqawi R, et al. Patients' perceptions and patient-reported outcomes in progressive-fibrosing interstitial lung diseases. Eur Respir Rev 2018;27(150):180075.

23. Weldring T, Smith SM. Patient-reported outcomes (PROs) and patient-reported outcome measures (PROMs). Health Serv Insights 2013;6:61–8.

24. Eakin EG, Resnikoff PM, Prewitt LM, et al. Validation of a new dyspnea measure: the UCSD shortness of breath questionnaire. University of California, san Diego. Chest 1998;113(3):619–24.

25. Maher TM, Corte TJ, Fischer A, et al. Pirfenidone in patients with unclassifiable progressive fibrosing interstitial lung disease: a double-blind, randomised, placebo-controlled, phase 2 trial. Lancet Respir Med 2020;8(2):147–57.

26. Swigris JJ, Yorke J, Sprunger DB, et al. Assessing dyspnea and its impact on patients with connective tissue disease-related interstitial lung disease. Respir Med 2010;104(9):1350–5.

27. Yorke J, Swigris J, Russell AM, et al. Dyspnea-12 is a valid and reliable measure of breathlessness in patients with interstitial lung disease. Chest 2011; 139(1):159–64.

28. Bestall JC, Paul EA, Garrod R, et al. Usefulness of the Medical Research Council (MRC) dyspnoea scale as a measure of disability in patients with chronic obstructive pulmonary disease. Thorax 1999;54(7):581–6.

29. Nishimura K, Izumi T, Tsukino M, et al. Dyspnea is a better predictor of 5-year survival than airway obstruction in patients with COPD. Chest 2002; 121(5):1434–40.

30. Mechanisms Dyspnea. , assessment, and management: a consensus statement. American Thoracic Society. Am J Respir Crit Care Med 1999;159(1):321–40.

31. Mahler DA, Wells CK. Evaluation of clinical methods for rating dyspnea. Chest 1988;93(3):580–6.

32. Missiuna C, Pollock N, Campbell WN, et al. Use of the Medical Research Council Framework to develop a complex intervention in pediatric occupational therapy: assessing feasibility. Res Dev Disabil 2012;33(5):1443–52.

33. Sato R, Handa T, Matsumoto H, et al. Clinical significance of self-reported cough intensity and frequency in patients with interstitial lung disease: a cross-sectional study. BMC Pulm Med 2019;19(1): 247.

34. Cheng JZ, Wilcox PG, Glaspole I, et al. Cough is less common and less severe in systemic sclerosis-associated interstitial lung disease compared to other fibrotic interstitial lung diseases. Respirology 2017;22(8):1592–7.

35. Birring SS, Prudon B, Carr AJ, et al. Development of a symptom specific health status measure for patients with chronic cough: Leicester Cough Questionnaire (LCQ). Thorax 2003;58(4):339–43.

36. Key AL, Holt K, Hamilton A, et al. Objective cough frequency in idiopathic pulmonary fibrosis. Cough 2010;6:4.

37. Bakker C, van der Linden S. Health related utility measurement: an introduction. J Rheumatol 1995; 22(6):1197–9.

38. Tsai APY, Hur SA, Wong A, et al. Minimum important difference of the EQ-5D-5L and EQ-VAS in fibrotic interstitial lung disease. Thorax 2020;76(1):37–43.

39. Rinciog C, Watkins M, Chang S, et al. A cost-effectiveness analysis of nintedanib in idiopathic pulmonary fibrosis in the UK. Pharmacoeconomics 2017;35(4):479–91.

40. Szentes BL, Kreuter M, Bahmer T, et al. Quality of life assessment in interstitial lung diseases:a comparison of the disease-specific K-BILD with the generic EQ-5D-5L. Respir Res 2018;19(1):101.

41. Ciaffi J, van Leeuwen NM, Liem SIE, et al. Lung function is associated with minimal EQ-5D changes over time in patients with systemic sclerosis. Clin Rheumatol 2020;39(5):1543–9.

42. Patel AS, Siegert RJ, Brignall K, et al. The development and validation of the King's Brief Interstitial Lung Disease (K-BILD) health status questionnaire. Thorax 2012;67(9):804–10.

43. Prior TS, Hilberg O, Shaker SB, et al. Validation of the King's brief interstitial lung disease questionnaire in idiopathic pulmonary fibrosis. BMC Pulm Med 2019;19(1):255.

44. Visca D, Mori L, Tsipouri V, et al. Effect of ambulatory oxygen on quality of life for patients with fibrotic lung disease (AmbOx): a prospective, open-label, mixed-method, crossover randomised controlled trial. Lancet Respir Med 2018;6(10):759–70.

45. Durheim MT, Hoffmann-Vold AM, Eagan TM, et al. ILD-specific health-related quality of life in systemic sclerosis-associated ILD compared with IPF. BMJ Open Respir Res 2020;7(1).

46. Cordier R, Brown T, Clemson L, et al. Evaluating the longitudinal item and category stability of the SF-36 full and summary scales using rasch analysis. Biomed Res Int 2018;2018:1013453.

47. Yorke J, Jones PW, Swigris JJ. Development and validity testing of an IPF-specific version of the St George's respiratory questionnaire. Thorax 2010; 65(10):921–6.

48. Yorke J, Spencer LG, Duck A, et al. Cross-Atlantic modification and validation of the A tool to assess quality of life in idiopathic pulmonary fibrosis (ATAQ-IPF-cA). BMJ Open Respir Res 2014;1(1):e000024.

49. de Kleijn WP, De Vries J, Wijnen PA, et al. Minimal (clinically) important differences for the Fatigue Assessment Scale in sarcoidosis. Respir Med 2011;105(9):1388–95.

50. Michielsen HJ, Drent M, Peros-Golubicic T, et al. Fatigue is associated with quality of life in sarcoidosis patients. Chest 2006;130(4):989–94.

51. Buysse DJ, Reynolds CF 3rd, Monk TH, et al. The Pittsburgh Sleep Quality Index: a new instrument for psychiatric practice and research. Psychiatry Res 1989;28(2):193–213.

52. Cho JG, Teoh A, Roberts M, et al. The prevalence of poor sleep quality and its associated factors in patients with interstitial lung disease: a cross-sectional analysis. ERJ Open Res 2019;5(3). 00062-2019.

53. Zigmond AS, Snaith RP. The hospital anxiety and depression scale. Acta Psychiatr Scand 1983; 67(6):361–70.

54. Bocerean C, Dupret E. A validation study of the Hospital Anxiety and Depression Scale (HADS) in a large sample of French employees. BMC Psychiatry 2014;14:354.

55. Holland AE, Fiore JF Jr, Bell EC, et al. Dyspnoea and comorbidity contribute to anxiety and depression in interstitial lung disease. Respirology 2014;19(8): 1215–21.

56. Hur SA, Guler SA, Khalil N, et al. Impact of psychological deficits and pain on physical activity of patients with interstitial lung disease. Lung 2019; 197(4):415–25.

57. Lee KK, Matos S, Evans DH, et al. A longitudinal assessment of acute cough. Am J Respir Crit Care Med 2013;187(9):991–7.

58. Swigris JJ, Brown KK, Behr J, et al. The SF-36 and SGRQ: validity and first look at minimum important differences in IPF. Respir Med 2010;104(2):296–304.

59. Raj AA, Pavord DI, Birring SS. Clinical cough IV:what is the minimal important difference for the Leicester Cough Questionnaire? Handb Exp Pharmacol 2009; 187:311–20.

60. Swigris JJ, Han M, Vij R, et al. The UCSD shortness of breath questionnaire has longitudinal construct validity in idiopathic pulmonary fibrosis. Respir Med 2012;106(10):1447–55.

61. Papiris SA, Daniil ZD, Malagari K, et al. The Medical Research Council dyspnea scale in the estimation of disease severity in idiopathic pulmonary fibrosis. Respir Med 2005;99(6):755–61.

62. Nolan CM, Birring SS, Maddocks M, et al. King's Brief Interstitial Lung Disease questionnaire: responsiveness and minimum clinically important difference. Eur Respir J 2019;54(3):1900281.

63. Smid DE, Franssen FM, Houben-Wilke S, et al. Responsiveness and MCID Estimates for CAT, CCQ, and HADS in Patients with COPD undergoing pulmonary rehabilitation: a prospective analysis. J Am Med Dir Assoc 2017;18(1):53–8.

Care Delivery Models and Interstitial Lung Disease
The Role of the Specialized Center

Jolene H. Fisher, MD, MSc[a], Vincent Cottin, MD, PhD[b],*

KEYWORDS

- Interstitial lung disease • Multidisciplinary team • Specialized center

KEY POINTS

- The goals of interstitial lung disease (ILD) care delivery models are multifaceted and centered around providing timely access to an accurate diagnosis and effective care plan.
- The specialized center plays an integral role in ILD care delivery, with key components including diagnosis, treatment, monitoring, care coordination, support/advocacy, education, and research.
- There are significant barriers to widespread access of specialized ILD care delivery, and innovative strategies that leverage technology are required to bridge these gaps.

INTRODUCTION

Interstitial lung disease (ILD) is rapidly evolving and multifaceted with patients that experience debilitating symptoms and poor prognosis. Care delivery models that use specialized centers with access to ILD-specific resources have emerged as a way to provide comprehensive care to these patients with complex diseases. The goals of the specialized center are multifold and centered around providing timely access to an accurate diagnosis and effective care plan. Other deliverables include management of treatment side effects and patient comorbidities, patient education and support groups, medical education of both practicing clinicians and trainees and access to clinical trials, lung transplant, and end-of-life care. A multidisciplinary team is integral to providing such complex care delivery and requires access to pulmonology, rheumatology, pathology, thoracic surgery/interventional pulmonology, radiology, palliative care, lung transplant, pharmacy, nursing, social work, and administrative support (both clinical and research), with ILD expertise

(**Fig. 1**). Universal access to these highly specialized centers with optimal resources and expertise remains a significant challenge that requires innovative strategies to overcome. The aims of this article are to (1) summarize the key components of ILD care, (2) describe the role of the specialized center in the delivery of each component of ILD care, and (3) identify the current challenges facing ILD care delivery models and propose viable strategies to overcome these gaps. Key messages are summarized in **Table 1**.

KEY COMPONENTS OF INTERSTITIAL LUNG DISEASE CARE AND THE ROLE OF THE SPECIALIZED CENTER IN DELIVERY
Diagnosis

ILD subtypes have variable epidemiology, clinical course, and management. A timely and accurate ILD diagnosis is critical for clinical decision-making, patient counseling, and advancing research. The current gold standard for ILD diagnosis is multidisciplinary discussion (MDD) between "experts" that integrate clinical, radiologic,

[a] Department of Medicine, University Health Network, University of Toronto, 9N-945 585 University Avenue, Toronto, Ontario M5G 2N2, Canada; [b] Department of Respiratory Medicine, National Coordinating Reference Center for Rare Pulmonary Diseases, Louis Pradel Hospital, Hospices Civils de Lyon, Claude Bernard University Lyon 1, INRAE, IVPC, RespiFil, Radico-ILD and ERN-LUNG, F-69008, UMR754, 28 Avenue Doyen Lepine, Lyon Cedex 69677, France
* Corresponding author.
E-mail address: vincent.cottin@chu-lyon.fr

Clin Chest Med 42 (2021) 347–355
https://doi.org/10.1016/j.ccm.2021.03.013
0272-5231/21/© 2021 Elsevier Inc. All rights reserved.

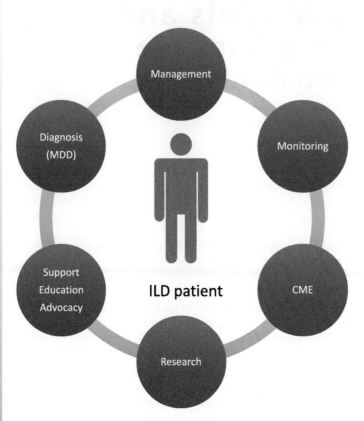

Fig. 1. Key components of interstitial lung disease care delivery. CME, continuing medical education; MDD, multidisciplinary discussion.

and where available, pathologic features in order to reach a consensus diagnosis.[1–4] Within the tripod of clinical, radiologic, and pathologic features, the MDD further incorporates a variety of information that contribute to diagnosis, including autoimmune serology, precipitins, clinical or molecular biology genetic information, molecular classifiers, or reports from other health care providers (eg, occupational medicine specialist, domiciliary visit looking for exposures that may cause hypersensitivity pneumonitis, etc.). Utilization of MDDs have been shown to improve diagnostic confidence and decrease interobserver variability.[5–8] MDDs, at minimum, include a pulmonologist and radiologist with ILD expertise and depending on the individual case, other specialty involvement, such as, pathology, and rheumatology.[9] Specialized diagnostic resources, including extensive autoimmune serology and histopathology obtained by videothoracoscopic surgical lung biopsy (SLB) or cryobiopsy, may be needed to make an accurate diagnosis. MDD groups that do not include all ILD-specific experts benefit from access to larger and more versed MDDs for their more complex cases, as the quality of MDD depends on experience.[10]

Widespread availability of safe and accurate diagnostic testing for ILD remains a significant challenge. Although decreased by the use of video-assisted techniques and appropriate patient selection, SLB is still associated with high morbidity and mortality,[11] particularly in centers with less experience.[12] In addition, there can be significant interobserver variability in histopathology interpretation.[13] Although less invasive, similar issues have been identified with the use of transbronchial lung cryobiopsy.[14–16] Such "volume-outcome" relationships have been described across a variety of medical and surgical specialties and used to support the regionalization of specialty care.[17,18] Awareness of the risk and limitations associated with SLB has contributed to efforts aimed at improving ILD diagnosis in its absence, such as developing the concept of a working/provisional diagnosis, the probable usual interstitial pneumonia definition, and a molecular classifier.[1,19–21] The expertise of an ILD center may reduce the number of cases in which a biopsy is contemplated and performed, as compared with centers with less ILD familiarity.

The complexities surrounding ILD diagnosis have led to increasing regionalization of care with a push to refer to expert centers. Although these regional, expert centers can increase diagnostic accuracy for ILDs, they can also be disadvantaged by limited accessibility. Delayed access to an ILD

Table 1 Summary of key messages	
Key Components of ILD Care and the Role of the Specialized Center in Delivery	
Care Delivery Component	**Key Messages**
Diagnosis	• Accurate and timely ILD diagnosis is a key component of ILD care. • MDD requires access to specialty resources that are typically only available at specialized ILD centers.
Management	• ILD management is multifaceted with pharmacologic and nonpharmacologic components. • Treatment decisions can be nuanced and are often guided by expert opinion, given that many cases do not fall into existing management guidelines. • The infrastructure needed to provide comprehensive ILD management is typically limited outside of the specialized center.
Longitudinal monitoring	• Longitudinal monitoring of patients with ILD is essential to informing management decision-making. • A "shared-care" model between local pulmonologists and ILD centers can facilitate timely access to care, minimize patient travel, and "off-load" specialty clinics.
Medical education	• ILD-related medical education for clinicians and trainees is a key component of ILD care delivery. • Additional research on ILD knowledge gaps and effective education strategies is required.
Patient education, support, and advocacy	• Patient education, support, and advocacy is a key component of ILD care delivery. • Specialized ILD clinics facilitate patient education, support, and advocacy through direct patient interaction and community engagement.
Research and access to clinical trials	• Access to clinical trials is an important part of ILD care delivery. • The infrastructure, momentum, and commitment to research required to conduct clinical trials in ILD is typically available at specialized centers.
Challenges and Solutions Facing ILD Care Delivery	
Challenge	**Key Messages**
Multidisciplinary discussion	• Limited access to an ILD center and a specialized MDD is a barrier to a timely diagnosis and effective treatment plan for patients with ILD. • Using virtual MDDs is a strategy to increase MDD access.
Longitudinal monitoring	• Remote monitoring and shared care models with local physicians can decrease travel burden for patients with ILD, provide timely access to care, offload specialized clinics, and contribute to the continuing medical education of referring physicians.
Racial, ethnic, and gender disparities and ILD care delivery	• Research on race, ethnic, and gender disparities in ILD care access and delivery is urgently needed.
Future of ILD care delivery	• International collaborations and networks are the future of ILD care delivery.

center is associated with increased mortality, independent of disease severity.[22] Disparate access varies widely and can result from geography, marginalization, and lack of health care resources. These specific barriers depend on jurisdiction with issues such as geography typically more relevant in places such as Canada and Australia as opposed to Europe. Innovative strategies are needed to overcome these barriers and increase access to MDDs and specialized diagnostic testing for patients with ILD.

Management

The comprehensive management of ILD is complex and rapidly evolving with both pharmacologic and nonpharmacologic components.[23–26] There are several reasons for this complexity. ILDs include multiple conditions with variable disease behavior and therefore different goals of therapy. Some of these conditions are potentially reversible or partially reversible such as nonfibrotic hypersensitivity pneumonitis, whereas others, such as idiopathic pulmonary fibrosis (IPF), are progressive. Treatment decisions regarding ILD medications can be nuanced, given that many therapies are aimed at slowing disease progression as opposed to disease reversal, necessitating careful consideration of the risk versus benefit profile in each patient. Although there has been a recent increase in quality data for the treatment of non-IPF ILD,[27,28] more is required, and treatment decisions for conditions such as hypersensitivity pneumonitis and unclassifiable ILD are often heavily influenced by "expert opinion." In the absence of management guidelines, decisions regarding treatment of connective tissue disease (CTD)-ILD are best done in conjunction with rheumatology to identify therapies that ideally treat both pulmonary and nonpulmonary disease manifestations.

Comprehensive management further includes access to pulmonary rehabilitation; lung transplant; symptom management/palliative care; advanced care planning; and patient education, support, and advocacy.[26,29,30] The infrastructure of specialized ILD centers are typically best equipped to deliver such comprehensive care, with access to the required resources often limited outside of these select programs.

Longitudinal Monitoring

Longitudinal monitoring of patients with ILD is central to informing management decisions.[3,25,31,32] Regular clinical assessments provide a mechanism to monitor symptoms, screen for disease progression, and identify treatment side effects and/or comorbidities. Information obtained from these interactions guide decisions related to treatment initiation, alteration, or discontinuation and appropriate timing of lung transplant referral, and/or end-of-life planning. In patients with provisional or working diagnoses, longitudinal monitoring provides an opportunity to reconsider the diagnosis that can become clearer overtime (eg, development of extrapulmonary CTD symptoms). Although the specialized center often plays an important role in the long-term monitoring of fibrotic ILD, access to a local pulmonologist has several advantages. Disease behavior is widely variable among patients with ILD, and access to an expedited clinical assessment is ideal in the event of acute deterioration. Shared-care models can facilitate faster access to appropriate expertise for patients. Local care providers can liaise with "expert" ILD centers on a patient's behalf in order to make timely care decisions. This type of care delivery model has the additional advantage of "off-loading" ILD centers with long waiting lists of some follow-up visits, allowing them to efficiently focus their expertise where it provides the most added value.

Medical Education

ILD-related continuing medical education for trainees, general practitioners, radiologists, pulmonologists, thoracic surgeons/interventional pulmonologists, pathologists, and rheumatologists is an essential component of ILD care delivery. Patients with ILD frequently report a lack of ILD awareness among their health care providers, which results in delayed specialist referral, diagnosis, and treatment.[33,34] "Real-world" registry data has shown high rates of SLBs (even in those with a definite usual interstitial pneumonia pattern on high-resolution computed tomography) and corticosteroid use with lower than expected rates of antifibrotic therapy in patients with IPF.[35] These findings are not necessarily surprising, given the complexity and rapid evolution of ILD diagnosis and management, and implies there is a need for ongoing ILD-related knowledge translation and dissemination to the medical community. There are data to support such endeavors, with a national French survey of physicians caring for patients with IPF showing improved knowledge and management of IPF after implementation of an education outreach program.[36] Specialized ILD centers are typically equipped with the necessary infrastructure, such as staff and accreditation, required to deliver these programs.

It is also important to recognize that clinical feedback to physicians referring to ILD centers provides a mechanism for informal medical education. For example, a referring pulmonologist would typically propose a first-choice diagnosis, which may or may not be modified by the MDD at the ILD center. These clinical feedback loops have important educational roles. The MDD has an additional training effect on participating physicians, whether trainees or more senior members.[8,10,37]

Ensuring pulmonology trainees gain competence in the diagnosis and management of ILD is an integral component of improving ILD care delivery. The specialty clinic plays an important role in trainee education, providing a mechanism for high-volume ILD clinical exposure. A survey of British Thoracic Society trainee members found that most of them thought their ILD training was inadequate.[38] Additional studies identifying specific barriers to trainee ILD education and mechanisms for improvement are required. The ILD specialty clinic is also a key component of ILD subspecialty clinical and research training programs.

Patient Education, Support, and Advocacy

Many ILDs are progressive conditions associated with poor quality of life and limited life expectancy. Patients with ILD and caregivers frequently report inadequate emotional and psychological support.[33] A survey of patient perspectives on the benefits of a specialized ILD center found patients placed a high value on gaining a better understanding of their disease and access to a specialized nurse that provided education and support,[39] reenforcing the importance of patient education, support, and advocacy as key components of ILD care delivery. Patients frequently search the Internet for information related to their disease, yet ILD Websites are often inaccurate and outdated.[40] Specialized ILD clinics can provide highly valued disease-related education to patients through many avenues, including direct discussion at clinic visits with an ILD physician and/or nurse educator, provision of disease-specific education handouts, lists of reliable online resources, and formal education programs. Specialized clinics can also facilitate patient and caregiver support groups that provide additional psychosocial and emotional support for patients and families dealing with ILD.

Specialized ILD clinics can promote community engagement through relationships with nonmedical partners, such as patient foundations or patient associations. ILD physicians or nurses from the specialized center may take an active role in the scientific committee of a patient foundation. Here the role of the ILD center goes beyond providing education to the patient during a clinic visit or a specific educational activity, by delivering important educational messages that will be conveyed by the patient foundation. These relationships are a key component of ILD care delivery and provide valuable platforms for education, fundraising, and research advancement. They also give the patient a seat at the table, helping identify and advocate for patient relevant outcomes.

Research and Access to Clinical Trials

There has been significant advancement in drug therapies for ILD and ongoing rapid development of new drugs that require rigorous testing. In many cases of fibrotic ILD, current therapies only offer a slowing of disease progression as opposed to reversal or cure. Subsequently, the ability to offer and effectively conduct clinical trials is a key component of ILD care delivery. Without this ability, drug development will be stifled and we will fall short of our ability to find effective therapies to advance the field of ILD. There are several barriers to physician and patient participation in clinical trials, including access to the required organizational structure, which is often only available at specialized centers. Components often needed include access to an MDD, research personnel (such as trial coordinators), institutional infrastructure (such as research ethics boards), and clinics with a high volume of patients with ILD.

Specialized ILD clinics can facilitate other important forms of research that require access to high volumes of patients with ILD, such as prospective patient registries. This "real world" data on epidemiology, disease course, treatments, and outcomes is especially valuable when studying heterogeneous and less common diseases such as ILDs. Large, national patient registries have published findings on ILD natural history, treatment, and outcomes that would be challenging to obtain by other research avenues.[35,41,42] In addition, registry research can give patients a voice[39] and provide opportunities to study and develop useful patient-centered outcomes.[43]

CHALLENGES FACING INTERSTITIAL LUNG DISEASE CARE DELIVERY MODELS AND PROPOSED SOLUTIONS

Specialized centers are generally highly appreciated by both referring physicians and patients, playing a central role in ILD care delivery. However, limitations of these models can include a lack of widespread and timely access for patients. Disparities in accessing the specialized center can exist due to long waiting lists, marginalization, and geography. Innovative strategies that leverage technology are required to bridge these gaps.

Multidisciplinary Discussion

Limited availability of MDD is a key barrier to accurate and timely ILD diagnosis. Access to MDD can be increased by using various virtual platforms, including remote chart and imaging review, telemedicine, and video conferencing. A retrospective, cross-sectional study from Canada showed that remotely accessed MDDs are feasible, decrease waiting time, and frequently lead to a change in diagnosis and management.[44] In addition, referring physicians report satisfaction with the process and improvement in their own assessment and management of patients with ILD. Although routine use of a remote MDD will benefit from additional study and validation, it is likely to have an increasing place in ILD care delivery. However, the organization of virtual MDD remains a barrier to use in many centers due to lack of secure virtual platforms for data sharing, the time commitment required, absence of remuneration/funding for this type of care model, and the importance of an in-person assessment for determining CTD features, antigenic exposures, and frailty. Virtual consultations with patients may overcome some of these barriers.

Virtual MDDs may not solve the issue of patient volume "overload" experienced at some ILD centers. Additional strategies to most efficiently use MDD resources can be considered in this setting. For example, ILD cases may be triaged to follow a specific MDD "path" according to complexity. Similar approaches have been successfully used in other disciplines, such as Oncology.[45] In the case of ILD, a patient with a usual interstitial pneumonia pattern, no identifiable cause for ILD, and older than 65 years may not require a full MDD discussion, in contrast to more complex cases, such as, unclassifiable ILD or fibrotic hypersensitivity pneumonitis without an identified antigen.

Longitudinal Monitoring

Longitudinal monitoring of patients with ILD solely at specialized centers has several disadvantages. First, many specialized centers do not have the capacity to see new referrals in a timely fashion and to conduct all follow-up visits. Second, attending ongoing follow-up visits can be a significant burden for patients who have to travel far distances. Third, it may be challenging (both for the patient and ILD clinic) to accommodate urgent assessments in the event of a clinical deterioration. Lastly, for successful collaboration, it is important to respect the preexisting patient-doctor relationship of referring physicians, who are intellectual and financial stakeholders in patient care. There are several viable strategies that can be used to circumvent some of these issues. Certain follow-up visits can be done remotely using phone or videoconference by the ILD physician or nurse. Blood work and pulmonary function testing can be done locally with results sent to specialized centers, and prescription renewals can be done remotely.

Home-based patient monitoring programs that incorporate home spirometry have emerged as viable vehicles for ILD care delivery.[46] These programs use eHealth technology to monitor patients remotely. Patient-reported outcomes and physiologic data, such as spirometry, are collected and transmitted real time to ILD care providers. Home spirometry has shown promise for detecting ILD progression and use as a clinical trial endpoint.[47,48] Home-based monitoring programs can decrease cumbersome travel for patients and empower them to take an active role in their disease management, while allowing their physicians to do more frequent monitoring.

In many cases, it is helpful for the patient to have a local pulmonologist who can alternate follow-up visits with the ILD center. There are several advantages to this model, including decreasing travel burden on patients, off-loading ILD centers with long waiting lists, and local access to an expedited assessment in the event of a clinical deterioration. Although the ILD center often plays a central role in confirming or changing the diagnosis and treatment plan, local pulmonologists can provide valuable ongoing monitoring and liaise with expert centers on behalf of their patient in the event of a clinical change. Some ILD centers provide expert opinions to local pulmonologists without directly seeing patients. The best care pathway and balance between remote, in-person and shared follow-up varies between centers and depends on local needs and priorities.

Racial, Ethnic, and Gender Disparities and Interstitial Lung Disease Care Delivery

Racial, ethnic, and gender disparities are well-described determinants of health and health care access.[49–51] It is not known how these characteristics influence access to specialized ILD care or its delivery. Patient gender has been shown to significantly influence whether a patient receives an IPF diagnosis, suggesting gender bias may exist among ILD physicians.[52] In addition, a patient's ILD care needs, expectations, and goals may vary according to culture and region of origin and are factors that need to be considered when delivering care.[30] Research studies evaluating the role that race, ethnicity, and gender play in how specialized ILD care is accessed and delivered are urgently required.

Future of Interstitial Lung Disease Care Delivery

With the exponential pace of knowledge generation, medicine is becoming increasingly subspecialized. ILD specifically has seen many changes in the past decade, with ongoing new discoveries. With such rapid advances, effective knowledge translation and dissemination becomes an increasingly daunting task as care delivery becomes more complex. As a field, the ILD community can leverage collective international expertise to continuously improve ILD care delivery. There are many opportunities for integrating both national and international expertise into local care delivery models. One example would be providing the ability to bring exceptional cases to a national or international MDD. The framework for these types of endeavors already exists in some places, with the European Research Network (ERN-LUNG, https://ern-lung.eu/) being one example. Such frameworks can be expanded on to include other jurisdictions. Infrastructure for national and international clinical care collaborations can also provide a mechanism for less formal interactions, such as asking for advice on a specific aspect of a case (ie, chest computed tomography or histopathology slides). These types of collaborations can increase access to highly specialized ILD care for both remote and marginalized communities and provide additional platforms for education and research. Establishing funding structures that support the time and resources needed to deliver this complex care is critical.

SUMMARY

In summary, comprehensive ILD care delivery has several key components including diagnosis, treatment, monitoring, support/advocacy, education, and research. The role of the specialized center in care delivery is multifaceted (see **Fig. 1**), with an overarching goal of improving patient care and advancing the field of ILD. The current role of the specialized center in ILD care delivery models faces significant feasibility and generalizability challenges. Creative and innovative strategies are needed to find ways to optimally deliver ILD care to the highest number of patients possible.

CLINICS CARE POINTS

- The specialized center plays an integral role in delivery of the multifaceted components of ILD care, including diagnosis, treatment, monitoring, care coordination, support/advocacy, education and research.

- Accurate and timely ILD diagnosis with access to a MDD is a key component of ILD care delivery. However, MDD requires specialty resources that are typically only available at ILD centers and innovative strategies are needed to overcome barriers to widespread MDD access.

- Strategies to improve access to ILD specialty care include virtual MDDs, remote monitoring and shared care models with local physicians and international collaborations and networks.

- ILD related medical education for clinicians and trainees is a key component of ILD care delivery and additional research on ILD knowledge gaps and effective education strategies are required.

- Patient education, support and advocacy is a key component of ILD care delivery and specialized ILD clinics can facilitate these through direct patient interaction and community engagement.

- Research on social, ethnic and gender disparities in ILD care access and delivery is urgently needed.

DISCLOSURE

J.H. Fisher reports no disclosures.

REFERENCES

1. Raghu G, Remy-Jardin M, Myers JL, et al. Diagnosis of idiopathic pulmonary fibrosis. An official ATS/ERS/JRS/ALAT clinical practice guideline. Am J Respir Crit Care Med 2018;198(5):e44–68.

2. Raghu G, Collard HR, Egan JJ, et al. An official ATS/ERS/JRS/ALAT statement: idiopathic pulmonary fibrosis: evidence-based guidelines for diagnosis and management. Am J Respir Crit Care Med 2011;183(6):788–824.

3. Travis WD, Costabel U, Hansell DM, et al. An official American Thoracic Society/European Respiratory Society statement: update of the international multidisciplinary classification of the idiopathic interstitial pneumonias. Am J Respir Crit Care Med 2013;188(6):733–48.

4. Johannson KA, Kolb M, Fell CD, et al. Evaluation of patients with fibrotic interstitial lung disease: a Canadian Thoracic Society position statement. Canadian Journal of Respiratory, Critical Care, and Sleep Medicine 2017;1(3):133–41.

5. Prasad JD, Mahar A, Bleasel J, et al. The interstitial lung disease multidisciplinary meeting: a position statement from the Thoracic Society of Australia and New Zealand and the Lung Foundation Australia. Respirology 2017;22(7):1459–72.

6. Jo HE, Corte TJ, Moodley Y, et al. Evaluating the interstitial lung disease multidisciplinary meeting: a survey of expert centres. BMC Pulm Med 2016;16:22.

7. Flaherty KR, King TE Jr, Raghu G, et al. Idiopathic interstitial pneumonia: what is the effect of a multidisciplinary approach to diagnosis? Am J Respir Crit Care Med 2004;170(8):904–10.

8. De Sadeleer LJ, Meert C, Yserbyt J, et al. Diagnostic ability of a dynamic multidisciplinary discussion in interstitial lung diseases: a retrospective observational study of 938 cases. Chest 2018;153(6): 1416–23.

9. Furini F, Carnevale A, Casoni GL, et al. The role of the multidisciplinary evaluation of interstitial lung diseases: systematic literature review of the current evidence and future perspectives. Front Med (Lausanne) 2019;6:246.

10. Cottin V, Castillo D, Poletti V, et al. Should patients with interstitial lung disease be seen by experts? Chest 2018;154(3):713–4.

11. Hutchinson JP, Fogarty AW, McKeever TM, et al. In-hospital mortality after surgical lung biopsy for interstitial lung disease in the United States. 2000 to 2011. Am J Respir Crit Care Med 2016;193(10): 1161–7.

12. Fisher JH, Shapera S, To T, et al. Procedure volume and mortality after surgical lung biopsy in interstitial lung disease. Eur Respir J 2019;53(2):1801164.

13. Lettieri CJ, Veerappan GR, Parker JM, et al. Discordance between general and pulmonary pathologists in the diagnosis of interstitial lung disease. Respir Med 2005;99(11):1425–30.

14. Johannson KA, Marcoux VS, Ronksley PE, et al. Diagnostic yield and complications of transbronchial lung cryobiopsy for interstitial lung disease. A systematic review and metaanalysis. Ann Am Thorac Soc 2016;13(10):1828–38.

15. Iftikhar IH, Alghothani L, Sardi A, et al. Transbronchial lung cryobiopsy and video-assisted thoracoscopic lung biopsy in the diagnosis of diffuse parenchymal lung disease. A meta-analysis of diagnostic test accuracy. Ann Am Thorac Soc 2017; 14(7):1197–211.

16. Sethi J, Ali MS, Mohananey D, et al. Are transbronchial cryobiopsies ready for prime time?: a systematic review and meta-analysis. J Bronchology Interv Pulmonol 2019;26(1):22–32.

17. Birkmeyer JD, Siewers AE, Finlayson EV, et al. Hospital volume and surgical mortality in the United States. N Engl J Med 2002;346(15):1128–37.

18. Halm EA, Lee C, Chassin MR. Is volume related to outcome in health care? A systematic review and methodologic critique of the literature. Ann Intern Med 2002;137(6):511–20.

19. Ryerson CJ, Corte TJ, Lee JS, et al. A standardized diagnostic ontology for fibrotic interstitial lung disease. An international working group perspective. Am J Respir Crit Care Med 2017;196(10):1249–54.

20. Lynch DA, Sverzellati N, Travis WD, et al. Diagnostic criteria for idiopathic pulmonary fibrosis: a Fleischner Society White Paper. Lancet Respir Med 2018; 6(2):138–53.

21. Raghu G, Flaherty KR, Lederer DJ, et al. Use of a molecular classifier to identify usual interstitial pneumonia in conventional transbronchial lung biopsy samples: a prospective validation study. Lancet Respir Med 2019;7(6):487–96.

22. Lamas DJ, Kawut SM, Bagiella E, et al. Delayed access and survival in idiopathic pulmonary fibrosis: a cohort study. Am J Respir Crit Care Med 2011; 184(7):842–7.

23. Assayag D, Camp PG, Fisher J, et al. Comprehensive management of fibrotic interstitial lung diseases: a Canadian Thoracic Society position statement. Can J Respir Crit Care Sleep Med 2018;2(4):234–43.

24. Richeldi L, Varone F, Bergna M, et al. Pharmacological management of progressive-fibrosing interstitial lung diseases: a review of the current evidence. Eur Respir Rev 2018;27(150):180074.

25. Wijsenbeek M, Cottin V. Spectrum of fibrotic lung diseases. N Engl J Med 2020;383(10):958–68.

26. Wijsenbeek MS, Holland AE, Swigris JJ, et al. Comprehensive supportive care for patients with fibrosing interstitial lung disease. Am J Respir Crit Care Med 2019;200(2):152–9.

27. Flaherty KR, Wells AU, Cottin V, et al. Nintedanib in progressive fibrosing interstitial lung diseases. N Engl J Med 2019;381(18):1718–27.

28. Maher TM, Corte TJ, Fischer A, et al. Pirfenidone in patients with unclassifiable progressive fibrosing interstitial lung disease: a double-blind, randomised, placebo-controlled, phase 2 trial. Lancet Respir Med 2020;8(2):147–57.

29. Jo HE, Troy LK, Keir G, et al. Treatment of idiopathic pulmonary fibrosis in Australia and New Zealand: a position statement from the Thoracic Society of Australia and New Zealand and the Lung Foundation Australia. Respirology 2017;22(7):1436–58.

30. Kreuter M, Bendstrup E, Russell AM, et al. Palliative care in interstitial lung disease: living well. Lancet Respir Med 2017;5(12):968–80.

31. Fisher JH, Johannson KA, Assayag D, et al. Long-term monitoring of patients with fibrotic interstitial

lung disease: a Canadian Thoracic Society Position Statement. Can J Respir Crit Care Sleep Med 2020; 1–9.

32. Wells AU. Any fool can make a rule and any fool will mind it. BMC Med 2016;14:23.

33. Bonella F, Wijsenbeek M, Molina-Molina M, et al. European IPF patient charter: unmet needs and a call to action for healthcare policymakers. Eur Respir J 2016;47(2):597–606.

34. Cosgrove GP, Bianchi P, Danese S, et al. Barriers to timely diagnosis of interstitial lung disease in the real world: the INTENSITY survey. BMC Pulm Med 2018; 18(1):9.

35. Behr J, Kreuter M, Hoeper MM, et al. Management of patients with idiopathic pulmonary fibrosis in clinical practice: the INSIGHTS-IPF registry. Eur Respir J 2015;46(1):186–96.

36. Cottin V, Bergot E, Bourdin A, et al. Adherence to guidelines in idiopathic pulmonary fibrosis: a follow-up national survey. ERJ Open Res 2015; 1(2):00032–2015.

37. De Sadeleer LJ, Wuyts WA. Response. Chest 2018; 154(3):714–5.

38. Sharp C, Maher TM, Welham S, et al. UK trainee experience in interstitial lung disease: results from a British Thoracic Society survey. Thorax 2015; 70(2):183.

39. McLean AEB, Webster SE, Fry M, et al. Priorities and expectations of patients attending a multidisciplinary interstitial lung disease clinic. Respirology 2021;26(1):80–6.

40. Fisher JH, O'Connor D, Flexman AM, et al. Accuracy and reliability of internet resources for information on idiopathic pulmonary fibrosis. Am J Respir Crit Care Med 2016;194(2):218–25.

41. Jo HE, Glaspole I, Grainge C, et al. Baseline characteristics of idiopathic pulmonary fibrosis: analysis from the Australian Idiopathic Pulmonary Fibrosis Registry. Eur Respir J 2017;49(2):1601592.

42. Jo HE, Glaspole I, Moodley Y, et al. Disease progression in idiopathic pulmonary fibrosis with mild physiological impairment: analysis from the Australian IPF registry. BMC Pulm Med 2018;18(1):19.

43. Tsai APY, Hur SA, Wong A, et al. Minimum important difference of the EQ-5D-5L and EQ-VAS in fibrotic interstitial lung disease. Thorax 2021;76(1):37–43.

44. Grewal JS, Morisset J, Fisher JH, et al. Role of a regional multidisciplinary conference in the diagnosis of interstitial lung disease. Ann Am Thorac Soc 2019;16(4):455–62.

45. Selby P, Popescu R, Lawler M, et al. The value and future developments of multidisciplinary team cancer care. Am Soc Clin Oncol Educ Book 2019;39: 332–40.

46. Moor CC, Mostard RLM, Grutters JC, et al. Home monitoring in patients with idiopathic pulmonary fibrosis. A randomized controlled trial. Am J Respir Crit Care Med 2020;202(3):393–401.

47. Russell AM, Adamali H, Molyneaux PL, et al. Daily home spirometry: an effective tool for detecting progression in idiopathic pulmonary fibrosis. Am J Respir Crit Care Med 2016;194(8):989–97.

48. Johannson KA, Vittinghoff E, Morisset J, et al. Home monitoring improves endpoint efficiency in idiopathic pulmonary fibrosis. Eur Respir J 2017;50(1): 1602406.

49. Bach PB, Pham HH, Schrag D, et al. Primary care physicians who treat blacks and whites. N Engl J Med 2004;351(6):575–84.

50. Medicine Io. Unequal treatment: confronting racial and ethnic disparities in health care. Washington, DC: The National Academies Press; 2003.

51. Shannon G, Jansen M, Williams K, et al. Gender equality in science, medicine, and global health: where are we at and why does it matter? Lancet 2019;393(10171):560–9.

52. Assayag D, Morisset J, Johannson KA, et al. Patient gender bias on the diagnosis of idiopathic pulmonary fibrosis. Thorax 2020;75(5):407–12.

Molecular Markers and the Promise of Precision Medicine for Interstitial Lung Disease

Chad A. Newton, MD, MSCS[a,*], Erica L. Herzog, MD, PhD[b]

KEYWORDS

- Interstitial lung disease • Biomarkers • Precision medicine • Omics

KEY POINTS

- Accurate classification of the interstitial lung diseases informs clinical management but is challenged by their overlapping and nonspecific nature.
- Omics-based investigations can efficiently query thousands of candidate molecules as potential biomarkers of clinically meaningful disease phenotypes.
- Discovery, validation, and implementation of clinically useful molecular biomarkers discovered through omics and other approaches will facilitate precision medicine in interstitial lung disease.

INTRODUCTION

The interstitial lung diseases (ILD) encompass diverse disorders characterized by parenchymal inflammation and fibrosis. Historically, the ILDs have been subdivided into seemingly discrete categories according to laborious, complex, and at times irreproducible clinical algorithms based on subjective interpretation of history, examination, imaging, or biopsy.[1,2] Although inflammatory ILDs are generally treated with immunosuppression, antifibrotic therapies are used for ILDs dominated by fibrosis.[3,4] Because of the potential for limited efficacy and off-target side effects of these therapies, the development of objective and reproducible diagnostic, prognostic, and theragnostic approaches would be valuable to patients and the clinicians who care for them.

Complex and heterogeneous conditions, such as ILD, are candidates for precision medicine, which couples clinical phenotypes with molecular endotypes to individualize care.[5] This process leverages objectively quantifiable measures, or "biomarkers," that are ideally noninvasive, accurate, precise, and reproducible. The quest to link ILD endotypes and phenotypes has yielded myriad biomarkers reflecting a convoluted pathobiology that may be deciphered by high-throughput "omics" discoveries. Accordingly, this review describes omics-based biomarker development in an extensively studied ILD, idiopathic pulmonary fibrosis (IPF). After describing the omics pipeline, the authors review representative biomarker discoveries in IPF genomics, epigenomics, transcriptomics, proteomics, and metabolomics. The benefits and limitations of omics and biomarkers are discussed, and the path to precision medicine in ILD will be proposed. The authors end with a series of actionable items to facilitate pursuit of this goal.

[a] Division of Pulmonary and Critical Care Medicine, Department of Internal Medicine, University of Texas Southwestern Medical Center, 5323 Harry Hines Boulevard, Dallas, TX 75390-8558, USA; [b] Section of Pulmonary, Critical Care, and Sleep Medicine, Department of Medicine, Yale School of Medicine, Yale University, 300 Cedar Street TAC441S, New Haven, CT 06520-8057, USA
* Corresponding author.
E-mail address: Chad.Newton@utsouthwestern.edu
Twitter: @cnewto (C.A.N.)

Clin Chest Med 42 (2021) 357–364
https://doi.org/10.1016/j.ccm.2021.03.011
0272-5231/21/© 2021 Elsevier Inc. All rights reserved.

OMICS PIPELINE

The term "omics" denotes the high-throughput and comprehensive assessment of similar molecules within biospecimens. This branch of science evaluates carefully constructed research questions using specimens obtained from explicitly defined cohorts. The general steps of high-quality omics-based analyses include molecular quantification, quality control, data normalization, computational and bioinformatics analysis, correlating molecular perturbations with disease phenotype, and validation of results across platforms and cohorts.[6] These studies have enabled discoveries linking the disciplines of genomics (DNA sequence), epigenomics (nonheritable changes in gene expression), transcriptomics (gene expression), proteomics (relative protein abundance), and metabolomics (metabolism-associated substances). Work in these domains frames IPF as a disease resulting from epithelial injury and overexuberant fibroblast activation that is modulated, but not initiated, by immune cells. Major omics-based discoveries as they relate to precision medicine in IPF are presented in later discussion.

GENOMICS

Genome-wide association studies identify single nucleotide polymorphisms (SNPs) in genomic DNA obtained from easily accessible specimens. These methods have advanced molecular understanding, if not clinical management, of IPF. Of the more than 20 SNPs associated with IPF susceptibility, the most common is an activating rs35705950 SNP located in the promoter region of *MUC5B*,[7–10] which augments MUC5B expression in the distal bronchiolar epithelium[7,11,12] and associates with improved survival.[13] Another SNP, the *TOLLIP* rs3750920, is also associated with IPF, but portends worse survival.[9] The ILD field has also been informed by genomic studies in patients with familial pulmonary fibrosis (FPF) identifying rare variants in surfactant (*SFTPC*) and telomere (*TERT, TERC, PARN, RTEL1, DKC1, NAF1, TINF2*) genes in 1% to 2% and 25% of FPF kindred, respectively.[14–18] These omics studies, many of which validated previous hypothesis-based work,[19–21] support the concept of repetitive lung injury and type II pneumocyte senescence as initiators of disease.[22] In addition, rare variants in telomere genes and short leukocyte telomere length (LTL) represent prognostic biomarkers that are associated with rapid lung function decline and poor survival in FPF and sporadic IPF patients.[23–26] Recently, a post hoc analysis of the landmark PANTHER study[27] demonstrated a harmful interaction between immunosuppression and short LTL,[28] suggesting an immunopathogenic connection to disease.[29] The PANTHER study also allowed the discovery of an interaction between the *TOLLIP* rs3750920 and *N*-acetylcysteine response,[30] which is being further explored in a prospective trial (NCT04300920). If validated, this SNP would represent the first ILD theragnostic biomarker and would demonstrate the utility of sharing well-curated clinical trial specimens within the IPF community.

To date, clinical genetic testing has generally been limited to FPF kindred to inform susceptibility risk. Although it is enticing to envision a genomic approach to ILD emulating the success of fields such as oncology and cystic fibrosis, these fields are not directly comparable. With rare exceptions, genomics-based personalized medicine in Oncology targets somatic mutations, whereas the approach in cystic fibrosis targets a monogenic germline mutation. As a complex disease that is thought to result from gene-environment interactions, IPF and related ILDs might be particularly suited to omics-based biomarker discovery. Therefore, clinical implementation will require prospectively conducted clinical trials incorporating genomic analyses to determine if, and how, genetic testing might influence clinical decision-making and patient care.

EPIGENOMICS

Epigenetic processes modulate gene expression without altering DNA sequence via DNA methylation, histone modification, and noncoding RNAs. Because the epigenome responds to external stimuli to produce disease phenotypes through gene-environment interactions, its study may identify biomarkers that inform the molecular impact of exposures on IPF development and behavior.

Differential DNA methylation and histone modifications regulate gene expression via conformational changes in promoters, enhancers, and repressors. Epigenome-wide assessment of IPF lung methylation patterns revealed that most differentially methylated regions occur within, or near, CpG islands, and hypomethylated regions were associated with increased expression of genes and transcription factors related to lung development.[31] Furthermore, although not discovered using an omics platform, altered expression of potentially targetable histone deacetylases within IPF lungs, which remove histone acetyl moieties causing chromatin condensation, resulted in fibroblast proliferation and differentiation into apoptosis-resistant myofibroblast within fibro-blastic foci.[32] Noncoding RNA species may represent prognostic biomarkers as specific IPF lung microRNAs have been associated with rapid progression.[33] Considering the limited information regarding these processes in extrapulmonary compartments and the difficulty in accessing ILD lung tissue, the development of clinically useful epigenomic markers will require identification of endotypes linked to epigenetic alterations in the cellular components of bronchoalveolar lavage (BAL) fluid and blood.

TRANSCRIPTOMICS

Transcriptomics involves the quantification of RNA transcripts, or transcriptome, within bio-specimens. This field represents a logical approach to biomarker development, as informative transcripts, or their corresponding proteins, can be directly quantified and potentially translated into clinical-grade tests. Over the last decade, transcriptional methods have evolved from bulk methods to single-cell technologies that, unlike genomics, provide compartment-specific information regarding disease pathogenesis and clinical management.

Transcriptomic studies of IPF lungs and BAL fluid leukocytes have demonstrated enrichment in cell adhesion, lung development, and extracellular matrix pathways,[34,35] suggesting that cross-compartment biomarkers may reflect disease progression and prognosis. Specifically, a 437-gene signature[36] and overlapping 134-gene signature[37] reflecting cellular mobilization, proliferation, and apoptosis were identified in IPF lung biopsies and predicted rapid progression. Moreover, a BAL cellular transcriptomic signature enriched for basal cell genes predicted worse mortality in IPF patients.[38] When viewed in light of the MUC5B data, these findings suggest a role for the distal airways in IPF pathogenesis.

The risk associated with lung biopsy and potential bias of studying end-stage explants have made peripheral blood an attractive and scalable transcriptomics option. As such, a rigorously validated peripheral blood mononuclear cell 52-gene signature reflecting activation of T-cell pathways has recently emerged.[39,40] This connection may be surprising given that IPF is a lung-specific disorder that lacks a primary immunopathogenesis. However, when coupled with preclinical models that suggest dysregulated T-cell responses exacerbate lung remodeling and fibrosis,[41] and the PANTHER data described above,[28,30] these observations may provide mechanistic insight that will require additional study before clinical use.

Bulk transcriptomics has several limitations, such as sampling of lung regions differentially affected by fibrosis[42] and the inability to determine the source of a particular expression pattern. These limitations are partially ameliorated by single-cell RNA sequencing (scRNA-seq), in which labeled cells or nuclei are sequenced and collapsed into large data sets. Cross-platform scRNA-seq studies have identified IPF-specific epithelial, endothelial, and extracellular matrix-producing mesenchymal cell populations.[43,44] These observations have refined the understanding of IPF and benefited from unprecedented data sharing through open access Web sites available to the scientific community.[45]

Although more studies are needed, transcriptomic studies have already produced clinically informative biomarkers. Recently, a 22-gene "UIP transcriptional signature" was translated into a first-in-class clinical-grade test amenable for transbronchial biopsy specimens.[46,47] Although it remains unclear how this classifier will impact clinical decision making in an era in which chest imaging supersedes histologic evaluation,[48] it demonstrates the power of transcriptomics to identify molecular endotypes that inform clinical management.

PROTEOMICS

As components of organ structure and biologic processes, proteins can be quantified via "Proteomics" measurements. In IPF lungs, this technology identified markers of unfolded protein response and ER stress pathway activation in perifibrotic type II pneumocytes,[49] recapitulating similar mechanistic alterations found in SFTPC mutation carriers.[20] Although mechanistically informative, lung biopsies raise concerns of safety, feasibility, and cost. In addition, proteomic analyses of lung tissues are challenged by specificity[50]; therefore, other compartments may be more clinically useful. For example, proteome-wide studies of BAL fluid from IPF patients have demonstrated markers of epithelial activation, matrix remodeling, and inflammation.[51] These proteins complement previously identified blood-based markers of IPF pathobiology, including epithelial injury (SP-A, KL6),[52,53] aberrant inflammation (CCL18),[54] and matrix turnover (MMP7, collagen neoepitopes).[55,56] More recently, proteome-wide studies of IPF patients' blood have revealed novel alterations within host defense, platelet and complement activation, and T-cell costimulation.[57] The concordance with the prognostic 52-gene transcriptomic profile[39,40] demonstrates cross-platform validity amenable for future study.

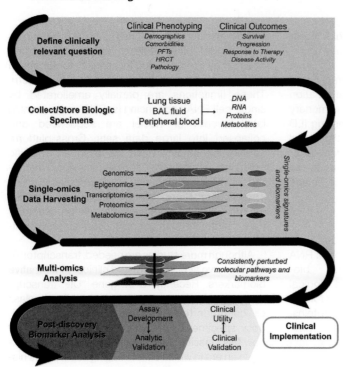

Fig. 1. Process for candidate biomarker development and implementation through single-omics data harvesting and layered multi-omics analysis. HRCT, high-resolution computed tomography of chest; PFTs, pulmonary function tests.

Although proteomics methods have yet to be used clinically, their potential clinical benefit was shown in preliminary findings from a phase 1 study of the TGF-β1 activator, αvβ6 integrin, in which BAL measurement of canonical TGF-β1 activation served as a surrogate for drug effect.[58] Thus, future studies of lung tissue, BAL, and blood may reveal novel biomarkers that in the latter 2 compartments might be leveraged for widespread clinical use.

METABOLOMICS

Metabolomics is the high-throughput assessment of signaling molecules reflecting cellular metabolism. Because mitochondrial dysfunction and glycolysis are linked to IPF,[59,60] unbiased studies of metabolism may be informative. Several small studies of IPF lungs have collectively identified disruptions in multiple metabolic pathways that may mediate fibrosis and remodeling.[61,62] For example, alterations in numerous metabolites, including sphingolipids, arginine, glucose and fatty acid metabolism, and the citric acid cycle, were identified using mass spectroscopy of explanted IPF lungs.[61] The internal validity of these observations was supported by concomitant microarray studies revealing commensurate changes in associated transcripts. However, the failure of these studies to replicate prior work attests to the difficulty in performing these types of studies on bulk tissues from end-stage lungs. When viewed in this light, it seems relevant that BAL and peripheral blood proteomic studies in IPF have revealed enrichment of proteins expected to impact metabolism.[51,57] Although it is attractive to speculate a pathobiologic contribution, the relatively small sample sizes, lack of replication cohorts, and difficulty integrating these finding with other omics-based results limit the utility of these observations.

A potential application of IPF metabolic profiling was highlighted in a recent phase 2 trial of an LPA1 antagonist in IPF.[63] LPA1 is a bioactive lipid metabolite implicated in lung injury responses.[64] In this trial, IPF patients randomized to the LPA1 antagonist experienced a reduced rate of FVC decline and reduced plasma concentrations of the LPA1 metabolite.[63] Although the relationship of these findings to drug response and clinical efficacy will require validation in larger cohorts with appropriate controls, they demonstrate the potential of metabolic monitoring in IPF care, which could be augmented by additional investigation using metabolomic platforms.

CHALLENGES AND OPPORTUNITIES IN OMICS-BASED BIOMARKER DEVELOPMENT

As most IPF omics-based investigations have aimed to advance knowledge of pathobiology, future studies could focus on translating key discoveries into informative biomarkers. Although the basic tenets of this transition are simple (**Fig. 1**), incorporation of biomarkers into ILD management will be complex. Clinical questions must be addressed using easily accessible bio-specimens obtained from well-phenotyped, longitudinal cohorts. Rigorous accounting for cross-platform validation, quality control, and normalization must be developed to allow creation of larger and more powerful data sets.[45] Multidimensionality and standardized integration must be adopted to allow merging of single-omics data into multi-omics data sets, where applicable, to identify pathway perturbations across omics layers. Good clinical practice requires analytical validation and technical reproducibility of all procedures, including sample collection, storage, preparation, and molecular measurements. Finally, cost, scale, and feasibility are important issues that cannot be ignored.

The lack of a "gold standard" for classification poses a unique challenge for precision medicine within ILD. Both the rarely used lung biopsy and widely used imaging and multidisciplinary discussions are all subject to interpreter bias and limited reproducibility. Therefore, comparing candidate diagnostic biomarker performance with these metrics is challenging, particularly because biomarker development occurs in cohorts of patients stratified according to these subjective classifications. In addition, because most ILD omics work has been performed in IPF, which primarily affects older white men, studies should be more inclusive of patients across the spectrum of ILD to identify endotypes that are independent of subjective classifications. The emergence of designations, such as "progressive-fibrosing ILD," which is based on disease behavior rather than morphology[65] and validated by response to anti-fibrotic therapies,[66] indicates that although current ILD classification schema rationally categorizes patients based on outward phenotypes, the underlying biology is unlikely to be as discrete.

A ROADMAP TO PRECISION MEDICINE IN INTERSTITIAL LUNG DISEASE

Plans to develop biomarker-driven precision strategies in ILD must recognize the benefits and challenges of this approach. In the short term, biomarkers are unlikely to supplant the cornerstones of ILD classification and management, such as history, examination, pulmonary function testing, and chest imaging. Therefore, an appropriate goal is to combine traditional clinical testing with molecular biomarkers to transform care. Baseline assessment of biomarkers may enable the classification of ILD patients into novel molecularly based endotypes that inform disease course and targeted therapies. Although

informative, lung tissue or BAL fluid biomarkers would be impractical, and the authors suggest focusing on compartments that are accessible in all patients, such as blood, or the less well-studied exhaled breath condensate, urine, and stool. The consideration of expense and practicality should be addressed by prioritizing low-cost assays that can be performed locally and with sufficient rapidity to enable their use in clinical care.

This transformative vision can be achieved through a series of actionable items. First, clinical grade candidate biomarkers should be developed and validated in numerous well-curated multicenter cohorts. Because the effort and cost required to generate these biobanks exceed the capabilities of a single investigator, concerted stakeholder collaboration is needed to achieve this goal. Second, well-controlled, randomized clinical trials will be required to ensure that the accuracy and precision of molecular biomarkers meaningfully exceed currently available methods. Finally, longitudinal impact analyses will be vital for ensuring that biomarkers enhance clinical decision making and translate into improved patient outcomes.

SUMMARY

The clinical heterogeneity of ILD offers numerous opportunities for biomarker-based precision medicine. Building up existing approaches, unbiased, omics-based methods could transform categorization and management of these disorders. Careful, practical, and collaborative approaches to biomarker discovery and validation may unveil new molecular endotypes and improve patient outcomes in this complex field.

CLINICS CARE POINTS

- Patients with interstitial lung disease experience highly variable morphology, disease course, and clinical outcomes which precludes precision medicine-based approaches to care.

- Layering omics-based studies with detailed phenotyping will inform pathobiology, identify endotypes, and provide opportunities for biomarker development for the interstitial lung diseases.

DISCLOSURE

C.A. Newton is supported by an NHLBI grant K23HL148498and has received consulting fees from Boehringer-Ingelheim. E.L. Herzog is supported by NHLBI grants R01HL109233, R01HL125850, R01HL152677, and U01HL112702, and grants from the Gabriel and Alma Elias Research Fund and the Greenwall Foundation.

REFERENCES

1. Travis WD, Costabel U, Hansell DM, et al. An official American Thoracic Society/European Respiratory Society statement: update of the International Multidisciplinary Classification of the Idiopathic Interstitial Pneumonias. Am J Respir Crit Care Med 2013; 188(6):733–48.
2. Walsh SLF, Wells AU, Desai SR, et al. Multicentre evaluation of multidisciplinary team meeting agreement on diagnosis in diffuse parenchymal lung disease: a case-cohort study. Lancet Respir Med 2016;4(7):557–65.
3. King TE Jr, Bradford WZ, Castro-Bernardini S, et al. A phase 3 trial of pirfenidone in patients with idiopathic pulmonary fibrosis. New Engl J Med 2014; 370(22):2083–92.
4. Richeldi L, du Bois RM, Raghu G, et al. Efficacy and safety of nintedanib in idiopathic pulmonary fibrosis. New Engl J Med 2014;370(22):2071–82.
5. Collins FS, Varmus H. A new initiative on precision medicine. New Engl J Med 2015;372(9):793–5.
6. Hasin Y, Seldin M, Lusis A. Multi-omics approaches to disease. Genome Biol 2017;18(1):83.
7. Seibold MA, Wise AL, Speer MC, et al. A common MUC5B promoter polymorphism and pulmonary fibrosis. New Engl J Med 2011;364(16):1503–12.
8. Fingerlin TE, Murphy E, Zhang W, et al. Genome-wide association study identifies multiple susceptibility loci for pulmonary fibrosis. Nat Genet 2013; 45(6):613–20.
9. Noth I, Zhang Y, Ma SF, et al. Genetic variants associated with idiopathic pulmonary fibrosis susceptibility and mortality: a genome-wide association study. Lancet Respir Med 2013;1(4):309–17.
10. Allen RJ, Porte J, Braybrooke R, et al. Genetic variants associated with susceptibility to idiopathic pulmonary fibrosis in people of European ancestry: a genome-wide association study. Lancet Respir Med 2017;5(11):869–80.
11. Nakano Y, Yang IV, Walts AD, et al. MUC5B promoter variant rs35705950 affects MUC5B expression in the distal airways in idiopathic pulmonary fibrosis. Am J Respir Crit Care Med 2016;193(4):464–6.
12. Conti C, Montero-Fernandez A, Borg E, et al. Mucins MUC5B and MUC5AC in distal airways and honeycomb spaces: comparison among idiopathic

pulmonary fibrosis/usual interstitial pneumonia, fibrotic nonspecific interstitial pneumonitis, and control lungs. Am J Respir Crit Care Med 2016;193(4): 462–4.
13. Peljto AL, Zhang Y, Fingerlin TE, et al. Association between the MUC5B promoter polymorphism and survival in patients with idiopathic pulmonary fibrosis. JAMA 2013;309(21):2232–9.
14. Lawson WE, Grant SW, Ambrosini V, et al. Genetic mutations in surfactant protein C are a rare cause of sporadic cases of IPF. Thorax 2004;59(11): 977–80.
15. Armanios MY, Chen JJ, Cogan JD, et al. Telomerase mutations in families with idiopathic pulmonary fibrosis. New Engl J Med 2007;356(13): 1317–26.
16. Tsakiri KD, Cronkhite JT, Kuan PJ, et al. Adult-onset pulmonary fibrosis caused by mutations in telomerase. Proc Natl Acad Sci U S A 2007;104(18): 7552–7.
17. Cronkhite JT, Xing C, Raghu G, et al. Telomere shortening in familial and sporadic pulmonary fibrosis. Am J Respir Crit Care Med 2008;178(7):729–37.
18. Diaz de Leon A, Cronkhite JT, Katzenstein AL, et al. Telomere lengths, pulmonary fibrosis and telomerase (TERT) mutations. PLoS One 2010;5(5):e10680.
19. Nogee LM, Dunbar AE 3rd, Wert SE, et al. A mutation in the surfactant protein C gene associated with familial interstitial lung disease. New Engl J Med 2001;344(8):573–9.
20. Mulugeta S, Nguyen V, Russo SJ, et al. A surfactant protein C precursor protein BRICHOS domain mutation causes endoplasmic reticulum stress, proteasome dysfunction, and caspase 3 activation. Am J Respir Cell Mol Biol 2005;32(6):521–30.
21. Katzen J, Wagner BD, Venosa A, et al. An SFTPC BRICHOS mutant links epithelial ER stress and spontaneous lung fibrosis. JCI insight 2019;4(6): e126125.
22. Alder JK, Barkauskas CE, Limjunyawong N, et al. Telomere dysfunction causes alveolar stem cell failure. Proc Natl Acad Sci U S A 2015;112(16): 5099–104.
23. Stuart BD, Lee JS, Kozlitina J, et al. Effect of telomere length on survival in patients with idiopathic pulmonary fibrosis: an observational cohort study with independent validation. Lancet Respir Med 2014;2(7):557–65.
24. Dai J, Cai H, Li H, et al. Association between telomere length and survival in patients with idiopathic pulmonary fibrosis. Respirology 2015;20(6):947–52.
25. Newton CA, Batra K, Torrealba J, et al. Telomere-related lung fibrosis is diagnostically heterogeneous but uniformly progressive. Eur Respir J 2016;48(6): 1710–20.
26. Newton CA, Oldham JM, Ley B, et al. Telomere length and genetic variant associations with

interstitial lung disease progression and survival. Eur Respir J 2019;53(4):1801641.

27. Idiopathic Pulmonary Fibrosis Clinical Research Network, Raghu G, Anstrom KJ, et al. Prednisone, azathioprine, and N-acetylcysteine for pulmonary fibrosis. N Engl J Med 2012;366(21):1968–77.

28. Newton CA, Zhang D, Oldham JM, et al. Telomere length and use of immunosuppressive medications in idiopathic pulmonary fibrosis. Am J Respir Crit Care Med 2018;200(3):336–47.

29. Cohen S, Janicki-Deverts D, Turner RB, et al. Association between telomere length and experimentally induced upper respiratory viral infection in healthy adults. JAMA 2013;309(7):699–705.

30. Oldham JM, Ma SF, Martinez FJ, et al. TOLLIP, MUC5B, and the response to N-acetylcysteine among individuals with idiopathic pulmonary fibrosis. Am J Respir Crit Care Med 2015;192(12): 1475–82.

31. Yang IV, Pedersen BS, Rabinovich E, et al. Relationship of DNA methylation and gene expression in idiopathic pulmonary fibrosis. Am J Respir Crit Care Med 2014;190(11):1263–72.

32. Rubio K, Singh I, Dobersch S, et al. Inactivation of nuclear histone deacetylases by EP300 disrupts the MiCEE complex in idiopathic pulmonary fibrosis. Nat Commun 2019;10(1):2229.

33. Oak SR, Murray L, Herath A, et al. A micro RNA processing defect in rapidly progressing idiopathic pulmonary fibrosis. PLoS One 2011;6(6):e21253.

34. Selman M, Pardo A, Barrera L, et al. Gene expression profiles distinguish idiopathic pulmonary fibrosis from hypersensitivity pneumonitis. Am J Respir Crit Care Med 2006;173(2):188–98.

35. Paplinska-Goryca M, Goryca K, Misiukiewicz-Stepien P, et al. mRNA expression profile of bronchoalveolar lavage fluid cells from patients with idiopathic pulmonary fibrosis and sarcoidosis. Eur J Clin Invest 2019;49(9):e13153.

36. Selman M, Carrillo G, Estrada A, et al. Accelerated variant of idiopathic pulmonary fibrosis: clinical behavior and gene expression pattern. PLoS One 2007;2(5):e482.

37. Boon K, Bailey NW, Yang J, et al. Molecular phenotypes distinguish patients with relatively stable from progressive idiopathic pulmonary fibrosis (IPF). PLoS One 2009;4(4):e5134.

38. Prasse A, Binder H, Schupp JC, et al. BAL cell gene expression is indicative of outcome and airway basal cell involvement in idiopathic pulmonary fibrosis. Am J Respir Crit Care Med 2019;199(5): 622–30.

39. Herazo-Maya JD, Noth I, Duncan SR, et al. Peripheral blood mononuclear cell gene expression profiles predict poor outcome in idiopathic pulmonary fibrosis. Sci Transl Med 2013;5(205):205ra136.

40. Herazo-Maya JD, Sun J, Molyneaux PL, et al. Validation of a 52-gene risk profile for outcome prediction in patients with idiopathic pulmonary fibrosis: an international, multicentre, cohort study. Lancet Respir Med 2017;5(11):857–68.

41. Birjandi SZ, Palchevskiy V, Xue YY, et al. CD4(+) CD25(hi)Foxp3(+) cells exacerbate bleomycin-induced pulmonary fibrosis. Am J Pathol 2016; 186(8):2008–20.

42. McDonough JE, Ahangari F, Li Q, et al. Transcriptional regulatory model of fibrosis progression in the human lung. JCI insight 2019;4(22):e131597.

43. Habermann AC, Gutierrez AJ, Bui LT, et al. Single-cell RNA sequencing reveals profibrotic roles of distinct epithelial and mesenchymal lineages in pulmonary fibrosis. Sci Adv 2020;6(28):eaba1972.

44. Adams TS, Schupp JC, Poli S, et al. Single-cell RNA-seq reveals ectopic and aberrant lung-resident cell populations in idiopathic pulmonary fibrosis. Sci Adv 2020;6(28):eaba1983.

45. Neumark N, Cosme C Jr, Rose KA, et al. The idiopathic pulmonary fibrosis cell atlas. Am J Physiol Lung Cell Mol Physiol 2020;319(6):L887–93.

46. Kim SY, Diggans J, Pankratz D, et al. Classification of usual interstitial pneumonia in patients with interstitial lung disease: assessment of a machine learning approach using high-dimensional transcriptional data. Lancet Respir Med 2015;3(6): 473–82.

47. Raghu G, Flaherty KR, Lederer DJ, et al. Use of a molecular classifier to identify usual interstitial pneumonia in conventional transbronchial lung biopsy samples: a prospective validation study. Lancet Respir Med 2019;7(6):487–96.

48. Lynch DA, Sverzellati N, Travis WD, et al. Diagnostic criteria for idiopathic pulmonary fibrosis: a Fleischner Society white paper. Lancet Respir Med 2018; 6(2):138–53.

49. Korfei M, Schmitt S, Ruppert C, et al. Comparative proteomic analysis of lung tissue from patients with idiopathic pulmonary fibrosis (IPF) and lung transplant donor lungs. J Proteome Res 2011;10(5): 2185–205.

50. Schiller HB, Mayr CH, Leuschner G, et al. Deep proteome profiling reveals common prevalence of MZB1-positive plasma B cells in human lung and skin fibrosis. Am J Respir Crit Care Med 2017; 196(10):1298–310.

51. Foster MW, Morrison LD, Todd JL, et al. Quantitative proteomics of bronchoalveolar lavage fluid in idiopathic pulmonary fibrosis. J Proteome Res 2015; 14(2):1238–49.

52. Kinder BW, Brown KK, McCormack FX, et al. Serum surfactant protein-A is a strong predictor of early mortality in idiopathic pulmonary fibrosis. Chest 2009;135(6):1557–63.

53. Yokoyama A, Kondo K, Nakajima M, et al. Prognostic value of circulating KL-6 in idiopathic pulmonary fibrosis. Respirology 2006;11(2):164–8.

54. Prasse A, Probst C, Bargagli E, et al. Serum CC-chemokine ligand 18 concentration predicts outcome in idiopathic pulmonary fibrosis. Am J Respir Crit Care Med 2009;179(8):717–23.

55. Rosas IO, Richards TJ, Konishi K, et al. MMP1 and MMP7 as potential peripheral blood biomarkers in idiopathic pulmonary fibrosis. Plos Med 2008;5(4):e93.

56. Jenkins RG, Simpson JK, Saini G, et al. Longitudinal change in collagen degradation biomarkers in idiopathic pulmonary fibrosis: an analysis from the prospective, multicentre PROFILE study. Lancet Respir Med 2015;3(6):462–72.

57. O'Dwyer DN, Norman KC, Xia M, et al. The peripheral blood proteome signature of idiopathic pulmonary fibrosis is distinct from normal and is associated with novel immunological processes. Sci Rep 2017;7:46560.

58. Raghu G, Mouded M, Culver DA, et al. Randomized, double-blind, placebo-controlled, multiple dose, dose-escalation study of BG00011 (former STX-100) in patients with Idiopathic Pulmonary Fibrosis (IPF). Am Thoracic Soc 2018;197:A7785.

59. Rangarajan S, Bernard K, Thannickal VJ. Mitochondrial dysfunction in pulmonary fibrosis. Ann Am Thorac Soc 2017;14(Supplement_5):S383–8.

60. Zank DC, Bueno M, Mora AL, et al. Idiopathic pulmonary fibrosis: aging, mitochondrial dysfunction, and cellular bioenergetics. Front Med (Lausanne) 2018;5:10.

61. Zhao YD, Yin L, Archer S, et al. Metabolic heterogeneity of idiopathic pulmonary fibrosis: a metabolomic study. BMJ Open Respir Res 2017;4(1):e000183.

62. Kang YP, Lee SB, Lee JM, et al. Metabolic profiling regarding pathogenesis of idiopathic pulmonary fibrosis. J Proteome Res 2016;15(5):1717–24.

63. Maher TM, van der Aar EM, Van de Steen O, et al. Safety, tolerability, pharmacokinetics, and pharmacodynamics of GLPG1690, a novel autotaxin inhibitor, to treat idiopathic pulmonary fibrosis (FLORA): a phase 2a randomised placebo-controlled trial. Lancet Respir Med 2018;6(8):627–35.

64. Tager AM, LaCamera P, Shea BS, et al. The lysophosphatidic acid receptor LPA1 links pulmonary fibrosis to lung injury by mediating fibroblast recruitment and vascular leak. Nat Med 2008;14(1):45–54.

65. Cottin V, Hirani NA, Hotchkin DL, et al. Presentation, diagnosis and clinical course of the spectrum of progressive-fibrosing interstitial lung diseases. Eur Respir Rev 2018;27(150):180076.

66. Flaherty KR, Wells AU, Cottin V, et al. Nintedanib in progressive fibrosing interstitial lung diseases. N Engl J Med 2019;381(18):1718–27.

Regenerative Medicine and the Hope for a Cure

Mareike Lehmann, PhD[a], Melanie Königshoff, MD, PhD[a,b,*]

KEYWORDS

- ILD • IPF • Regeneration • Translation • Aging • Cellular senescence • Developmental pathways

KEY POINTS

- Idiopathic pulmonary fibrosis (IPF) is a disease of regenerative failure with impaired stem cell function, particularly, epithelial cells.
- Aging is a major contributor to failure of regeneration in IPF.
- Recent research findings highlight the potential of the human diseased lung to regenerate.
- Human translational models are needed to understand regenerative process in the IPF lung.
- Earlier diagnosis and earlier intervention targeting regenerative processes are ultimate goals to reverse fibrotic changes.

REGENERATIVE POTENTIAL OF THE (DISEASED) LUNG

Introduction

Regeneration of the human diseased lung represents an exciting and ambitious approach to treat chronic lung disease. For the longest time, the lung has been regarded as a highly quiescent organ, with limited regenerative capacity. Over the past years, however, both the understanding of general regenerative processes in the lung and insight into the pathobiology of diseases, such as fibrotic lung diseases, have been tremendously enhanced. Recent research in rodents highlights that the lung possesses a substantial reparative capacity, in which the resident progenitor cell populations proliferate and differentiate into diverse cell types during homeostasis or after injury.[1] Notably, a few cases have reported regrowth of the human lung in adults.[2] Only recently, with the generation of novel human tissue-based translational models of chronic lung disease, the potential of the chronically diseased human lung to initiate the repair process has been shown explicitly.[3,4]

Based on this knowledge, the concepts for the development of novel treatments changed, and therapies targeting repair and regenerative processes are emerging. These therapies include ways to boost endogenous regeneration, a process essentially driven by stem cell populations in the lung. These cells are tightly regulated by distinct signaling pathways as well as the surrounding cellular and extracellular niche. In addition, exogenous approaches, in which stem cells are administered to the diseased lung, are explored. Given the age-dependent demographics of idiopathic pulmonary fibrosis (IPF), it is important to note that alterations in progenitor cells along with increased inflammation in the aged lung impair regenerative processes. Multiple cellular mechanisms, such as cellular senescence and inflammaging, have been described to act as roadblocks to regeneration and must be targeted by therapies aiming at regenerating the aged fibrotic lung.[5–7]

In IPF, injury and reprogramming of the distal lung epithelium, including lung stem cell populations, have been identified as key pathomechanisms for disease development and are suggested to be early process driving disease.[8] Aberrant cell phenotypes and increased activities of developmental pathways support the notion that

[a] Research Unit Lung Repair and Regeneration, Helmholtz Zentrum München, German Center of Lung Research (DZL), Max-Lebsche-Platz 31, München 81377, Germany; [b] Division of Pulmonary, Allergy and Critical Care Medicine, Department of Medicine, University of Pittsburgh, Pittsburgh, PA, USA
* Corresponding author. UPMC Montefiore NW628, 3459 Fifth Avenue, Pittsburgh, PA 15213.
E-mail address: koenigshoffm@upmc.edu

Clin Chest Med 42 (2021) 365–373
https://doi.org/10.1016/j.ccm.2021.03.012

regenerative mechanisms are not completely silenced in IPF, but rather impaired and/or misdirected, causing a progressive destruction of functional lung tissue.[9] Currently approved therapeutics have been shown to slow down the progression of disease; however, these do not lead to reversal of the disease processes.[10] The ultimate aim for future therapies must be the restoration of lung architecture and function, and thus, curing the disease.[10] The advancement in the understanding of regenerative processes and disease pathobiology, along with better and earlier diagnosis, is an essential pillar that moves the field forward and paves the way for this ambitious, but imperative goal.

Within the following paragraphs, the authors outline the current knowledge on lung stem cell function and signaling pathways involved in lung regeneration. They describe the current evidence for an impaired regenerative capacity in IPF and outline novel approaches in regenerative therapies for IPF.

Lung Epithelial Stem Cells

The human respiratory system comprises different epithelial cell populations, mesenchymal cells, and immune cells in a well-defined spatial composition along the respiratory tract.[11] Especially within the epithelium, several cells have been identified to have stem/progenitor cell function. Although many functional stem cell studies have been conducted in animal models, recent single-cell analysis approaches have shed light onto potential stem and progenitor cells in the human (IPF) lung.[12–17]

The proximal airways from the trachea to the bronchioles are composed of a pseudostratified epithelium with serous goblet, club, and basal cells.[1,18–20] Basal cells are well-described airway stem cells giving rise to nearly all epithelial cells within the airway. In the distal lung, the human airway epithelium becomes thinner and largely consists of club cells, with fewer basal and goblet cells. Club cells have been shown to serve as progenitor cells and potentially give rise to more distal alveolar epithelial cells. Neuroendocrine cells are further found along the airway[21] and are suggested to contribute to epithelial repair by supporting the maintenance of epithelial progenitor cell populations in the lung.[21,22] The alveoli are covered by squamous alveolar epithelial cells type I (ATI cells), the main site for gas exchange, and cuboidal ATII cells that are critical for the synthesis of surfactant lipids to reduce surface tension.[18,19,23–25] ATII cells are the best described progenitor cells in the distal lung, giving rise to ATI cells. Furthermore, in mice, the presence of bronchioalveolar stem cells present at the bronchoalveolar duct junctions has been described.[11,26–28]

Novel Methods to Study Lung Stem Cells and Regeneration

Given the constant exposure of the lung to multiple exogenous factors over the lifetime, the existence and plasticity of residing progenitor populations seem highly likely in the human lung. Analysis of human tissue and cells has generated a significant amount of knowledge and is essential not only to enable investigations to relevant environmental exposures but also to take several genetic alterations and aging into account.[19,29] It is important to note that the functional role of these stem cells has been largely described during lung development and during response to experimental injuries in rodents, which have a different cellular composition and lung physiology. However, recent advances in 3-dimensional (3D) models, such as precision-cut lung slices or organoid models, have pushed the investigation of human primary cells and tissue.[30] Using chronic obstructive pulmonary disease–derived tissue and cells, regenerative processes, such as activation of ATII cells and organoid formation, have been investigated.[4,31] These methodological advances also enable the study of functional properties of epithelial stem cells within their niche, including signals from surrounding cells, such as mesenchymal cells and extracellular matrix. Moreover, these methods also allow the analysis of signaling pathways that control stem cell function. Ample evidence exists documenting the impact of developmental signaling pathways, such as the Wnt/β-catenin or Notch signaling, on lung stem cells.[32] Activity of these pathways in lung stem cells is tightly regulated, and thus, endogenous lung regeneration approaches need to be based on a deep understanding of lung stem cells and their regulatory pathways in homeostasis as well as in disease.[33]

In addition, recent single-cell analysis approaches, such as RNA sequencing of single cells, highlight the complexity of cell types and cell states in the mouse and human lung during homeostasis.[12–17] These studies led to the identification of novel epithelial, stromal, immune, and endothelial cell types, such as ionocytes,[34,35] and a novel transient ATII cell population, among others.[12] In the future, these approaches will allow the comparison of cellular composition of the lung at different stages of life and with different genetic backgrounds, studies that have been performed already partially in rodents.[36,37] These investigations have been extended to include studies of human interstitial lung disease (ILD)/IPF tissue,[13–17] which is discussed later.

IDIOPATHIC PULMONARY FIBROSIS AS A DISEASE OF IMPAIRED REGENERATION
Current Research: Lung Epithelial Cell Injury and Reprogramming

IPF is thought to result from aberrant and continuous activation of injured alveolar and bronchial epithelial cells resulting in massive change in cellular phenotypes and functions. Ongoing exposure to cigarette smoke, inhaled toxins, gastroesophageal reflux, or infections, possibly in a genetically predisposed background, leads to alveolar and airway epithelial (stem) cell damage and impaired injury response. Genetic alterations include mutations in the surfactant protein (Sftp) C or Sftp-A2 genes, relevant for ATII cell function, or in the telomerase complex, which most likely impacts aging processes in the lung.[38] Profibrotic mediators secreted by these "reprogrammed" cells lead to the activation and proliferation of mesenchymal and immune cell populations and further contribute to increased deposition of extracellular matrix, dysregulated wound repair, and persistent lung remodeling.[38,39]

It has been proposed that this abnormal wound-healing process after repetitive insults to the epithelium might compromise the regenerative potential of the lung.[29,40] Given the complexity of the lung, a plethora of different factors together probably contributes to this impairment; however, signal alteration of developmental core pathways and aging-related mechanisms, such as cellular senescence, have emerged as major contributors and potential targets to initiate lung regeneration.[5]

Current Research: Developmental Pathways in Idiopathic Pulmonary Fibrosis

During lung development, several signaling pathways must act in a tight spatiotemporal interplay to successfully achieve proper organ development.[41,42] These pathways include the Wnt, Notch, sonic hedgehog, and transforming growth factor (TGF) signaling families, among others. Notably, ample evidence revealed that many of these classical developmental, or "generative," pathways are dysregulated in ILDs, including IPF.[43–45] For example, Wnt/β-catenin signaling, a well-known driver of cellular proliferation, differentiation, and stem cell function, has been demonstrated to be active in IPF.[45] Similar findings have been reported for other ILDs.[44] Based on these data, the fibrotic response is characterized by a noncontrolled or misdirected activation of developmental pathways. As these developmental pathways are tightly regulated to ensure proper regular tissue repair in nonfibrotic conditions, the current data point to the fact that the parallel (nonregulated) activity of several core pathways, including TGF-β signaling as an essential remodeling pathway, at the same time, leads to altered signaling outcomes.[46–49] This hypothesis is in line with histologic features of the IPF lungs, which shows many similarities with developmental/premature lungs and diseases of prematurity, such as bronchopulmonary dysplasia.[40,50,51] Overall, these early findings sparked the idea to therapeutically target impaired repair and to induce proper tissue restoration and regeneration in IPF.

Current Research: Impaired Stem Cells in Idiopathic Pulmonary Fibrosis

Developmental pathways play a major role in determining the function of stem cells. As outlined earlier, several studies over the last few years have provided evidence for alterations in ATII cells, which are well-known alveolar stem cells. More recently, novel single-cell analysis approaches allowed a mapping of the cellular composition of IPF lungs in unprecedented depth.[13–17] These studies identified IPF-specific subpopulations in different cellular compartments, including mesenchymal, immune, and epithelial cells. Notably, a distinct epithelial cell cluster, with stem cell marker as well as fibrosis marker, was identified in at least 2 different studies.[13,14] These newly termed "basaloid" cells showed enriched gene expression for cellular senescence, extracellular matrix proteins, mesenchymal markers, and integrin signaling pathways, further corroborating that epithelial cells are majorly affected in IPF, contributing to a variety of features known in fibrogenesis and remodeling. The emergence of reprogrammed epithelial cells in the IPF lungs also points to an impaired stem cell capacity of epithelial cells as an important feature of the disease. These studies also found several alterations in immune and mesenchymal cell populations, thus highlighting the importance of impaired cellular crosstalk and cell-ECM crosstalk, which creates a profibrotic and potentially antiregenerative niche in IPF.

Only recently, in order to start to functionally characterize stem cell behavior and impaired cellular crosstalk in IPF, novel 3D models that are based on primary (human) cells, so-called organoids, have been applied.[52] Most studies have been performed using cells derived from murine experimental fibrosis models showing that ATII cells derived from fibrotic lungs exhibit a reduction in colony-forming efficiency,[53] thus reduced stem cell function. Similar results have been reported in first studies using IPF-derived ATII cells.[37,54] Although these models currently are largely limited to epithelial/fibroblasts interaction, they have the potential to be further developed to include immune or endothelial cells, which would improve our ability to model the recent findings from IPF lungs in its complexity.

Notably, stem cell exhaustion/failure is a common hallmark of aging, and organoid studies as outlined above have also been performed using aged ATII cells, resulting in similar reduced stem cell function in organoids assays.[55,56]

Current Research: Aging in Idiopathic Pulmonary Fibrosis: Cellular Senescence

Aging is a major risk factor for many ILDs, including IPF.[29] Several hallmarks of aging, such as telomere biology, inflammaging, stem cell exhaustion, and cellular senescence, are evident in IPF and have been shown to contribute to disease development and progression, thus supporting a close connection between premature aging, impaired regenerative capacity, and fibrosis.[5,6] Cellular senescence is one of the best described age-related changes in the fibrotic lung, and senescence-based antiaging therapies are explored for the treatment of IPF patients. Cellular senescence describes a permanent cell-cycle arrest, along with resistance to apoptosis and the secretion of specific proteins (the senescence-associated secretory phenotype [SASP]).[57] The SASP contributes to systemic proinflammatory conditions, known as inflammaging. Inflammaging is characterized by the activation of the innate immune system, with a dominant role of myeloid cells secreting several proinflammatory cytokines, such as interleukin-6 (IL-6), IL-8, lymphotoxin β, and IL-1β[58]; many of these are increasingly expressed in ILDs, including IPF. Although it remains largely unknown how inflammaging affects major structural effector cells in IPF, it is well described that SASPs components are able to induce cellular senescence in vitro, suggesting a mechanism by which senescence and inflammation are reinforced.[59,60]

Notably, the effect of senescence on organ health can be highly variable depending on the affected organ, cell type, and microenvironment. Initially known as a tumor suppressive mechanisms, nonproliferating senescent cells can be cleared by an (intact) immune system, by natural killer cells or macrophages,[57,61–63] and thus preventing the spread of senescence within the tissue, known as secondary senescence.[64] Under pathologic conditions, such as chronic damage

or premature aging, senescent cells accumulate and persist in the tissue, where they contribute to impaired regeneration observed in lung aging and disease.[65–68] How these cells evade the clearance mechanisms is not fully understood yet; however, it is proposed that age-related immune system dysfunction or differences in the SASP might be responsible for the accumulation of senescent cells.[69–71]

Senescence is a well-recognized feature of lung fibrosis, and all evidence points toward a pathologic role of senescence in IPF. Patients with mutations in telomere genes, which causes replicative senescence, develop familial forms of IPF, indicating that senescence causally contributes to the development of lung fibrosis.[72] Cellular senescence was also observed in nonfamilial IPF.[66,67,73–76] With respect to impaired regenerative capacity, it is important to highlight that senescence is a prominent feature of impaired epithelial cellular phenotypes in IPF, specifically, in lung stem cells, such as ATII cells or basal cells.[67,74–78] Recent data from genetically engineered mice with ATII cell senescence provided evidence that senescence is indeed a driving factor for fibrosis development in the lung, rather than a bystander phenomenon.[79,80] In addition to the major role of senescent ATII cells in fibrosis, other cell types, such as (myo)fibroblasts and bone marrow–derived mesenchymal stem cells, show increased cellular senescence in IPF,[81–83] further contributing to an impaired repair response. Notably also, other epithelial stem cell populations have been demonstrated to be senescent. Recent single-cell RNA sequencing studies that dissected the cellular composition of IPF lungs and identified the aberrant basaloid cells in irreversibly remodeled IPF lungs also found a clear senescence signature in these cells.[13,14] Their data confirmed that the previously described aberrant epithelial cells show prominent expression of senescence markers.[75] Similar aberrant lung stem cell populations have been found in experimental models of pulmonary fibrosis.[55,84,85] Overall, these are compelling data that outline a mechanisms by which these cells drive a failed repair attempt in IPF.[6]

THERAPEUTIC INTERVENTION
Targeting Endogenous Lung Regeneration

Therapeutic drug discovery and approaches for IPF have evolved over the past years with a focus initially on anti-inflammatory drugs, which shifted to (myo-)fibroblast biology and IPF as a fibroproliferative disease as a main focus for drug discovery over recent years. As 1 successful result, nintedanib and pirfenidone have been the first Food and Drug Administration–approved drugs for IPF, and both are thought to predominantly affect (myo-)fibroblast function.[44,86] Both treatments are able to slow down the progression of disease; however, none of these drugs has been reported to halt or even reverse the disease process. Several recent studies have further advanced the understanding of IPF pathogenesis and lung epithelial cell injury and damage, with subsequent reprogramming, and failure of lung epithelial (stem) cells has crystalized not only as a major disease process but also as an early fibrosis event. This knowledge is of importance, as potential intervention at earlier stages of the disease process would be a major advantage to reverse disease processes and be able to achieve restoration of lung tissue and function, thus curing the disease.

As outlined earlier, current data suggest that regenerative mechanisms are not completely silenced in IPF, but rather impaired and/or misdirected. Thus, targeting endogenous regeneration, in particular, the impaired function of the lung epithelium, has lately become a promising focus to develop novel therapies for IPF. Preclinical data strongly support the potential to redirect regeneration in the fibrotic lung. Several studies have been performed with novel compounds that target epithelial cell-driven processes and led to significant antifibrotic effects.[87–89] The hope is that targeting earlier, epithelial cell-driven processes will not only restore epithelial cell function but also prevent further profibrotic mechanisms or, quite likely, also have a direct effect on the profibrotic permissive niche, including other cell types, such as fibroblasts and macrophages, and matrix components.

Targeting Aging/Cellular Senescence

In the field of regenerative antiaging therapies, approaches largely aim to eliminate senescent cells and thus "release" the proper regenerative function of the remaining lung cells. Consistently, depletion of senescent cells using senolytic drugs or genetic models showed a protective effect against fibrosis, which improved epithelial cell function, lung function, and physical health.[66,67] Importantly, first-in-human clinical trials haven been performed, confirming senolytics as a viable therapeutic option for the treatment of IPF.[90] A major concern for antiaging/regenerative therapies is the potential to cause "too much" regeneration and even initiate neoplastic disease. It is important to consider that treatment regimens for regenerative drugs can be developed under a

"hit-and-run" concept, with only a few doses that boost and/or redirect a regenerative process within an endogenously primed lung, such as in IPF. These first-in-human trial of senolytics was based on intermittent application of the preclinically tested combination of the senolytic compounds dasatinib and quercetin for 3 days per week for 3 weeks.[66,67,80] This dosing regimen resulted in improved physical performance in IPF patients as compared with baseline.[90] It is important to highlight that although this further supports senolytics as a potential therapeutic approach, bigger placebo-controlled clinical trials are needed to prove their efficacy. Of note, although preclinical studies have demonstrated that senolytics target lung epithelial cells,[67,80] it is not known whether a similar mechanism is the basis for the results seen in humans.

Overall, these initial data are promising and strengthen the field of regenerative medicine. They open up a novel exciting research focus aiming to better understand potential cell-specific senescence, which would enable more targeted therapies. It remains unknown whether disease-induced senescence is congruent to normal age-induced senescence and why some senescent cells are required for homeostasis.[91,92] Also, other approaches to target senescence are explored, such as inhibition of the SASP, with the idea to further inhibit other aberrant functions, such as increased ECM protein expression and rescue proper lung stem cell function and thus allow for tissue restoration. A better characterization of the SASP could also serve to identify (bio)markers for aging and regeneration.[90] The abundance of SASP factors in the blood is low and it might be difficult to detect changes in minimal invasive diagnostics; however, SASP analysis of BAL might be worth considering.

In general, we need to generate a better toolbox with specific readouts and potential biomarkers to assess aging as well as lung regeneration in the human diseased lung and thus be able to critically evaluate future therapeutic approaches to redirect lung regeneration.

CONCLUSION AND FUTURE OUTLOOK

The lung was once thought to be a quiescent organ, but ample research over the last decade has revealed a previously underappreciated regenerative capacity of the lung, not only in rodents but also in human diseased lung tissue. Several endogenous lung stem cell populations have been identified, and light has been shed onto the regulation of these cells and their niche. In parallel to these advances, the understanding of IPF pathomechanisms has also further evolved, demonstrating the accumulation of aberrant epithelial (stem) cell phenotypes in IPF, which are thought to result from an attempted but failed regenerative process in the aged IPF lung. Most recently, these disease features have been the focus of (pre)clinical studies, and first data on regenerative therapy for treatment of IPF leave us with hope for a cure. The next steps to enable successful translation into the clinic should focus on adapting and applying clinically relevant human disease models that will inform about the regenerative potential in the human lung as well as the discovery of regenerative parameters that are needed for clinical evaluation of future therapies.[30] Especially in the context of regeneration, we must take into consideration that most IPF patients are elderly, which impairs regenerative capacity of lung progenitor cells per se. However, current approaches aim to overcome these hurdles, and there is hope that we can redirect regeneration also in an aged lung. The timeframe in which we are still capable of inducing regeneration in a diseased lung is currently unknown; it is, however, fair to speculate that it will be challenging to do this in end-stage disease. Stem cell failure is likely an early event in disease pathogenesis, and developing biomarker and companion diagnostic tools based on stem cell failure is of great importance for the translation of regenerative medicine approaches.

CLINICS CARE POINTS

- Current treatments for IPF slow down progression of disease but do not halt or let alone reverse disease.
- Therapies enabling lung regeneration might offer novel approaches.
- The extend of human lung regeneration in a fibrotic lung is currently unknown.
- Adapted treatment regimen for antiaging/regenerative drugs ("hit and run") need to be explored and might reduce side and off-target effects.
- Developing biomarker and companion diagnostic tools based on regenerative failure is required.

DISCLOSURE

The authors have nothing to disclose.

REFERENCES

1. Basil MC, Katzen J, Engler AE, et al. The cellular and physiological basis for lung repair and regeneration: past, present, and future. Cell Stem Cell 2020;26(4):482–502.
2. Butler JP, Loring SH, Patz S, et al. Evidence for adult lung growth in humans. N Engl J Med 2012;367(3):244–7.
3. Alsafadi HN, Staab-Weijnitz CA, Lehmann M, et al. An ex vivo model to induce early fibrosis-like changes in human precision-cut lung slices. Am J Physiol Lung Cell Mol Physiol 2017;312(6):L896–902.
4. Uhl FE, Vierkotten S, Wagner DE, et al. Preclinical validation and imaging of Wnt-induced repair in human 3D lung tissue cultures. Eur Respir J 2015;46(4):1150–66.
5. Melo-Narvaez MC, Stegmayr J, Wagner DE, et al. Lung regeneration: implications of the diseased niche and ageing. Eur Respir Rev 2020;29(157):200222.
6. Meiners S, Lehmann M. Senescent cells in IPF: locked in repair? Front Med 2020;7(1002):606330.
7. Mora AL, Rojas M, Pardo A, et al. Emerging therapies for idiopathic pulmonary fibrosis, a progressive age-related disease. Nat Rev Drug Discov 2017;16(11):810.
8. Selman M, Pardo A. The leading role of epithelial cells in the pathogenesis of idiopathic pulmonary fibrosis. Cell Signal 2020;66:109482.
9. Konigshoff M, Eickelberg O. WNT signaling in lung disease: a failure or a regeneration signal? Am J Respir Cell Mol Biol 2010;42(1):21–31.
10. Lederer DJ, Martinez FJ. Idiopathic pulmonary fibrosis. N Engl J Med 2018;378(19):1811–23.
11. Lee RE, Miller SM, Randell SH. Adult pulmonary epithelial stem cells and their niches. In: Reis RL, editor. Encyclopedia of tissue engineering and regenerative medicine. Oxford (England): Academic Press; 2019. p. 319–36.
12. Travaglini KJ, Nabhan AN, Penland L, et al. A molecular cell atlas of the human lung from single-cell RNA sequencing. Nature 2020;587(7835):619–25.
13. Adams TS, Schupp JC, Poli S, et al. Single-cell RNA-seq reveals ectopic and aberrant lung-resident cell populations in idiopathic pulmonary fibrosis. Sci Adv 2020;6(28):eaba1983.
14. Habermann AC, Gutierrez AJ, Bui LT, et al. Single-cell RNA sequencing reveals profibrotic roles of distinct epithelial and mesenchymal lineages in pulmonary fibrosis. Sci Adv 2020;6(28):eaba1972.
15. Carraro G, Mulay A, Yao C, et al. Single-cell reconstruction of human basal cell diversity in normal and idiopathic pulmonary fibrosis lungs. Am J Respir Crit Care Med 2020;202(11):1540–50.

16. Reyfman PA, Walter JM, Joshi N, et al. Single-cell transcriptomic analysis of human lung provides insights into the pathobiology of pulmonary fibrosis. Am J Respir Crit Care Med 2019;199(12):1517–36.

17. Morse C, Tabib T, Sembrat J, et al. Proliferating SPP1/MERTK-expressing macrophages in idiopathic pulmonary fibrosis. Eur Respir J 2019;54(2):1802441.

18. Kotton DN, Morrisey EE. Lung regeneration: mechanisms, applications and emerging stem cell populations. Nat Med 2014;20(8):822–32.

19. Navarro S, Driscoll B. Regeneration of the aging lung: a mini-review. Gerontology 2017;63(3):270–80.

20. Morrisey EE. Basal cells in lung development and repair. Dev Cell 2018;44(6):653–4.

21. Song H, Yao E, Lin C, et al. Functional characterization of pulmonary neuroendocrine cells in lung development, injury, and tumorigenesis. Proc Natl Acad Sci U S A 2012;109(43):17531–6.

22. Reynolds SD, Giangreco A, Power JH, et al. Neuroepithelial bodies of pulmonary airways serve as a reservoir of progenitor cells capable of epithelial regeneration. Am J Pathol 2000;156(1):269–78.

23. Desai TJ, Brownfield DG, Krasnow MA. Alveolar progenitor and stem cells in lung development, renewal and cancer. Nature 2014;507(7491):190–4.

24. Ahmad S, Ahmad A. Chapter 6 - epithelial regeneration and lung stem cells. In: Sidhaye VK, Koval M, editors. Lung epithelial biology in the pathogenesis of pulmonary disease. Boston: Academic Press; 2017. p. 91–102.

25. Cho SJ, Stout-Delgado HW. Aging and lung disease. Annu Rev Physiol 2020;82(1):433–59.

26. Kim CFB, Jackson EL, Woolfenden AE, et al. Identification of bronchioalveolar stem cells in normal lung and lung cancer. Cell 2005;121(6):823–35.

27. Chen F, Fine A. Stem cells in lung injury and repair. Am J Pathol 2016;186(10):2544–50.

28. Liu Q, Liu K, Cui G, et al. Lung regeneration by multipotent stem cells residing at the bronchioalveolar-duct junction. Nat Genet 2019;51(4):728–38.

29. Meiners S, Eickelberg O, Königshoff M. Hallmarks of the ageing lung. Eur Respir J 2015;45(3):807–27.

30. Alsafadi HN, Uhl FE, Pineda RH, et al. Applications and approaches for three-dimensional precision-cut lung slices. Disease modeling and drug discovery. Am J Respir Cell Mol Biol 2020;62(6):681–91.

31. Conlon TM, John-Schuster G, Heide D, et al. Publisher correction: inhibition of LTβR signalling activates WNT-induced regeneration in lung. Nature 2021;589(7842):E6.

32. Nabhan AN, Brownfield DG, Harbury PB, et al. Single-cell Wnt signaling niches maintain stemness of alveolar type 2 cells. Science 2018;359(6380):1118–23.

33. Rock J, Konigshoff M. Endogenous lung regeneration: potential and limitations. Am J Respir Crit Care Med 2012;186(12):1213–9.

34. Montoro DT, Haber AL, Biton M, et al. A revised airway epithelial hierarchy includes CFTR-expressing ionocytes. Nature 2018;560(7718):319–24.

35. Plasschaert LW, Zilionis R, Choo-Wing R, et al. A single-cell atlas of the airway epithelium reveals the CFTR-rich pulmonary ionocyte. Nature 2018;560(7718):377–81.

36. Angelidis I, Simon LM, Fernandez IE, et al. An atlas of the aging lung mapped by single cell transcriptomics and deep tissue proteomics. Nat Commun 2019;10(1):963.

37. Liang J, Huang G, Liu X, et al. Single-cell transcriptomics identifies dysregulated metabolic programs of aging alveolar progenitor cells in lung fibrosis. bioRxiv 2020.

38. Chilosi M, Poletti V, Rossi A. The pathogenesis of COPD and IPF: distinct horns of the same devil? Respir Res 2012;13(1):3.

39. King TE Jr, Pardo A, Selman M. Idiopathic pulmonary fibrosis. Lancet 2011;378(9807):1949–61.

40. Plataki M, Koutsopoulos AV, Darivianaki K, et al. Expression of apoptotic and antiapoptotic markers in epithelial cells in idiopathic pulmonary fibrosis. Chest 2005;127(1):266–74.

41. Morrisey EE, Hogan BL. Preparing for the first breath: genetic and cellular mechanisms in lung development. Dev Cell 2010;18(1):8–23.

42. Hogan BL, Barkauskas CE, Chapman HA, et al. Repair and regeneration of the respiratory system: complexity, plasticity, and mechanisms of lung stem cell function. Cell Stem Cell 2014;15(2):123–38.

43. Stabler CT, Morrisey EE. Developmental pathways in lung regeneration. Cell Tissue Res 2017;367(3):677–85.

44. Distler JHW, Gyorfi AH, Ramanujam M, et al. Shared and distinct mechanisms of fibrosis. Nat Rev Rheumatol 2019;15(12):705–30.

45. Burgy O, Konigshoff M. The WNT signaling pathways in wound healing and fibrosis. Matrix Biol 2018;68-69:67–80.

46. Zhang J, Tian XJ, Xing J. Signal transduction pathways of EMT induced by TGF-beta, SHH, and WNT and their crosstalks. J Clin Med 2016;5(4):41.

47. Borggrefe T, Lauth M, Zwijsen A, et al. The Notch intracellular domain integrates signals from Wnt, Hedgehog, TGFbeta/BMP and hypoxia pathways. Biochim Biophys Acta 2016;1863(2):303–13.

48. Cigna N, Farrokhi Moshai E, Brayer S, et al. The hedgehog system machinery controls transforming growth factor-beta-dependent myofibroblastic differentiation in humans: involvement in idiopathic pulmonary fibrosis. Am J Pathol 2012;181(6):2126–37.

49. Burgy O, Fernandez Fernandez E, Rolandsson Enes S, et al. New players in chronic lung disease identified at the European Respiratory Society

International Congress in Paris 2018: from micro-RNAs to extracellular vesicles. J Thorac Dis 2018; 10(Suppl 25):S2983–7.

50. Chilosi M, Poletti V, Zamo A, et al. Aberrant Wnt/beta-catenin pathway activation in idiopathic pulmonary fibrosis. Am J Pathol 2003;162(5):1495–502.

51. Sucre JMS, Deutsch GH, Jetter CS, et al. A shared pattern of beta-catenin activation in bronchopulmonary dysplasia and idiopathic pulmonary fibrosis. Am J Pathol 2018;188(4):853–62.

52. Barkauskas CE, Chung MI, Fioret B, et al. Lung organoids: current uses and future promise. Development 2017;144(6):986–97.

53. Chen H, Matsumoto K, Brockway BL, et al. Airway epithelial progenitors are region specific and show differential responses to bleomycin-induced lung injury. Stem Cells 2012;30(9):1948–60.

54. Liang J, Zhang Y, Xie T, et al. Hyaluronan and TLR4 promote surfactant-protein-C-positive alveolar progenitor cell renewal and prevent severe pulmonary fibrosis in mice. Nat Med 2016;22(11):1285–93.

55. Choi J, Park JE, Tsagkogeorga G, et al. Inflammatory signals induce AT2 cell-derived damage-associated transient progenitors that mediate alveolar regeneration. Cell Stem Cell 2020;27(3):366–82.e7.

56. Lehmann M, Hu Q, Hu Y, et al. Chronic WNT/beta-catenin signaling induces cellular senescence in lung epithelial cells. Cell Signal 2020;70:109588.

57. Munoz-Espin D, Serrano M. Cellular senescence: from physiology to pathology. Nat Rev Mol Cell Biol 2014;15(7):482–96.

58. Franceschi C, Garagnani P, Parini P, et al. Inflammaging: a new immune-metabolic viewpoint for age-related diseases. Nat Rev Endocrinol 2018; 14(10):576–90.

59. Ortiz-Montero P, Londono-Vallejo A, Vernot JP. Senescence-associated IL-6 and IL-8 cytokines induce a self- and cross-reinforced senescence/inflammatory milieu strengthening tumorigenic capabilities in the MCF-7 breast cancer cell line. Cell Commun Signal 2017;15(1):17.

60. Kuilman T, Michaloglou C, Vredeveld LC, et al. Oncogene-induced senescence relayed by an interleukin-dependent inflammatory network. Cell 2008;133(6):1019–31.

61. Kang TW, Yevsa T, Woller N, et al. Senescence surveillance of pre-malignant hepatocytes limits liver cancer development. Nature 2011;479(7374):547–51.

62. Krizhanovsky V, Yon M, Dickins RA, et al. Senescence of activated stellate cells limits liver fibrosis. Cell 2008;134(4):657–67.

63. Rhinn M, Ritschka B, Keyes WM. Cellular senescence in development, regeneration and disease. Development 2019;146(20):dev151837.

64. Kirschner K, Rattanavirotkul N, Quince MF, et al. Functional heterogeneity in senescence. Biochem Soc Trans 2020;48:765–73.

65. Munoz-Espin D, Canamero M, Maraver A, et al. Programmed cell senescence during mammalian embryonic development. Cell 2013;155(5):1104–18.

66. Schafer MJ, White TA, Iijima K, et al. Cellular senescence mediates fibrotic pulmonary disease. Nat Commun 2017;8:14532.

67. Lehmann M, Korfei M, Mutze K, et al. Senolytic drugs target alveolar epithelial cell function and attenuate experimental lung fibrosis ex vivo. Eur Respir J 2017;50(2):1602367.

68. Martin-Medina A, Lehmann M, Burgy O, et al. Increased extracellular vesicles mediate WNT-5A signaling in idiopathic pulmonary fibrosis. Am J Respir Crit Care Med 2018;198(12):1527–38.

69. Shehata HM, Hoebe K, Chougnet CA. The aged nonhematopoietic environment impairs natural killer cell maturation and function. Aging Cell 2015; 14(2):191–9.

70. Ovadya Y, Landsberger T, Leins H, et al. Impaired immune surveillance accelerates accumulation of senescent cells and aging. Nat Commun 2018; 9(1):5435.

71. Pereira BI, Devine OP, Vukmanovic-Stejic M, et al. Senescent cells evade immune clearance via HLA-E-mediated NK and CD8+ T cell inhibition. Nat Commun 2019;10(1):2387.

72. Arish N, Petukhov D, Wallach-Dayan SB. The role of telomerase and telomeres in interstitial lung diseases: from molecules to clinical implications. Int J Mol Sci 2019;20(12):2996.

73. Alvarez D, Cardenes N, Sellares J, et al. IPF lung fibroblasts have a senescent phenotype. Am J Physiol Lung Cell Mol Physiol 2017;313(6):L1164–73.

74. Barnes PJ, Baker J, Donnelly LE. Cellular senescence as a mechanism and target in chronic lung diseases. Am J Respir Crit Care Med 2019;200(5):556–64.

75. Minagawa S, Araya J, Numata T, et al. Accelerated epithelial cell senescence in IPF and the inhibitory role of SIRT6 in TGF-beta-induced senescence of human bronchial epithelial cells. Am J Physiol Lung Cell Mol Physiol 2011;300(3):L391–401.

76. Parimon T, Yao C, Stripp BR, et al. Alveolar epithelial type II cells as drivers of lung fibrosis in idiopathic pulmonary fibrosis. Int J Mol Sci 2020;21(7):2269.

77. Disayabutr S, Kim EK, Cha SI, et al. miR-34 miRNAs regulate cellular senescence in type II alveolar epithelial cells of patients with idiopathic pulmonary fibrosis. PLoS One 2016;11(6):e0158367.

78. Chilosi M, Carloni A, Rossi A, et al. Premature lung aging and cellular senescence in the pathogenesis of idiopathic pulmonary fibrosis and COPD/emphysema. Transl Res 2013;162(3):156–73.

79. Borok Z, Horie M, Flodby P, et al. Grp78 loss in epithelial progenitors reveals an age-linked role for endoplasmic reticulum stress in pulmonary fibrosis. Am J Respir Crit Care Med 2020;201(2):198–211.

80. Yao C, Guan X, Carraro G, et al. Senescence of alveolar type 2 cells drives progressive pulmonary fibrosis. Am J Respir Crit Care Med 2020;203(6):707–17.

81. Cárdenes N, Álvarez D, Sellarés J, et al. Senescence of bone marrow-derived mesenchymal stem cells from patients with idiopathic pulmonary fibrosis. Stem Cell Res Ther 2018;9(1):257.

82. Paxson JA, Gruntman A, Parkin CD, et al. Age-dependent decline in mouse lung regeneration with loss of lung fibroblast clonogenicity and increased myofibroblastic differentiation. PLoS One 2011;6(8):e23232.

83. Yanai H, Shteinberg A, Porat Z, et al. Cellular senescence-like features of lung fibroblasts derived from idiopathic pulmonary fibrosis patients. Aging 2015;7(9):664–72.

84. Kobayashi Y, Tata A, Konkimalla A, et al. Persistence of a regeneration-associated, transitional alveolar epithelial cell state in pulmonary fibrosis. Nat Cell Biol 2020;22(8):934–46.

85. Strunz M, Simon LM, Ansari M, et al. Alveolar regeneration through a Krt8+ transitional stem cell state that persists in human lung fibrosis. Nat Commun 2020;11(1):3559.

86. Spagnolo P, Kropski JA, Jones MG, et al. Idiopathic pulmonary fibrosis: disease mechanisms and drug development. Pharmacol Ther 2020;222:107798.

87. Konigshoff M, Kramer M, Balsara N, et al. WNT1-inducible signaling protein-1 mediates pulmonary fibrosis in mice and is upregulated in humans with idiopathic pulmonary fibrosis. J Clin Invest 2009;119(4):772–87.

88. Bueno M, Lai YC, Romero Y, et al. PINK1 deficiency impairs mitochondrial homeostasis and promotes lung fibrosis. J Clin Invest 2015;125(2):521–38.

89. Yu G, Tzouvelekis A, Wang R, et al. Thyroid hormone inhibits lung fibrosis in mice by improving epithelial mitochondrial function. Nat Med 2018;24(1):39–49.

90. Justice JN, Nambiar AM, Tchkonia T, et al. Senolytics in idiopathic pulmonary fibrosis: results from a first-in-human, open-label, pilot study. EBioMedicine 2019;40:554–63.

91. Grosse L, Wagner N, Emelyanov A, et al. Defined p16(High) senescent cell types are indispensable for mouse healthspan. Cell Metab 2020;32(1):87–99.e6.

92. de Mochel NR, Cheong KN, Cassandras M, et al. Sentinel p16INK4a+ cells in the basement membrane form a reparative niche in the lung. bioRxiv 2020.

Looking Ahead
Interstitial Lung Disease Diagnosis and Management in 2030

Kerri A. Johannson, MD, MPH[a,b,*], Harold R. Collard, MD[c],
Luca Richeldi, MD, PhD[d]

KEYWORDS

- Pulmonary fibrosis • Mobile health • Diagnosis • Biomarkers • Patient centered

KEY POINTS

- Based on tremendous progress, the diagnosis and management of patients with interstitial lung disease (ILD) is expected to change substantially over the next decade.
- Immediately actionable items include improving access to ILD specialty care, understanding and addressing barriers to evidence-based therapies, and prioritizing patient-centered domains into clinical care and research.
- Future work should focus on screening of at-risk individuals; biomarker development for diagnosis and treatment; and classification systems rooted in genotypic, phenotypic, and theranostic features.

INTRODUCTION

As shown earlier in this issue, tremendous progress has been realized in interstitial lung disease (ILD). These developments provide optimism for earlier diagnoses, improved clinical care delivery, and the availability of regenerative, even curative, therapies. Intentional, collaborative efforts should focus on implementing key scientific advancements detailed herein and meeting the remaining unmet needs. Looking ahead to 2030, important changes are anticipated that will positively affect patients living with ILD, their family members, and their care partners.

This article outlines what the authors hope to see achieved over the next decade. The first half summarizes strategies that we believe are ready for immediate implementation, building on recent scientific evidence. The second half outlines a list of priorities that we hope will be realized in the upcoming decade. This list was developed in conjunction with the Third International Summit for Interstitial Lung Disease (ISILD-3), held in Erice, Italy, in December 2019. The authors are deeply grateful to these 64 ILD expert participants, representing 16 countries, who are listed as collaborators in the acknowledgments of this article.

Actionable Items

Early diagnosis

Early recognition and diagnosis improve clinical outcomes for patients with ILD.[1] However, the current reality is that ILD is often recognized at late stages, in some cases years after the development of the patients' first symptoms.[2] At such late stages, the disease process may be slowed but frequently quality of life (QoL) is already severely impaired. Such late diagnosis contributes to the grim prognosis for many patients with ILD, in particular those with idiopathic pulmonary fibrosis (IPF), which still carries a median prognosis of 3 to

[a] Department of Medicine, University of Calgary, Calgary, Alberta, Canada; [b] Department of Community Health Sciences, University of Calgary, Calgary, Alberta, Canada; [c] Department of Medicine, University of California San Francisco, 490 Illinois Street, 6thFloor, San Francisco, CA 94158, USA; [d] Department of Medical and Surgical Sciences, Università Cattolica del Sacro Cuore, Largo Agostino Gemelli 1, Roma 001168, Italy
* Corresponding author. Pulmonary Diagnostics, 4448 Front Street Southeast, Calgary, Alberta T3M-1M4, Canada.
E-mail address: kerri.johannson@ahs.ca

Clin Chest Med 42 (2021) 375–384
https://doi.org/10.1016/j.ccm.2021.03.014

5 years from diagnosis.[3] Improving outcomes for patients with fibrotic ILD requires early disease recognition, prompt mitigation of risk factors, immediate initiation of disease-modifying therapy, and, where appropriate, early referral to a lung transplant program.

The reasons for diagnostic delays in ILD are multifactorial, but include low awareness of ILD by health care providers and patients alike. IPF is still considered an orphan or rare disease, a label that may serve to facilitate drug regulatory approvals, but that belies its increasing prevalence and impact. Epidemiologic studies indicate that the most common forms of ILD are increasing in incidence and prevalence globally, with close to 1 in 200 septuagenarians affected in some studies.[4–6] There seems to be both increasing disease occurrence and increasing recognition of disease caused by widespread use of chest computed tomography (CT) imaging and greater disease awareness.[7] Critically, access to effective treatments in the last decade may be reversing the widespread therapeutic nihilism that for decades has argued against the need for an accurate ILD diagnosis, or the referral of suspected patients with ILD to a specialty clinic.

Disease awareness campaigns have been launched that target the general public and health care providers. Given that many patients with ILD receive 2 or more alternative diagnoses before their final diagnosis,[2] such awareness campaigns are intended to empower patients whose respiratory symptoms are not responding to inhalers, or whose cardiac investigations are normal to push for continued diagnostic evaluation. Educational resources for clinicians are also increasingly available, through conferences, webinars, seminars, and talks. Education efforts and campaigns on social media may also increase awareness of these diagnoses. Some online resources endorse non–evidence-based recommendations for patients with ILD, whereas others achieve congruence with an evidence-based approach to diagnosis and management.[8,9] One comparative study showed that, over a 5-year period, information found online increased in accuracy, suggesting that, over time, resources are improving in quality.[10]

Action items
- Early diagnosis should be promoted as a top priority in the care of patients with ILD through partnerships between clinicians, scientists, health care providers, industry, and patient advocacy organizations.
- The ILD community should push funding agencies to support studies of care pathways and diagnostic algorithms that improve early diagnosis.
- Researchers and clinicians should partner with health systems to successfully implement proven approaches to early ILD diagnosis and codify standard of practice through societal guidelines and continuing medical education.

Proactive disease management

Pharmacologic therapy In 2021, effective therapies exist to treat a wide range of ILDs, including immunomodulatory and antifibrotic medications. Robust and reproducible data from clinical trials, administrative cohorts, and real-life registries support these drugs' ability to affect lung function and slow the rate of disease progression.[11–16] Despite their approval by regulatory and funding agencies and evidence of efficacy, their real-world uptake, or effectiveness, has failed to reach its full potential. Recent data from a large US-based administrative claims dataset suggest that only one-quarter of patients with IPF are receiving an antifibrotic therapy.[17]

A 2016 survey of 290 physicians from 5 European countries found that more than half of patients with IPF did not receive treatment with an approved antifibrotic therapy.[18] Early funding approvals for antifibrotics in some regions limited their access to populations defined in the sentinel clinical trials, thus excluding patients with too mild or too severe disease from drug coverage. The individual preferences of the treating clinician may also affect drug prescription, with certain patients less likely to be offered therapy based on perceived need or anticipated benefit, as determined by the physician. The US-based administrative study identified significant out-of-pocket costs associated with antifibrotics, indicating that, for some patients, financial constraints are likely at play.[17] Understanding and overcoming barriers to medication usage is an important and immediate goal.

Management of comorbidities Although precision medicine approaches in the treatment of ILD may not yet be ready for prime time, many specific and potentially effective interventions are being underused. Some may be appropriate for certain subsets of patients but not broadly applicable to all. Applied phenotyping of individuals can be achieved while considering each patient's unique circumstances and drivers of disease behavior. Specific interventions to consider include smoking cessation, occupational remediation of exposures, and domestic and avocational exposure abatement. Ongoing work in these areas will help identify patients at highest likelihood of benefit, in the pursuit of personalized care.

Management of comorbidities and complications associated with ILD is of high importance and recent data can guide changes in approaches. For example, targeting abnormal gastroesophageal reflux with fundoplication surgery may have an impact on disease progression in patients with IPF.[19,20] Several other comorbidities are associated with worse outcomes in patients with ILD, including heart disease, cancer, and sleep disordered breathing.[21,22] It is unknown whether targeted treatment of these comorbidities improves outcomes, but the authors believe they should be proactively identified and managed as part of comprehensive clinical care for ILD.

Supplemental oxygen therapy The role of supplemental oxygen in patients with ILD with resting or isolated exertional hypoxemia has been clarified with recent works focused on providing evidence-based guidance.[23] An international Delphi survey found agreement among experts that patients with ILD with severe resting hypoxemia, or isolated exertional hypoxemia with functional limitation or symptoms, should be offered supplemental oxygen therapy.[24] Most recently, an evidence-based clinical practice guideline recommended oxygen therapy for patients with ILD with severe resting hypoxemia, or severe exertional hypoxemia.[25] These data can be used to guide prescription and funding policies, as well as informing target saturations for patients during activity and exercise. Data-guided policies should serve to optimize and standardize care for patients with ILD, given the largely discrepant historical use of supplemental oxygen in this patient population.[26,27]

Exercise and disease education Formal exercise and disease education intervention through what has been termed pulmonary rehabilitation remains one of few interventions shown to improve health-related QoL in patients with ILD, and its access should widen so that all patients can realize these benefits, regardless of where they live. Online platforms have been instrumental for many programs to reach patients at a distance and can be further refined moving forward to foster participation by as many patients as possible.

Action items
- A focus on data-driven, evidence-based care implementation in everyday clinical encounters is imperative to ensure all patients are receiving optimal care.
- Barriers to accessing pharmacologic therapies for ILD should be identified and removed,

leveraging implementation science methodology and quality improvement initiatives.
- Affordable, portable, high-flow supplemental oxygen therapy should be made available to all patients with ILD with symptomatic exertional hypoxemia through innovations in technology and improvements in cost and coverage.
- Digital exercise and education programs for patients with ILD should be developed, taking advantage of patient-generated data (eg, wearables) and technology (eg, Zoom) to broaden the reach and impact of pulmonary rehabilitation.

Patient-centered research and care
Patient-centered care and research values metrics and outcomes as defined by the patient experience. Such an approach to ILD care is increasingly valued, and by extension is becoming more accurately defined in order to ensure robustness and reliability in clinicians' approaches. As outlined in Alyson W. Wong and Sonye K. Danoff's article, "Providing patient-centered care in interstitial lung disease," elsewhere in this issue, this is of critical importance. Under the umbrella of patient-centered research are patient-centered outcome metrics and patient-reported outcome metrics (PROMs). Several PROMs exist for use in ILD, and these should be prioritized and incorporated into clinical trials and clinical management pathways. Composite outcome metrics that combine physiology, symptoms, health-related QoL, and meaningful outcomes such as hospitalization or acute exacerbation should be used in trials of interventions and therapeutics in ILD.

Patients with ILD prioritize research into the treatment of cough and the development of portable, lighter, and efficient oxygen delivery systems.[28] Ongoing clinical trials of drugs to treat ILD-related cough should better inform the management approach to this at times debilitating symptom, and the field must continue to advocate for active research in this area. Beyond symptom management, patients and caregivers express a consistent desire for more information about their disease and better understanding of what to expect as the disease progresses.[29] Palliative care and end-of-life support can and should be provided more broadly to patients with ILD, many of whom have a known life-limiting illness with no cure.[30] Many patients with ILD die in hospital, although it has been found that most patients would prefer to stay in their homes at the end of life, if accommodations can be made. Understanding each patient's unique circumstances, from a sociocultural standpoint, is also imperative, in order to provide individualized support at the end of life.[30] Collaborative approaches that include ILD experts, palliative clinicians, primary care providers, expert nursing teams, social workers, and other allied health partners are essential for patient-centered care at the end of life. These pathways have been defined, but challenges in implementation (financial and logistic) may prevent patients from accessing them even when indicated.

Action items:
- Patients with ILD should be involved in the development and conduct of research, and in clinical care pathway development through the principles of community and stakeholder engagement.
- Palliative and supportive care should be offered to patients with ILD early on in the disease course, with support services available as patients decline, and discussions to determine the safest location for the patient that is consistent with their wishes.
- Multidisciplinary ILD care teams should be established to coordinate end-of-life care as part of the routine ILD care algorithm.

Technological advancements

A revolution in remote monitoring and wearable technologies has enabled home-based assessments for patients with ILD. As the general population becomes increasingly technology-connected, this broadens the potential applications of mobile health for ILD patient care.

Wearable and remote monitoring technologies have been shown to be feasible, informative, and beneficial in patients with ILD.[31,32] The largest program started in the Netherlands, where the team collaboratively developed their platform with patients who provided iterative feedback. Their remote monitoring program incorporates home handheld spirometry, symptom surveys, QoL questionnaires, medication monitoring, and access to virtual consultations with the care team.[33] In a prospective randomized controlled trial of home monitoring versus usual care, use of the home-monitoring program was associated with improved domains of QoL, closer monitoring of medication side effects leading to medication adjustments, and early identification of warning signals for clinical deterioration. Patients found the program beneficial and not burdensome. Other studies have shown home spirometry to be feasible and informative to identify early changes in lung function heralding acute exacerbations or disease progression.[34] These tools are ready for implementation in health systems and patient populations with sufficient resources and capacity. It is anticipated that home monitoring of spirometry, oximetry, and PROMs will evolve with improved accuracy of measures, reliability of data, and ease of use. Innovative modalities of measuring and transmitting established clinical parameters, such as digital recording of lung sounds,[35] are likely to be incorporated in future protocols for telemonitoring of patients with ILD. These protocols will provide important, patient-centric tools that can facilitate disease monitoring and management.

Clinical trials of therapeutics in patients with ILD are frequently limited by low patient numbers or limited access to clinical trials, which are typically conducted at large urban-based ILD referral centers. This limitation is problematic for several reasons. Clinical trials are not equally accessible to all patients, leading to disparate access to care and opportunity. Clinical trial populations may not be generalizable to the larger population given the selection bias in trial recruitment. Further, for diseases with low prevalence, this presents challenges for recruitment and sample size. With increasing numbers of trials competing for patients, and effective therapies that make it harder to detect changes in the primary outcome, innovative trial designs are needed. Remote monitoring of physiology, function, symptoms, and QoL can be integrated into clinical trial design. There have been challenges with this, particularly with concerns about the reliability of home spirometry data.[36] However, ongoing work is ensuring that the platforms are increasingly reliable and easy to use. Such integrated systems to measure lung function and PROMs should facilitate virtual trial cohorts with large and representative patient populations, revolutionizing the clinical trial landscape.

Electronic health records (EHRs) are now widespread in many parts of the world and provide a transformative opportunity to clinicians and researchers in rare diseases such as ILD.[37] Health care systems can now use their EHRs and associated data technology resources to integrate patient-generated data, administrative data, encounter-generated data, procedural data (eg, pulmonary function test results, CT scan images), biospecimen-generated data (eg, laboratory values, genetics, omics profiles), external data elements (eg, guideline recommendations or decision aids), and other electronic assets into a single point-of-care portal for use by clinicians and researchers in the care and study of patients with ILD. These collective data can also be deidentified and provided to researchers, enabling immediate access to thousands of patients with ILD with well-characterized clinical and biological profiles.[38,39] Research that took years to accomplish because of the limited size and slow construction of single-center research datasets (or was simply too challenging to contemplate) can now be conducted in a matter of months.[40]

Telehealth programs have evolved in the outpatient ambulatory care world to facilitate access to subspecialty care for patients who may live far from the clinics or who, for myriad reasons, may be unable to travel for appointments. This situation has become a prevalent reality for many health systems during the severe acute respiratory syndrome coronavirus-2 (SARS-CoV-2) pandemic, because medical clinics were limited for routine visits because of concerns for viral transmission during in-person care.[41] Most ILD subspecialty clinics are located in urban hospital settings, and may not be equitably accessible to all ILD patients depending on travel time or distance to clinic, and/or socio-economic factors. Improving access to subspecialty ILD clinics through virtual health can expand the gold standard of care for large numbers of patients and reduce disparate access.[42]

Technological advances can be capitalized on to disseminate information to regions where ILD expertise may be lacking, including rural communities and low to middle income countries. Knowledge translation can occur through virtual education systems, consultations, and through social media platforms. The infrastructure exists for data sharing across registries and research platforms, opening the potential for international sharing of data. Collaborative approaches to science should be encouraged by ensuring safe and secure data storage, sharing, and analysis. The technology exists to enable this, but the infrastructure and logistics must continue to be developed by academic institutions and governments in order to foster collaboration.

Action items
- Handheld spirometry and other home management approaches to ILD management should be implemented and studied by ILD centers of excellence to ensure added benefit to patients and patient care.
- Health systems should invest in creating clinician and researcher–facing information portals in their EHRs that integrate multisource digital information to improve patient care and scientific discovery.
- Telehealth visits should be routinely offered to patients who are geographically or otherwise prohibited from in-person visits. Comparative effectiveness researchers should evaluate telehealth and in-person visits to establish standard-of-care practices (**Table 1**).

Table 1
Action items for immediate implementation

Objective	Action
Improve ILD awareness	• Engage with patients, care partners, clinicians, pulmonary societies, and industry to increase awareness of ILD
Standardize care for patients with ILD	• Build capacity for remote care, telehealth, virtual MDD • Identify and address financial, social, geographic barriers to accessing care at ILD specialty clinics • Reduce financial or informational barriers to medication usage
Prioritize patient-centered metrics	• Integrate patient-centered metrics into research and clinical care • Include patients as key stakeholders
Leverage technology	• Develop remote clinical care tools • Integrate mobile health into clinical trials • Build capacity for collaborative research, including registries and biological samples
Prevention	• Advocate for smoking cessation, safe workplaces, reduced air pollution
Management	• Support clinical trials for cough • Develop portable, less-burdensome oxygen delivery systems • Increase access to pulmonary rehabilitation

Abbreviation: MDD, multidisciplinary discussion.

Priorities for Development

Prevention

Aging or a genetic predisposition to pulmonary fibrosis are not modifiable. However, minimizing exposure to known risks associated with ILD may prevent, slow, or delay the onset of pulmonary fibrosis in some patients. Cigarette smoking is an established risk factor for several different ILDs. Worldwide tobacco use has declined markedly over the past 20 years, but e-cigarette use and vaping are increasingly reported among youth and young adults,[43] with their long-term impacts unknown. Notably, data suggest that vaping may increase the likelihood of cigarette smoking in young people.[44] E-cigarette/vaping–induced lung injury (EVALI) is a new but serious hazard of vaping, indicating the potential for inhalational injury.[45] It remains unknown whether vaping or e-cigarette use is a risk factor for fibrotic lung disease. Evidence-based policy decisions to protect the lung health of future generations are paramount to prevent more people from dying of pulmonary fibrosis in the upcoming decade.

Beyond smoking, other inhaled environmental and occupational risk factors can be mitigated. Several occupational exposures cause lung fibrosis, whereas others are less directly causal but are implicated along the disease pathway.[46,47] Occupational health and safety guidelines should strive to achieve the most stringent safety measures to prevent work-related lung diseases in all forms. Implementation and enforcement of workplace regulations could prevent future lung fibrosis in at-risk and exposed individuals. Air pollution exposure has also been associated with risk of developing IPF,[48] and disease progression or exacerbation in patients with IPF.[49–51] Environmental policy and air quality guidelines should consider the preventive impacts when establishing safety standards.

Diagnosis

Early identification of disease or of preclinical ILD requires targeted screening of at-risk populations. Screening programs may incorporate clinical evaluation alone with physical examination, lung function testing, and CT chest, or may include genetic testing.[52,53] For maximum efficiency, screening programs should be tailored toward at-risk individuals. Identifying those at risk can be accomplished by understanding the pathobiology of disease, including genetic and environmental/occupational risks, and how lung aging correlates with disease. Advancements in these areas will inform the approach to risk stratification and targeted screening programs.

Worldwide, there are differing approaches to ILD screening of first-degree family members of patients with known pulmonary fibrosis. If the individual patient has undergone genetic testing, family members may subsequently be able to undergo testing for the specific mutations of the proband case, if such resources are clinically available. Alternatively, at-risk family members may undergo clinical evaluation with physical examination, pulmonary function testing, and high-resolution CT chest imaging. By 2030, genetic testing may be routinely offered to patients with ILD and their family members, in contrast with now, when only a few select centers worldwide offer routine genetic counseling and testing to patients with ILD. Many programs currently exist for research purposes but do not feed clinical data back to the patients or physicians to guide management strategies. Further data are needed to understand whether the identification of genetic risks for ILD lead to improved outcomes for affected individuals, or whether such information could have negative psychological, physical, or financial (ie, insurance eligibility) impacts. The impact of earlier identification of asymptomatic or preclinical disease needs clarification before the widespread initiation of screening programs.

Increasing data inform the inhaled environmental and occupational risks associated with the development of pulmonary fibrosis. Targeted screening of individuals working in high-risk occupations may become the norm. For example, farmers, bird fanciers, pigeon breeders, metal workers, sandblasters, or those working in dusty environments may undergo occupational or avocational screening programs to identify early signs of disease. However, it should be clearly noted that the priority should remain to minimize harmful exposures and optimize working and recreational conditions to protect the lung health of all, not just those identified as potentially at risk.

Artificial intelligence and algorithmic approaches to identifying interstitial lung abnormality (ILA) or ILD based on chest imaging, or combinations of clinical testing and CT findings, may become routinely available.[54] Artificial intelligence algorithms are currently being developed to recognize ILAs and ILD and prompt clinicians to refer patients for ILD assessment. Models to predict the presence of fibrotic lung disease, supported by health services for clinical evaluation and treatment, may lead to increasing identification of disease in patients that may previously not have been recognized through usual care pathways.

Biomarkers and disease classification

Perhaps one of the most dynamic areas in ILD is biomarker development, with the potential to enable reliable and meaningful measurements of disease pathobiology and responses to therapy (theranostics). Molecular blood markers of lung inflammation and fibrosis could be combined with clinical and radiological data to characterize the fibrotic lung diseases and permit precision medicine–based approaches to diagnosis and care. Identifying blood correlates to pulmonary disease activity could obviate lung biopsy and its associated risks. Simple blood tests could provide information data on disease activity and prognosis, with clinically relevant information beyond the morphologic features from lung biopsy. This possibility is within the realm of reality, with several groups worldwide working toward such goals.

It is hoped that the long-standing debates on terminology for the fibrotic lung diseases may be settled by 2030. Although decades of work to understand the pathobiology behavior and trajectory of the ILDs have led to the current framework, the authors anticipate that subsequent classification systems will be based on precise genotypic, phenotypic, and disease activity features. Perhaps the word idiopathic will be retired from the IPF disease entity,[55] with entities regrouped by their shared behavioral and theranostic characteristics.

It is hoped that the CTD-ILDs will be similarly reclassified to reflect the biological drivers of disease and responses to therapy. Rather than the current silo of IPF, patients may, for example, be diagnosed with telomere-related progressive fibrosis with high MMP-7 level. Treatable traits and informative features will inform the preferred ontology for ILDs.

Treatment

In the upcoming decade, treatment of fibrotic lung disease is anticipated to evolve toward targeted biomarker-informed therapy. Molecular biomarkers will inform disease targets, akin to current approaches in lung cancer therapy. Multiple novel or existent compounds could be delivered simultaneously in 1 well-tolerated form. Tools will exist to measure bioavailability to minimize dose and side effects while optimizing efficacy. Theranostic biomarkers will indicate that treatments are working as expected to inhibit the targeted pathways. The authors further anticipate the discovery of treatments that stop, or even reverse, lung fibrosis, through several potential pathways. As outlined elsewhere in this issue, this goal seems feasible (**Table 2**).

Table 2
Research priorities for continued progress in interstitial lung disease

Objective	Areas of Research
Earlier diagnosis and prevention	• Identify additional genetic risks for ILD • Characterize the impact of screening on at-risk individuals • Characterize the behavior of preclinical ILD and ILA for risk stratification • Improve access to genetic testing and counseling
Personalized care	• Develop AI for chest imaging • Integrate AI into clinical assessment • Develop biomarkers of disease activity and response to therapy
Reverse or cure lung fibrosis	• Develop targeted therapies to halt or reverse lung fibrosis • Regenerative therapies for lung fibrosis
Meaningful classification systems	• Integrate genotype, phenotype, and treatable traits to classify patients with ILD

Abbreviation: AI, artificial intelligence.

SUMMARY

Recent developments in ILD should guide the current approaches to clinical care and research. Where data exist to inform optimal pathways, clinicians should now focus on implementation. The discoveries of the upcoming decade will likely transform the field, and the authors remain optimistic that these innovations will improve the lives of patients living with pulmonary fibrosis.

ACKNOWLEDGMENTS

The Third Erice International Summit for ILD (ISILD-3) Collaborators: Carlo Albera, Goksel Altinisik, Katerina M. Antoniou, Kjetil Ask, Elisabetta Balestro, Elena Bergagli, Elisabeth Bendstrup, Marialuisa Bocchino, Francesco Bonella, Martina Bonifazi, Giulia Cacopardo, Mariarosaria Calvello, Diego M. Castillo, Nazia Chaudhuri, Ulrich Costabel, Vincent Cottin, Bruno Crestani, Manuela Funke-Chambour, Jack Gauldie, Peter M. George, Johannes C. Grutters, Sergio Harari, Richard G. Jenkins, Kerri A. Johannson, Mark G. Jones, Meena Kalluri, Michael P. Keane, Maria A. Kokosi, Michael Kreuter, Donato Lacedonia, Brett Ley, Alessandro Libra, Fabrizio Luppi, Toby M. Maher, Georgios Margaritopoulos, Fernando J. Martinez, Jelle Miedema, Nesrin Mogulkoc, Maria Molina-Molina, Philip L. Molyneaux, Julie Morisset, Stefano Palmucci, Mauro Pavone, Ganesh R. Raghu, Elisabetta A. Renzoni, Luca Richeldi, Gianluca Sambataro, Alfredo Sebastiani, Paolo Spagnolo, Giulia Maria Stella, Martina Sterclova, Irina Strambu, Sara Tomassetti, Sebastiano Torrisi, Jacopo Simonetti, Eliza Tsitoura, Haluk Turktas, Argyrios Tzouvelekis, Claudia Valenzuela, Ada Vancheri, Carlo Vancheri, Francesco Varone, Patrizio Vitulo, Athol U. Wells, Marlies S. Wijsenbeek, Wim A. Wuyts.

DISCLOSURE

Dr. Collard is supported by the National Institute of Health (NIH). The other authors have nothing to disclose.

REFERENCES

1. Lamas DJ, Kawut SM, Bagiella E, et al. Delayed access and survival in idiopathic pulmonary fibrosis: a cohort study. Am J Respir Crit Care Med 2011; 184(7):842–7.
2. Cosgrove GP, Bianchi P, Danese S, et al. Barriers to timely diagnosis of interstitial lung disease in the real world: the INTENSITY survey. BMC Pulm Med 2018; 18(1):9.
3. Raghu G, Remy-Jardin M, Myers JL, et al. Diagnosis of idiopathic pulmonary fibrosis. an official ATS/ERS/ JRS/ALAT clinical practice guideline. Am J Respir Crit Care Med 2018;198(5):e44–68.
4. Fernandez Perez ER, Kong AM, Raimundo K, et al. Epidemiology of hypersensitivity pneumonitis among an insured population in the United States: a claims-based cohort analysis. Ann Am Thorac Soc 2018;15(4):460–9.
5. Hutchinson J, Fogarty A, Hubbard R, et al. Global incidence and mortality of idiopathic pulmonary fibrosis: a systematic review. Eur Respir J 2015; 46(3):795–806.
6. Harari S, Madotto F, Caminati A, et al. Epidemiology of idiopathic pulmonary fibrosis in Northern Italy. PLoS One 2016;11(2):e0147072.
7. Harari S, Davì M, Biffi A, et al. Epidemiology of idiopathic pulmonary fibrosis: a population-based study in primary care. Intern Emerg Med 2020;15(3):437–45.
8. Fisher JH, O'Connor D, Flexman AM, et al. Accuracy and reliability of internet resources for information on idiopathic pulmonary fibrosis. Am J Respir Crit Care Med 2016;194(2):218–25.
9. Goobie GC, Guler SA, Johannson KA, et al. YouTube videos as a source of misinformation on idiopathic pulmonary fibrosis. Ann Am Thorac Soc 2019; 16(5):572–9.
10. Grewal JS, Fisher JH, Ryerson CJ. An updated assessment of online information on idiopathic pulmonary fibrosis. Ann Am Thorac Soc 2021. [Epub ahead of print].
11. King TE Jr, Bradford WZ, Castro-Bernardini S, et al. A phase 3 trial of pirfenidone in patients with idiopathic pulmonary fibrosis. N Engl J Med 2014; 370(22):2083–92.
12. Richeldi L, du Bois RM, Raghu G, et al. Efficacy and safety of nintedanib in idiopathic pulmonary fibrosis. N Engl J Med 2014;370(22):2071–82.
13. Tashkin DP, Roth MD, Clements PJ, et al. Mycophenolate mofetil versus oral cyclophosphamide in scleroderma-related interstitial lung disease (SLS II): a randomised controlled, double-blind, parallel group trial. Lancet Respir Med 2016;4(9):708–19.
14. Flaherty KR, Wells AU, Cottin V, et al. Nintedanib in progressive fibrosing interstitial lung diseases. N Engl J Med 2019;381(18):1718–27.
15. Dempsey TM, Sangaralingham LR, Yao X, et al. Clinical effectiveness of antifibrotic medications for idiopathic pulmonary fibrosis. Am J Respir Crit Care Med 2019;200(2):168–74.
16. Moon SW, Kim SY, Chung MP, et al. Longitudinal changes in clinical features, management, and outcomes of idiopathic pulmonary fibrosis: a nationwide cohort study. Ann Am Thorac Soc 2020. https://doi. org/10.1513/AnnalsATS.202005-451OC.
17. Dempsey TM, Payne S, Sangaralingham L, et al. Adoption of the anti-fibrotic medications pirfenidone

and nintedanib for patients with idiopathic pulmonary fibrosis. Ann Am Thorac Soc 2021. https://doi.org/10.1513/AnnalsATS.202007-901OC.

18. Maher TM, Molina-Molina M, Russell AM, et al. Unmet needs in the treatment of idiopathic pulmonary fibrosis-insights from patient chart review in five European countries. BMC Pulm Med 2017;17(1):124.

19. Raghu G, Pellegrini CA, Yow E, et al. Laparoscopic anti-reflux surgery for the treatment of idiopathic pulmonary fibrosis (WRAP-IPF): a multicentre, randomised, controlled phase 2 trial. Lancet Respir Med 2018;6(9):707–14.

20. Johannson KA, Barnes H, Bellanger AP, et al. Exposure assessment tools for hypersensitivity pneumonitis. an official American Thoracic Society Workshop Report. Ann Am Thorac Soc 2020; 17(12):1501–9.

21. Wälscher J, Gross B, Morisset J, et al. Comorbidities and survival in patients with chronic hypersensitivity pneumonitis. Respir Res 2020;21(1):12.

22. Wong AW, Lee TY, Johannson KA, et al. A cluster-based analysis evaluating the impact of comorbidities in fibrotic interstitial lung disease. Respir Res 2020;21(1):322.

23. Visca D, Mori L, Tsipouri V, et al. Effect of ambulatory oxygen on quality of life for patients with fibrotic lung disease (AmbOx): a prospective, open-label, mixed-method, crossover randomised controlled trial. Lancet Respir Med 2018;6(10):759–70.

24. Lim RK, Humphreys C, Morisset J, et al. Oxygen in patients with fibrotic interstitial lung disease: an international Delphi survey. Eur Respir J 2019;54(2): 1900421.

25. Jacobs SS, Krishnan JA, Lederer DJ, et al. Home oxygen therapy for adults with chronic lung disease. an official American Thoracic Society Clinical practice guideline. Am J Respir Crit Care Med 2020; 202(10):e121–41.

26. Johannson KA, Pendharkar SR, Mathison K, et al. Supplemental oxygen in interstitial lung disease: an art in need of science. Ann Am Thorac Soc 2017;14(9):1373–7.

27. Khor YH, Goh NS, McDonald CF, et al. Oxygen therapy for interstitial lung disease: a mismatch between patient expectations and experiences. Ann Am Thorac Soc 2017;14(6):888–95.

28. Tikellis G, Tong A, Lee JYT, et al. Top 10 research priorities for people living with pulmonary fibrosis, their caregivers, healthcare professionals and researchers. Thorax 2020. https://doi.org/10.1136/thoraxjnl-2020-215731.

29. Overgaard D, Kaldan G, Marsaa K, et al. The lived experience with idiopathic pulmonary fibrosis: a qualitative study. Eur Respir J 2016;47(5):1472–80.

30. Kreuter M, Bendstrup E, Russell AM, et al. Palliative care in interstitial lung disease: living well. Lancet Respir Med 2017;5(12):968–80.

31. Marcoux V, Wang M, Burgoyne SJ, et al. Mobile health monitoring in patients with idiopathic pulmonary fibrosis. Ann Am Thorac Soc 2019;16(10):1327–9.

32. Moor CC, Wapenaar M, Miedema JR, et al. A home monitoring program including real-time wireless home spirometry in idiopathic pulmonary fibrosis: a pilot study on experiences and barriers. Respir Res 2018;19(1):105.

33. Moor CC, Mostard RLM, Grutters JC, et al. Home monitoring in patients with idiopathic pulmonary fibrosis. a randomized controlled trial. Am J Respir Crit Care Med 2020;202(3):393–401.

34. Russell AM, Adamali H, Molyneaux PL, et al. Daily home spirometry: an effective tool for detecting progression in idiopathic pulmonary fibrosis. Am J Respir Crit Care Med 2016;194(8):989–97.

35. Sgalla G, Larici AR, Sverzellati N, et al. Quantitative analysis of lung sounds for monitoring idiopathic pulmonary fibrosis: a prospective pilot study. Eur Respir J 2019;53(3):1802093.

36. Maher TM, Corte TJ, Fischer A, et al. Pirfenidone in patients with unclassifiable progressive fibrosing interstitial lung disease: a double-blind, randomised, placebo-controlled, phase 2 trial. Lancet Respir Med 2020;8(2):147–57.

37. Farrand E, Anstrom KJ, Bernard G, et al. Closing the evidence gap in interstitial lung disease. the promise of real-world data. Am J Respir Crit Care Med 2019; 199(9):1061–5.

38. Ley B, Urbania T, Husson G, et al. Code-based diagnostic algorithms for idiopathic pulmonary fibrosis. case validation and improvement. Ann Am Thorac Soc 2017;14(6):880–7.

39. Farrand E, Iribarren C, Vittinghoff E, et al. Impact of idiopathic pulmonary fibrosis on longitudinal healthcare utilization in a community-based cohort of patients. Chest 2021;159(1):219–27.

40. Farrand E, Vittinghoff E, Ley B, et al. Corticosteroid use is not associated with improved outcomes in acute exacerbation of IPF. Respirology 2020;25(6):629–35.

41. Nakshbandi G, Moor CC, Wijsenbeek MS. Home monitoring for patients with ILD and the COVID-19 pandemic. Lancet Respir Med 2020;8(12):1172–4.

42. Grewal JS, Morisset J, Fisher JH, et al. Role of a regional multidisciplinary conference in the diagnosis of interstitial lung disease. Ann Am Thorac Soc 2019;16(4):455–62.

43. Besaratinia A, Tommasi S. Vaping: a growing global health concern. EClinicalMedicine 2019;17:100208.

44. Quick facts on the risks of E-cigarettes for kids, teens, and young adults. Centers for Disease Control; 2020. Available at: https://www.cdc.gov/tobacco/basic_information/e-cigarettes/Quick-Facts-on-the-Risks-of-E-cigarettes-for-Kids-Teens-and-Young-Adults.html. Accessed January 15, 2021.

45. Koslow M, Petrache I. A Finale on EVALI?: the abated but not forgotten outbreak of acute

respiratory illness in individuals who vape. JAMA Netw Open 2020;3(11):e2019366.

46. Glazer CS, Newman LS. Occupational interstitial lung disease. Clin Chest Med 2004;25(3):467–78.

47. Abramson MJ, Murambadoro T, Alif SM, et al. Occupational and environmental risk factors for idiopathic pulmonary fibrosis in Australia: case-control study. Thorax 2020;75(10):864–9.

48. Conti S, Harari S, Caminati A, et al. The association between air pollution and the incidence of idiopathic pulmonary fibrosis in Northern Italy. Eur Respir J 2018;51(1):1700397.

49. Johannson KA, Vittinghoff E, Lee K, et al. Acute exacerbation of idiopathic pulmonary fibrosis associated with air pollution exposure. Eur Respir J 2014;43(4):1124–31.

50. Sese L, Nunes H, Cottin V, et al. Role of atmospheric pollution on the natural history of idiopathic pulmonary fibrosis. Thorax 2017;73(2):145–50.

51. Winterbottom CJ, Shah RJ, Patterson KC, et al. Exposure to Ambient particulate matter is associated with accelerated functional decline in idiopathic pulmonary fibrosis. Chest 2017;153(5):1221–8.

52. Cottin V, Richeldi L. Neglected evidence in idiopathic pulmonary fibrosis and the importance of early diagnosis and treatment. Eur Respir Rev 2014;23(131):106–10.

53. Kropski JA, Young LR, Cogan JD, et al. Genetic evaluation and testing of patients and families with idiopathic pulmonary fibrosis. Am J Respir Crit Care Med 2017;195(11):1423–8.

54. Walsh SLF, Humphries SM, Wells AU, et al. Imaging research in fibrotic lung disease; applying deep learning to unsolved problems. Lancet Respir Med 2020;8(11):1144–53.

55. Wolters PJ, Blackwell TS, Eickelberg O, et al. Time for a change: is idiopathic pulmonary fibrosis still idiopathic and only fibrotic? Lancet Respir Med 2018;6(2):154–60.

Moving?

Make sure your subscription moves with you!

To notify us of your new address, find your **Clinics Account Number** (located on your mailing label above your name), and contact customer service at:

Email: journalscustomerservice-usa@elsevier.com

800-654-2452 (subscribers in the U.S. & Canada)
314-447-8871 (subscribers outside of the U.S. & Canada)

Fax number: 314-447-8029

Elsevier Health Sciences Division
Subscription Customer Service
3251 Riverport Lane
Maryland Heights, MO 63043

*To ensure uninterrupted delivery of your subscription, please notify us at least 4 weeks in advance of move.

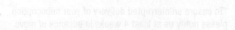

Printed and bound by CPI Group (UK) Ltd, Croydon, CR0 4YY

08/05/2025

01864692-0011